OXFORD MEDICAL PUBLICATIONS

Elimination or Reduction
of Diseases?

Editorial board

ALAN J. SILMAN
*Senior Lecturer, Department of Clinical Epidemiology,
The London Hospital, London*

SHANE P.A. ALLWRIGHT
*Lecturer, Department of Community Health,
University of Dublin, Dublin*

LUCIEN KARHAUSEN
*Officer of the Commission of the EEC,
Brussels*

SUSIE STEWART
Technical Editor, Glasgow

ELIMINATION OR REDUCTION OF DISEASES?

Opportunities for Health Service Action in Europe

Edited by

Alan J. Silman

*Senior Lecturer,
Department of Clinical Epidemiology,
The London Hospital*

and

Shane P.A. Allwright

*Lecturer,
Department of Community Health,
University of Dublin*

OXFORD   NEW YORK   TOKYO
OXFORD UNIVERSITY PRESS
1988

Oxford University Press, Walton Street, Oxford OX2 6DP
Oxford   New York   Toronto
Delhi   Bombay   Calcutta   Madras   Karachi
Petaling Jaya   Singapore   Hong Kong   Tokyo
Nairobi   Dar es Salaam   Cape Town
Melbourne   Auckland
and associated companies in
Berlin   Ibadan

Oxford is a trade mark of Oxford University Press

Published in the United States
by Oxford University Press, New York

© ECSC-EEC-EAEC, Brussels-Luxembourg, 1988
Publication No. EUR 10855 of the
Commission of the European Communities,
Directorate-General Telecommunications, Information
Industries and Innovation, Luxembourg

LEGAL NOTICE
Neither the Commission of the European Communities nor any person
acting on behalf of the Commission is responsible for the use which
might be made of the following information.

All rights reserved. No part of this publication may be reproduced,
stored in a retrieval system, or transmitted, in any form or by any means,
electronic, mechanical, photocopying, recording, or otherwise, without
the prior permission of Oxford University Press

British Library Cataloguing in Publication Data
Elimination or reduction of diseases:
opportunities for health service action in Europe.
1. Western Europe. Preventive medicine
I. Silman, Alan J.   II. Allwright, Shane P.A.
614.4'4'094
ISBN 0-19-261700-1

Library of Congress Cataloging in Publication Data
Elimination or reduction of diseases?: opportunities for health service action in
Europe/edited by Alan J. Silman and Shane P.A. Allwright.
(Oxford medical publications)
Includes index.
1. Diseases——Europe——Prevention.   2. Preventive health services——Europe.
3. Medical screening——Europe.   4. Diseases——Europe.
I. Silman, Alan J.   II. Allwright, Shane P.A.   III. Series.
[DNLM: 1. Epidemology——Europe.   2. Health Policy——Europe.
3. Public Health——Europe.]
RA483.E45   1988   362.1'094——dc 19   88-5110
ISBN 0-19-261700-1

Typeset by Colset Private Limited, Singapore
Printed and bound in Great Britain by
Biddles Ltd, Guildford and King's Lynn

Acknowledgements

We would like to thank Professor Walter Holland, Professor Edward Bennett, and members of the Panel of Social Medicine and Epidemiology of the Commission of the European Communities for their advice and encouragement during the preparation of this book. We also acknowledge the Directorate-General of Employment, Social Affairs and Education of the EEC for financial support and for organizing a seminar for contributors in Luxembourg from 17–19 September 1986. We are likewise very grateful to numerous colleagues, and particularly Professor Nick Wald, for constructive comments on the early draft submissions to this volume. We also extend our appreciation to Ruth Silman for help in translation and to Joanne Walton for many hours of secretarial assistance.

Contents

List of contributors — ix

Prospects for elimination — xi
Alan J Silman

Section I
Primary prevention — 1

A   Infectious diseases — 3

Introduction — 5
Shane Allwright

1 Congenital rubella — 8
Philippe De Wals and Michel Lechat

2 Whooping cough — 26
Shane Allwright

3 Measles — 46
Norman Noah

4 Mumps — 60
Norman Noah

5 Hepatitis B — 65
Jens Ole Nielsen

6 Tuberculosis — 77
Matthijs A Bleiker and Karel Styblo

B   Non-infectious disorders — 99

7 Vitamin D deficiency — 101
Mark Baker

8 Iodine deficiency and goitre — 115
Claude H Thilly, Beatrice Swennen, and Raphael Lagasse

9 Iron deficiency — 126
Peter C Elwood

10 Dental caries and periodontal disease   140
    Martin Hobdell and Gerard Gavin

11 Occupational cancers   157
    Franco Merletti and Nereo Segnan

Section II
Screening to eliminate childhood morbidity   179

12 Down syndrome and neural tube defects   181
    Janine Goujard

13 Thalassaemia   211
    Eleni Petridou and Dimitris Loukopoulos

14 Congenital hypothyroidism   226
    Takis Panayotopoulos

15 Congenital hip dislocation   243
    Christos Bartsocas

Section III
Preventable fetal and infant loss   255

16 Perinatal mortality   257
    Valerie Dowding

17 Post-neonatal mortality   287
    Elizabeth Watson

Section IV
Screening to reduce morbidity and mortality from cancer   309

18 Cervical cancer   311
    Franco Berrino

19 Breast cancer   328
    Christopher D Frost

Appendix I.   Summary of main conclusions for the
              topics considered   350

Appendix II. Theoretical prerequisites for elimination   356

Index   362

Contributors

Ms Shane P.A. Allwright
Department of Community Health, University of Dublin, Trinity College, Dublin 2, Ireland.

Professor Mark Baker
Bradford Health Authority, Daisy Bank, 109 Duckworth Lane, Bradford, West Yorkshire BD9 6RL, England.

Dr Christos S. Bartsocas
Department of Pediatrics, 'P and A Kyriakou' Children's Hospital, 11527 Athens, Greece.

Dr Franco Berrino
Lombardy Cancer Registry, Epidemiology Unit, Istituto Nazionale Tumori, Via Venezian 1, Milan, Italy.

Dr Matthijs A. Bleiker
International Tuberculosis Surveillance Centre, Post Box 146, 2501 CC The Hague, The Netherlands.

Dr Philippe De Wals
Department of Epidemiology, School of Public Health, Catholic University of Louvain, Clos-Chapelle-aux-Champs 30, 1200 Brussels, Belgium.

Dr Valerie Dowding
Department of Community Health, University of Dublin, Trinity College, Dublin 2, Ireland.

Dr Peter C. Elwood
MRC Epidemiology Unit, 4, Richmond Road, Cardiff, Wales.

Mr Christopher D. Frost
Department of Environmental and Preventive Medicine, The Medical College of St Bartholomew's Hospital, Charterhouse Square, London EC1M 6BQ, England.

Dr Gerard T. Gavin
Department of Community Dental Health, Preventive Dentistry and General Practice, University of Dublin, Trinity College, Dublin 2, Ireland.

Dr Janine Goujard
INSERM, Unité de Recherches Epidémiologiques sur la Mère et l'Enfant, 123 Boulevard de Port Royal, 75014 Paris, France.

Professor Martin Hobdell
Department of Community Dental Health, Preventive Dentistry and General Practice, University of Dublin, Trinity College, Dublin 2, Ireland.

Contributors

Dr Raphael Lagasse
Laboratoire d'Epidémiologie et de Médecine Sociale, Ecole de Santé Publique, University of Brussels, CPI 590, Route de Lennik 808, 1070 Brussels, Belgium.

Professor Michel Lechat
Department of Epidemiology, School of Public Health, Catholic University of Louvain, Clos-Chapelle-aux-Champs 30, 1200 Brussels, Belgium.

Dr Dimitris Loukopoulos
School of Medicine, University of Athens, 11527 Athens (Goudi), Greece.

Dr Franco Merletti
Department of Biomedical Sciences and Human Oncology, University of Torino, Via Santena 7, 10126 Turin, Italy.

Dr Jens Ole Nielsen
Department of Infectious Diseases, University of Copenhagen, Hvidovre Hospital 144, 2650 Hvidovre, Denmark.

Dr Norman Noah
PHLS Communicable Disease Surveillance Centre, 61 Colindale Avenue, London NW9 5EQ, England.

Dr Takis Panayotopoulos
Foundation for Research in Childhood, Amalias Str 42, Athens 10558, Greece.

Dr Eleni Petridou
School of Medicine, University of Athens, 11527 Athens (Goudi), Greece.

Dr Nereo Segnan
Unit of Epidemiology, National Health Service, Via San Francesco da Paola 31, 10123 Turin, Italy.

Dr Alan J. Silman
Department of Clinical Epidemiology, The London Hospital Medical College, Turner Street, London E1 2AD, England.

Dr Karel Styblo
Tuberculosis Surveillance Research Unit, Post Box 146, 2501 CC The Hague, The Netherlands.

Dr Beatrice Swennen
Laboratoire d'Epidémiologie et de Médecine Sociale, Ecole de Santé Publique, University of Brussels, CPI 590, Route de Lennik 808, 1070 Brussels, Belgium.

Professor Claude Thilly
Laboratoire d'Epidémiologie et de Médecine Sociale, Ecole de Santé Publique, University of Brussels, CPI 590, Route de Lennik 808, 1070 Brussels, Belgium.

Dr Elizabeth Watson
Department of Clinical Epidemiology, The London Hospital Medical College, Turner Street, London E1 2AD, England.

Prospects for elimination

Alan J. Silman

Lessons from history

Disease elimination implies a reduction in the incidence of a disease until it is no longer a public health problem, although isolated cases may still occur. In Western Europe such a state is restricted to relatively few disorders, the majority of which are infectious in aetiology. Historically one can point to plague, cholera, and other similar disorders which affected whole communities. More recently scarlet fever and rheumatic fever have followed the same path, although it is salutary to remember that in parts of Africa, for example, rheumatic fever remains as the main antecedent cause of heart disease. The reason for these public health successes probably lies less with specific health intervention programmes and more with a combination of improvement in socio-economic and environmental conditions leading to increased host resistance on the one hand, and a decline in pathogen load and organism virulence on the other, together with various specific factors in each individual case.

In contrast, however, smallpox (world-wide) and bovine tuberculosis (some countries) have been eliminated as a result of a direct programme of action; immunization in the former and the treatment of herds and pasterization of milk in the latter. There have been other recent successes too. Widespread immunization against diphtheria and polio have reduced these disorders to medical rarities in Western society. Likewise widespread early neonatal screening for phenylketonuria has virtually eliminated the occurrence of mental handicap from this cause.

Despite a successful programme of primary prevention, changes in the antecedent causes of some disorders have resulted in little change in disease incidence. Hence the virtual disappearance of tuberculosis of the adrenal gland has not resulted in the elimination of Addison's disease; in Western societies the latter now mainly results from auto-immune destruction of the gland. Similarly the decline in acute post-streptococcal glomerulonephritis has been matched by a rise in the more chronic, again auto-immune, forms.

Rationale for this volume

It is widely held that there are disorders whose incidence can be reduced substantially by the direct intervention of programmes based on the health service. It is our purpose to consider targets for such programmes within Western Europe and to consider how likely it is for the stated intervention to achieve a worthwhile reduction in disease in the next decade or so. The main criteria for inclusion in this volume is that, although mechanisms with which to achieve disease reduction are thought to exist for given disorders, their potential is not being reached. The reasons for this failure are varied. In some instances, despite widespread beliefs to the contrary, there is no scientific proof of efficacy for the intervention. Alternatively, the intervention might be successful in an empirical clinical trial, but fails in the general population because of low public and professional acceptability and lack of compliance. Furthermore, demonstration that a programme is effective does not necessarily result in its general implementation. In the reviews that follow, the lack of organization and commitment to running a successful programme are a recurring theme. There are a number of reasons for this. Cost, interestingly, is of less importance than other factors. Thus the costs of measles immunization or iodine supplementation are negligible in relation to the benefits; it is administrative inertia that has often impeded progress. There are also political and other constraints—the fluoridation of water is a classic example of how governments have been apprehensive about introducing a cheap and effective programme against the wishes of an articulate and emotional minority.

What are the targets?

The selection of topics to be included was based primarily on the concept of potential for reduction, where the introduction of a *specific health service programme* can be expected to achieve a quantifiable result. Hence there is no place for those disorders which rely on achieving changes in human behaviour. Cigarette smoking, excessive alcohol intake, excess food or energy intake, and sexual promiscuity are under individual control. Although the potential for the reduction of diseases directly caused by these aspects of lifestyle is vast, recent history suggests that health service interventions *per se* have little to offer. The decline in cigarette smoking in many Western European countries (Greece being a notable exception) has probably resulted from social and economic pressures in addition to raised health awareness. The health education programmes, however, seem to have been relatively ineffectual. Similarly, the desire to limit energy intake results more from perceptions about body image than any anxiety about diabetes or osteoarthritis. Our aim is not to minimize the importance of a sustained health education campaign in these areas, but rather to exclude this group where the intervention—health education—is both low in efficacy, unpredictable in effect, and operates primarily by inducing life-style changes. Also not considered are specific health interventions where the evidence for major reductions in disease incidence is lacking. Hence, although the link between hypertension and stroke is strong, and the widespread screening and treatment of detected hypertensives is effective for a few, the impact on total stroke incidence is likely to be modest at best.

In selecting topics for inclusion a broad view has been taken of the remit of health services. Thus, in addition to screening and immunization programmes, we have included, for example, the control of fortification and supplementation of food and water supplies.

The chapters are arranged in four groups according to the *principal strategy* of prevention proposed. Elimination of a disorder normally requires identification and removal of its causes(s), a strategy we refer to as primary prevention. Hence the demonstration of a micro-organism, nutritional deficiency, or occupational exposure as the single primary cause of a disease should lead swiftly to its elimination by immunization, dietary supplementation, or withdrawal from exposure, respectively. Section I is devoted to this group of disorders and is divided into infectious and non-infectious categories. It may be such programmes are only cost-effective when aimed at certain high-risk subgroups. Hence a programme of immunizing high-risk groups against hepatitis B is acceptable in cost terms and immunizing the general population is not.

A second and less ideal strategy is to identify, by screening, those with early or reversible disease, and here the aim is to eliminate further morbidity from that disorder. Section II considers a number of such possibilities for the elimination of childhood morbidity. In the prenatal period disease elimination is based on the early identification and termination of an affected pregnancy. Such a programme is less than ideal, and for some cultures, unacceptable. For those disorders discussed in this volume—Down syndrome, neural tube defects, and thalassaemia—there is also a contribution from primary prevention, for example, by genetic counselling (especially in thalassaemia) and avoidance of high-risk conceptions. The results of further research may obviate the need for prenatal screening. In the neonatal period screening aims to detect markers of subsequent serious morbidity. We have included the detection of a biochemical marker (low thyroid hormone concentrations) as a strategy to prevent physical and mental handicap from hypothyroidism; and of a clinical marker (subluxable hip) as a strategy to prevent locomotor disability from congenital dislocation of the hip.

In the third section we consider the prospects for reduction of perinatal and post-neonatal mortality. In the past 50 years the reduction in both, in Western Europe, has been dramatic, but, as discussed in these chapters, the rates and trends are not equal within and between European countries. The most successful countries have argued against the concept of an irreducible minimum. It is thus reasonable to consider the reasons for the differences between populations and to discuss the role health services played in the observed declines. Such a role covers the full range of preventive strategies from primary prevention aimed at avoiding high-risk conceptions, to perinatal screening, and tertiary prevention in resuscitating asphyxiated neonates.

The final section in this volume is devoted to two cancers where, since primary prevention is not feasible with current knowledge, the aim is the identification of disease at a stage where intervention might improve the prognosis and reduce morbidity and, particularly, mortality. The objectives of the two programmes considered, differ. Thus cervical cancer screening aims to detect pre-cancerous pathology, whereas screening for breast cancer aims to detect early cancer and prevent morbidity and mortality. Recent trials have provided some optimism for this latter possibility and indeed a significant reduction in mortality could be achieved. However, in contrast to cervical cancer, where an 80 per cent reduction in *incidence* is proposed, for breast cancer, even under the most optimal assessment of screening efficacy, a reduction of less than half that amount in the target group's *mortality* is probably the maximum benefit attainable.

Our classification into four sections is necessarily imperfect because the programmes proposed for many of the disorders considered comprise elements of different levels of prevention. Further, within each of the four sections, as suggested above, there are considerable variations in the likelihood of achieving elimination with the recommended programmes. The identification of feasible goals is discussed for the disorders for which elimination is unlikely.

Two disorders are included for which there is widespread professional and public belief that elimination is feasible, but for which the scientific evidence underlying those beliefs is lacking or contradictory. This volume thus comes out against both iron fortification to prevent anaemia (Chapter 9) and against formal screening programmes to prevent disability from congenital dislocation of the hip (Chapter 15). New evidence may come to light which might alter these conclusions, but to proceed with either, on current evidence, would be premature.

Chapter format

We have attempted to follow a consistent and logical pattern. Hence for each disorder the medical context of the problem is stated and is followed by an estimate of its size within Western Europe, where available. Where relevant, the presence of specific target or at-risk groups is noted. The basis for the proposed intervention is then identified—be it the elimination of a specific cause (primary prevention), or the early detection by screening of a reversible precursor of the targeted disorder (when secondary prevention may be achieved by further intervention). The nature of the intervention is described and evidence for its efficacy, from controlled studies, and for its effectiveness, from population experience, discussed. The effectiveness of an intervention may be much lower than the efficacy because of constraints such as lack of population acceptability, unwanted side-effects, political inertia, or cost. The relative contribution of each of these factors to the current status is described and this is followed by recommendations for a programme of action. Such programmes should include a system for monitoring and evaluation, and most of the chapters discuss this feature.

The major findings are summarized, at the end of the volume, in Appendix I (p. 350). In a second appendix (p. 356) we have attempted to draw up, for each disorder, a list of theoretical prerequisites for elimination. While these lists are obviously an over-simplified extrapolation of complex issues described in the individual chapters, we thought it a useful way of highlighting reasons why expectations for elimination are not being met. In some cases, the prerequisites listed would not be acceptable ethically, politically, or financially, in present-day Europe. For these disorders, elimination is simply not a realistic goal; and reduction of morbidity and/or mortality would appear to be the best that can be hoped for at present. For other disorders, although the prerequisites would appear in general to be acceptable, they are not being satisfied.

For the future?

The development of new interventions will pose new challenges, but, for the present, we have restricted analyses to currently available programmes. It is perhaps only a question of time, for example, before the sequencing of DNA will permit the detection *in utero* of single gene disorders at a time when termination can be considered. A future volume may need to tackle the realistic proposition that Duchenne muscular dystrophy and cystic fibrosis can be eliminated. Similarly we have not attempted to discuss the acquired immunedeficiency syndrome (AIDS) despite its rise to prominence, in public and political terms, as a major public health problem. The development of an effective vaccine would alter the decision about its inclusion, but, for the present, intervention is based on health education towards 'safer sex'. There are other gaps—some have advocated population screening for colorectal cancer using occult blood testing, for glaucoma using tonometry or ophthalmoscopy, and for secretory otitis media (glue ear) using audiography; there are probably many others. In our judgement the population effectiveness of these procedures has not been sufficiently evaluated to merit inclusion.

There is a demand for programmes of disease prevention within the countries of the European Economic Community. We hope that this volume will help those in a position to influence the implementation of such programmes to focus their attention on the realistic advances that can be made in disease prevention, and also to highlight the fact that in some areas current expectations are unrealistic.

Section I

Primary prevention

A Infectious diseases

Introduction

Shane Allwright

Prospects for the elimination of a variety of common infectious diseases are considered in this section. Immunization is the primary tool for the prevention of most of these. The aim of any immunization programme should be clearly identified in terms of the possible goals: eradication, elimination, or containment (control). These options differ widely both in their effectiveness, and their efficiency—that is, their ability to provide an effective intervention at an acceptable cost.

Eradication refers to a situation where the disease and its causal agent have been completely and permanently removed, as is the current situation with smallpox. Eradication is expensive and requires a complete global strategy. Once achieved, however, eradication may be maintained with little further effort or cost so that, in the long term, it may be the most cost-effective choice.

Elimination refers to a situation where virtually the entire population is resistant to the disease, but the causal agent remains—for example, polio and diphtheria in Northern Europe, and measles in Czechoslovakia. Elimination thus reduces morbidity to negligible levels, but maintenance of elimination requires ongoing expenditure (for continued vaccination programmes, surveillance, and prompt intervention in outbreaks). It is, therefore, a very costly option both in the long and short term. However, even when the characteristics of a particular disease and its intervention favour eradication, elimination of an infectious disease may be the best that can be achieved by an individual country in the absence of world-wide co-operative effort.

Containment (or control) of the disease may be defined as the point at which the disease, although not eradicated or eliminated, no longer constitutes a significant public health problem (Noah 1983). The definition is deliberately vague as the point at which a country is satisfied with its immunization programme will vary considerably and will be related to opportunity costs. Containment is not necessarily a second best option and could be the natural aim of an immunization programme. Control does not necessarily imply action to the whole population and may be concentrated for example on selective immunization for high-risk groups. An example of this is hepatitis B which is discussed in chapter 5. Although in theory selective immunization is the most efficient strategy, there are major practical difficulties in identifying the target groups and achieving sufficiently high immunization uptake in them.

The success or effectiveness of an immunization programme lies in its ability to reduce incidence of a disease in a community. This in turn depends on vaccine efficacy and its uptake (Noah 1983). Vaccine efficacy is the ability of a vaccine, under ideal conditions, to protect immunized individuals from infection. Efficacy is never 100 per cent, but many vaccines are more than 95 per cent efficacious. The length of time for which vaccine-induced immunity lasts must also be considered. The level of vaccine uptake required to achieve the aims of the programme is dictated by factors such as the communicability of the infection, the nature (demographic, social, geographical) of the target population, the type of vaccine, and the world incidence of infection. In practice, the level of vaccine uptake achieved depends largely on the vaccine's acceptability to both the general public and the medical profession. Acceptability, in turn, depends on the 'danger' of the disease as perceived by the public, and is naturally much affected by the level of side-effects (real or perceived) attributable to the vaccine.

Table Characteristics of smallpox and smallpox vaccine favouring eradication

Smallpox	Smallpox vaccine
Low infectivity	Immunity after immunization is of relatively long duration
High average age at infection	
Disease transmitted person-to-person (no animal or insect reservoir)	Immunity produced after one injection
	Evidence of vaccine immunity detectable (vaccine scar)
Characteristic clinical disease, easily diagnosed	
Few or no sub-clinical cases	Vaccine is:
No long-term carrier states	safe, few side-effects
Only one causative agent or serotype	stable, resists physical and genetic change
Short period of infectivity pre- and post-disease	inexpensive to produce or purchase
	simple to administer
Immunity after disease is:	
of long duration	
not subject to reinfection or reactivation	
decreases or eliminates excretion of organism	
Evidence of immunity is usually visible (scars)	
Disease is seasonal (permitting vaccine strategies)	
Disease has significant impact on economy	

Adapted from Evans (1985).

The successful planned eradication of smallpox from the world has provided a model against which to assess the likelihood of eradication of other infectious diseases. Both smallpox and the smallpox vaccine possessed certain features which favoured eradication and these are summarized in the Table.

References

Evans, A.S. (1985). The eradication of communicable diseases: myth or reality? *Am. J. Epidemiol.* **122**, 199–207.

Noah, N.D. (1983). The strategy of immunization. *Comm. Med.* **5**, 140–7.

1
Congenital rubella

Philippe De Wals and Michel Lechat

SUMMARY

Rubella is a world-wide viral disease. It is transmitted by close person-to-person contact, has a short period of infectiousness, and is usually a mild and sometimes asymptomatic illness. Contracted during early pregnancy, however, the virus can cause serious damage to the developing fetus. Outcomes of fetal infection include spontaneous abortion, stillbirth, birth of an infant with congenital rubella syndrome (CRS), or birth of a normal infant who may remain normal or may develop late manifestations of the disease. Serological surveys indicate that 5-15 per cent of pregnant women lack specific antibodies against rubella. A safe, effective vaccine exists for rubella alone and for rubella in combination with measles and mumps. Eradication of the rubella infection is thus possible and attractive, both from a human and a cost-benefit point of view. In reality, however, the elimination of congenital rubella syndrome, either by a 'selective' or 'mass' strategy of immunization, remains the stated objective of all control programmes established throughout the world. Recommendations include improvement in health education on the dangers of rubella to increase acceptance of vaccination, improved training and motivation of health workers involved, proper evaluation of preventive programmes, and the establishment of an effective health information system on rubella in every country.

Defining the problem

Epidemiology of rubella infection

Rubella is a world-wide viral disease. No animal reservoir has been described. The virus is shed from the nasopharynx of infected individuals and is conveyed in droplets into the environment. As the virus is fragile and does not persist in the environment, close person-to-person contact is necessary for transmission. When infected droplets are inhaled by a susceptible contact, the virus contaminates the respiratory tract and spreads to regional lymph nodes where replication occurs. After 1 week of incubation, viraemia develops and the mucosae of the respiratory tract are invaded. The period of infectiousness is usually short, lasting no more than 2 weeks (Hortsmann 1982).

Typical clinical rubella is a mild illness characterized by enlargement of the cervical lymph nodes, a maculopapular rash, and general signs of infection. Many infections are asymptomatic. Complications of rubella in children and adults are exceptional. Joint manifestations of arthralgia and arthritis are mostly seen in adolescent and adult females. Thrombocytopenic purpura, which is more frequent in children than in adults, has an incidence of approximately 1 in 3000 cases. The prognosis is usually good. Encephalitis, the most serious complication, occurs in approximately 1 in 5000 cases. The overall case-fatality rate of encephalitis is 20 per cent (Heggie and Robbins 1969).

In temperate climates, rubella is an endemic disease with a seasonal peak during spring. Epidemics usually occur at intervals of 5–9 years. Most cases occur in the 5–9 year age group. Local outbreaks are seen in military recruits, in boarding schools, and in other confined populations (Witte et al. 1969; Assad and Ljungars-Esteves 1985).

Infection stimulates a lasting protective immunity although reinfection has been described in 1.5–3.4 per cent of those with naturally acquired immunity exposed to the virus (Preblud et al. 1980). Results of serological surveys indicate a uniform pattern of age-related immunity in most parts of the world. The proportion of individuals with rubella antibodies increases with age, reaching more than 80 per cent in adults (Cockburn 1969).

Teratogenic action of rubella virus

In 1941, Gregg reported an epidemic of 78 cases of congenital cataract in newborn babies in Australia. In 44 cases, the eye malformation was associated with a cardiac defect. By calculating back from the date of birth of affected babies, it was estimated that the early period of pregnancy corresponded with an epidemic of rubella. In all but 10 cases of the series, there was a history of rubella infection in the mother.

The nature of fetal damage caused by intrauterine rubella infection is mainly determined by the stage in pregnancy at which infection takes place. The virus circulates in the mother's blood, crosses the placenta, and localizes in the developing and differentiating cells, causing destruction. The virus survives in the fetus and can be excreted for some months after birth (Hortsmann 1982).

Outcomes of fetal infection include spontaneous abortion, stillbirth, birth of an infant with congenital rubella syndrome, or birth of a normal infant who may remain normal or may develop late manifestations of the disease. The clinical manifestations of congenital rubella can be grouped in two categories: the transient manifestations of infection and the permanent structural and developmental defects (Cooper 1985).

The transient manifestations of congenital rubella are seen in newborn and young infants. They are intrauterine growth retardation, thrombocytopenic purpura, haemolytic anaemia, generalized adenopathy, hepatitis, meningoencephalitis, pneumonia, myocarditis, and radiographic bone lesions. The disease can result in infant death or in recovery with or without permanent sequelae.

Permanent structural manifestations may be detected at birth or may be recognized later during infancy. They include deafness which is the most common manifestation of congenital rubella, heart malformation such as patent ductus arteriosus or pulmonary stenosis, eye anomalies such as cataract, microphthalmia, glaucoma, and retinopathy, inguinal hernia, and cryptorchidism. Other manifestations are less frequent. Infection of the central nervous sytem results in developmental disturbances such as mental retardation which is characteristically severe and profound, spastic diplegia, and behavioural disorders. If progressive rubella panencephalitis is to occur, it usually develops during the second or third decade of life in patients with previously stable congenital rubella syndrome. The late appearance of endocrine disorders such as hyperthyroidism, hypothyroidism, or diabetes mellitus has also been described.

Size of the problem

Serological surveys indicate that 5–15 per cent of pregnant women lack specific antibodies against rubella and are at risk of infection (Cockburn 1969). In any country, however, a larger proportion of susceptible women can be found in particular population groups, such as ethnic minorities (Peckham *et al.* 1983). In the United States, a prospective survey of pregnant women showed that the incidence of clinical rubella was between 4–8 per 10 000 women, during an endemic period (White *et al.* 1969), and rose to approximately 20 cases per 10 000 women during an epidemic (Sever *et al.* 1969). The real incidence of rubella infection should be 1.5–3 times higher since 33–66 per cent of infections are sub-clinical (Bisno *et al.* 1969; Sever *et al.* 1969).

The risk to the fetus after maternal rubella during pregnancy was estimated from a prospective survey of 1016 serologically confirmed cases in the United Kingdom (Miller *et al.* 1982). Of the 966 women for whom the outcome of pregnancy was known, 54 per cent had therapeutic abortions and 4 per cent had spontaneous abortions. Among pregnancies that continued to term,

Table 1.1 Risk of congenital infection and of permanent congenital rubella syndrome (CRS) according to the stage of pregnancy at which maternal rubella occurs.

Stage of pregnancy (weeks)	Livebirths infected (%)	CRS in livebirths infected (%)	CRS in livebirths infected and not infected (%)
<11	90	100	90
11–12	67	50	33
13–14	67	17	11
15–16	47	50	24
17–18	39	0	0
>18	40	0	0

Adapted from Miller *et al.* (1982).

there were 2 per cent of stillbirths, about twice the expected frequency. Fetal infection was diagnosed in 43 per cent of liveborn babies. Congenital malformations or developmental defects compatible with congenital rubella syndrome were observed in 20 per cent of infants with proven infection. The risk of fetal infection and of congenital rubella syndrome is clearly related to the stage of pregnancy at which the maternal disease occurs (Table 1.1).

The exact frequency of congenital rubella syndrome in a population is difficult to assess. Terminations of pregnancy as a result of maternal disease or contact are certainly decreasing the frequency of the condition among livebirths. In many cases, the congenital syndrome is not clinically apparent at birth and is only detected during childhood when confirmation of diagnosis by laboratory investigation is difficult to establish (Orenstein *et al.* 1985). In the absence of control measures, estimates of the frequency of congenital rubella syndrome vary from 0.2 cases per 1000 births in a non-epidemic period to 2.0 cases per 1000 births during an epidemic (Knox 1980; Stray-Pedersen 1982). In the United Kingdom, before immunization began, it was estimated that 15 per cent of all cases of sensorineural deafness (Peckham *et al.* 1979) and 2 per cent of all cases of congenital heart disease (Campell 1965) were attributable to congenital rubella.

Nature of intervention

Vaccine against rubella

The rubella virus was isolated in 1961 (Parkman *et al.* 1962; Weller and Neva

1962), beginning successful research to find an effective vaccine based on a live, attenuated strain. In 1969, the first vaccines were licensed in Europe, Japan, and the United States. The vaccine is produced in monovalent form (rubella only) and in combination (measles–rubella, rubella–mumps, and measles–mumps–rubella vaccines) (Perkins 1985).

Although natural infection with wild rubella virus induces a more vigorous immune response than the vaccine, 95 per cent or more of susceptible persons, receiving a single dose of vaccine, seroconvert. Long-term follow-up, for almost 15 years after immunization, indicates loss of detectable serum antibodies in less than 10 per cent of those immunized who seroconverted initially. Vaccine-induced immunity usually protects against both clinical illness and viraemia after natural exposure. Reinfection of persons with vaccine-induced immunity has been described, but the risk to the fetus of a woman with rubella reinfection seems to be very low (Morgan-Capner et al. 1985). Similarly, the risk of transmission of virus from reinfected individuals to susceptible contacts is low (Preblud et al. 1980; Schiff et al. 1985).

Occasionally rubella vaccine can cause rubella-like symptoms in recipients. Transient rheumatic side-effects occur in 10–40 per cent of susceptible women, but are less frequent in children. In exceptional cases, side-effects can be recurrent or chronic. They are never associated with serious disability (Preblud et al. 1980).

Rubella vaccine virus can cross the placenta and infect the fetus. Review of the outcome of women who received rubella vaccine shortly before or after conception did not reveal one confirmed case of congenital rubella syndrome (Bart et al. 1985b; Sheppard et al. 1986). However, since the actual risk may not be zero, women known to be pregnant should not be immunized, and conception should be avoided for 3 months after immunization. Accidental immunization of a pregnant woman is not considered as an indication for abortion.

Objectives of rubella immunization

Rubella infection and the vaccine fulfil most of the criteria that make worldwide eradication theoretically possible (Table 1.2). It has been shown in mathematical models that transmission of the virus should be completely interrupted when systematic immunization of young children achieves a high level of artificially induced immunity in the population (Knox 1980; Anderson and May 1983; Hethcote 1983).

The cost–benefit of eradication is an important factor to consider. In a cost–benefit analysis, an attempt is made to translate all the costs and benefits from a programme into financial terms. Direct costs of rubella eradication include the cost of the vaccine, its administration, serological tests for the identification of immunity (if they are performed), and treatment of

Table 1.2 Biological factors favouring eradication of rubella

Biological factor	Applicability to rubella
Infection and disease limited to human host and transmitted person to person (no animal or insect reservoir)	Yes
Characteristic clinical disease, usually serious, and easily diagnosed	No
Few or no sub-clinical cases	No
No long-term carrier states	Yes
Only one causative agent or serotype	Yes
Short period of infectivity pre- and post-disease	Yes
Immunity after disease or immunization is:	
of long duration	Yes
not subject to reinfection or reactivation	Yes
decreases or eliminates excretion of organism	Yes
evidence of vaccine immunity detectable	Yes
Disease has seasonality (permitting vaccine strategies)	Yes
Characteristics of vaccine needed:	
simulates natural infection	Yes
stable: resists physical and genetic change	Yes

Adapted from Evans (1985).

vaccine complications. Benefits are defined as the expenditure saved by not having to diagnose, treat, rehabilitate, and educate children with congenital rubella syndrome, and not having to prevent the birth of affected babies by therapeutic abortion (direct benefits), and the gain in production by not having disabled individuals or people who die prematurely (indirect benefits). Cost–benefit analyses of different programmes in different industrialized western countries always show that eradication would be largely cost-saving (Elo 1974; Schoenbaum et al. 1976; Stray-Pedersen 1982; Gudnadottir 1985). The benefits of eradication are largely the prevention of costs associated with special schooling for deaf and blind children and the institutionalization of mentally retarded individuals.

Eradication is also attractive since it could prevent the human tragedy associated with the birth of an abnormal infant and the anxiety caused by the threat of infection during pregnancy. The acceptability of the rubella vaccine to the public and health professionals is high since it is particularly safe and easy to administer. The possibility of integrating rubella immunization in other preventive programmes such as immunization against measles is another argument favouring the strategy of eradication.

There are, however, two important factors that make the prospect of world-wide eradication unlikely in the near future. First, the impact of congenital rubella syndrome on public opinion and on the economy of industrialized countries is not sufficient to induce strong political will for eradication. Second, in many developed countries, the disease is at the bottom of the list of health priorities and the limited resources available cannot be diverted into a specific surveillance and immunization programme against rubella. As a result, the elimination of congenital rubella syndrome, not the eradication of rubella infection, remains the stated objective of all control programmes established throughout the world (Begg and Noah 1985; Hinman 1985).

Strategies for immunization

There are two main immunization strategies for preventing rubella infection during pregnancy. The 'selective' approach aims to protect susceptible women of childbearing age without interfering with the transmission of the virus in the child population and the acquisition of natural immunity. This policy was adopted in all European countries in the early 1970s. The 'mass' strategy aims to interrupt the spread of rubella in the population by the immunization of all children. Thus non-immunized women are protected from exposure itself (herd immunity) rather than from the effects of exposure. This second policy leads also to direct protection when the cohort of immunized girls reaches childbearing age. The mass strategy was adopted in the United States and Canada. Variants of these two strategies are described in Table 1.3 (Stray-Pedersen 1982). Eventually, the two approaches can be combined as in Sweden where all 18-month-old children are vaccinated with combined rubella–measles–mumps vaccine and girls are revaccinated at the age of 12 years (Christenson *et al.* 1983).

Effectiveness of immunization programmes

The relative effectiveness of the two main strategies in preventing congenital rubella syndrome and epidemics of rubella disease in the population can be evaluated *a priori* in simulation models. There is agreement in the conclusions reached by different models applied to the epidemiological situation of rubella in industrialized countries (Knox 1980; Anderson and May 1983; Hethcote 1983; Knox 1985).

The effectiveness of the selective strategy in preventing congenital rubella syndrome is proportional to the immunization rate in the target population. Elimination of congenital rubella syndrome will only be achieved if 100 per cent of susceptible women are immunized using a vaccine that is 100 per cent effective. This strategy has little impact on the frequency and severity of

Table 1.3 Immunization strategies for the control of congenital rubella syndrome

Permanent running programmes
I Immunization of all infants (at 15 months or older): 'mass' strategy
II Immunization of girls in puberty (at 11–15-years-old): 'selective' strategy
   1. Immunization of all girls
   2. Immunization of susceptible (non-immunized) girls after serological screening for rubella antibodies

Supplementary programmes
III Immunization of women in the immediate postpartum period
   1. Immunization of all women
   2. Immunization of non-immunized women after serological screening in pregnancy
   3. Serological screening of paired sera in the first trimester, collected preferentially in the sixth and thirteenth gestational week, combined with therapeutic abortions of risk pregnancies and immunization of non-immunized women
IV Premarital serological screening and immunization of non-immunized women
V Selective immunization of women especially at risk of exposure (nursery and kindergarten staff, school teachers, health care providers)

Adapted from Stray-Pedersen (1982).

rubella epidemics. The maximum effect of an immunization programme for teenage girls will only be reached 20 years after its start. A more rapid effect could, however, be achieved when the programme is supplemented by immunization of the population of women of childbearing age.

In the mass strategy, there is no linear relationship between the vaccination rate and the magnitude of effects. If a high rate of immunization (more than 80 per cent) can be achieved among children, the mass strategy will be theoretically more effective than the selective strategy in reducing the number of cases of congenital infection, and this effect will manifest earlier. Epidemics of rubella infection in the whole population will also be prevented. With this strategy, there is, however, a danger of *increasing* the frequency of congenital rubella syndrome if the immunization rate in children is low. In such circumstances, rubella epidemics are not prevented and the reduction in the transmission of virus among children postpones the age of first exposure among the non-immunized increasing the risk of disease in pregnant women. On the other hand, mass immunization could interrupt the transmission of the virus in the population and achieve complete elimination of fetal infection, provided high immunization rates are sustained.

There seems to be something to be gained from adopting a strategy combining the two approaches, as long as a high level of immunization of young children is achieved (Anderson and Grenfell 1985; Knox 1987). Systematic immunization of teenage girls with supplementary child immunization in excess of 70–80 per cent uptake will provide substantial long-term benefits. With lower uptake rates in young children, the benefits will be marginal, if any, and there is a risk of inducing oscillations in the subsequent incidence of rubella and fetal infection. Knox (1987) has pointed out that, as the two approaches are based on opposing principles, use of combined programmes without an underlying commitment to elimination may do more harm than good.

The relative cost of different strategies is another important element in decision-making. The effectiveness, costs, and benefits of three immunization programmes were estimated by Schoenbaum *et al.* in 1976 (Table 1.4). This model is based on the assumption that the immunization of young children does not reduce the risk of exposure in pregnant women as a result of herd immunity. Induced abortions after confirmed maternal infection or contact were not taken into account in the analysis. Assuming a compliance rate of 80 per cent in immunization of the target population, the combined approach is the more effective in reducing the number of cases of congenital rubella syndrome, but this is also the most expensive policy. The cheapest strategy is based on the use of a combined measles–rubella vaccine in young children who are given measles vaccine anyway. However, this model shows that the maximum benefit is obtained from the selective strategy—that is, the immunization of 12-year-old girls. This is mainly because this strategy gives results more rapidly than immunization at a younger age and, thus, a more rapid return on investment. To determine accurately the value of a programme, all costs and benefits to occur in the future should be discounted to their present value, since a sum of money is worth more today than it will be in the future (Holland 1983). Stray-Pedersen (1982) and Gudnadottir (1985) reached the same conclusion that the immunization of 12-year-old girls is more cost-effective and cost-beneficial than the systematic immunization of all young children even if the rubella vaccine is integrated in a control programme against measles. Immunization of teenage girls with or without previous testing for immunity should be decided according to the relative cost of the test and of the vaccine, which may differ from country-to-country (Gudnadottir 1985).

The practical feasibility of an immunization programme is, perhaps, the most important criterion for selecting a strategy. As any strategy is largely cost-beneficial and as every industrialized Western country can easily afford the more expensive of the proposed programmes, the final choice is determined essentially by the capability of the existing health care facilities to reach the target population and achieve a satisfactory immunization rate.

Table 1.4 Estimated epidemiological and economic effects of various rubella immunization strategies[a]

Effect	Immunization of 12-year-old girls[b]	Immunization of 2-year-old children both sexes[c]	Immunization of 12-year-old girls and of 2-year-old children both sexes
Natural infections prevented (%)	10.1	75.9	78.5
Births with congenital rubella prevented (%)	81.3	73.7	95.9
Benefits of prevention of acute rubella and congenital rubella[d]	64.1	36.6	46.1
Costs of immunization[d]	2.4	1.6	2.9
Benefits–costs ratio	27:1	23:1	16:1
Net benefits[d]	61.7	35.0	43.2
Benefits per case of congenital rubella prevented[d]	0.052	0.029	0.028

[a]Costs and benefits are calculated on the basis of immunization of a target population of one million females with 80 per cent compliance.
[b]Immunization without previous screening for immunity.
[c]Using a combined measles–rubella vaccine and assuming that measles vaccine would have been given anyway.
[d]In million dollars, 1975 value.
Adapted from Schoenbaum *et al.* (1976).

Monitoring immunization programmes

The collection of epidemiological data on rubella is essential for planning and evaluating any immunization programme. The indicators which should be measured for monitoring the implementation and the impact of programmes are the immunization rate, the incidence of rubella disease, the prevalence of immune status, and the frequency of congenital rubella syndrome including therapeutic abortions (Orenstein *et al.* 1985). In many countries, the total number of vaccines distributed is the only indicator available for evaluating programme progress. A comprehensive system for the surveillance of rubella and the monitoring of control programmes exists in only a few countries.

In the United Kingdom (Tobin *et al.* 1985), information on acquired rubella is obtained from routinely collected reports from public health laboratories, from weekly reports of clinical cases submitted by selected general practitioners, and by notification of clinical disease from selected health authorities. Information on congenital rubella syndrome is collected in a special registry to which confirmed or suspected cases are passively notified. The national surveillance system of abortions provides the number of rubella-associated terminations of pregnancy. Data are also available on the immunization rate among schoolgirls, and special surveys are conducted periodically, in population groups such as students or pregnant women, in order to monitor the prevalence of immunity in the adult population.

In the United States (Centers for Disease Control 1976), epidemiological information on rubella is centralized at the Centers for Disease Control, Atlanta. Acquired rubella has been a nationally reportable disease since 1966. In 1969, a national registry was established for collecting detailed reports on cases of congenital rubella syndrome. A comparison of the different sources of information provides an accurate picture of the epidemiology of rubella and of the impact of control measures.

Impact of continuing programmes

The effectiveness of rubella control programmes has been evaluated in a number of countries including: Australia (Menser *et al.* 1985); Israel (Swartz *et al.* 1985); Japan (Kono *et al.* 1985); the United States (Bart *et al.* 1985a); Canada (Furesz *et al.* 1985); Iceland (Gudnadottir 1985), the United Kingdom (Dudgeon 1985); Finland (Peltola *et al.* 1986); and Sweden (Christenson *et al.* 1983). In most European countries, information is scarce.

In the United Kingdom, the selective immunization of girls aged 11–14 years was the preventive strategy adopted in 1970 (Dudgeon 1985). No previous serological testing of immunity was done. The immunization acceptance rate among schoolgirls is currently 85 per cent. The programme was reinforced by a recommendation to immunize all susceptible women of childbearing age. The short-term results of the programme do not indicate a change in the epidemiology of natural rubella or a major decline in the incidence of fetal infection (Table 1.5). It appears, however, that the incidence of congenital rubella in children born to mothers who belong to the first cohorts eligible for immunization is much lower than in children born to older women. Results of serological surveys in 18-year-old girls indicate an increase in the proportion of seropositive individuals from approximately 80 per cent in the early 1970s to 95 per cent in the early 1980s (Tobin *et al.* 1985).

In the United States, a universal immunization programme started in 1969, first by mass immunization of children below the age of puberty and then by systematic immunization of all children of one year of age. In 1978–79, the programme was reinforced to achieve better coverage and the use of combined measles–mumps–rubella vaccine was encouraged. Increased emphasis was also placed on immunizing susceptible women of childbearing

Table 1.5 Notified cases of rubella, of congenital rubella syndrome, and rubella-associated terminations of pregnancy in the United Kingdom from 1970 to 1983.

Year	Mean weekly number of cases of clinical rubella per 100 000	Number of laboratory reports of rubella infection	Number of cases of congenital rubella syndrome	Number of cases of termination of pregnancy for rubella disease
1970	2.70	491	52	a
1971	5.50	815	85	a
1972	6.15	1117	70	a
1973	4.40	1667	85	a
1974	4.45	1722	59	512
1975	4.45	1578	45	406
1976	2.05	929	14	144
1977	2.25	760	21	118
1978	6.75	4154	86	659
1979	4.45	3548	41	431
1980	2.75	731	13	153
1981	3.45	557	18[b]	88
1982	4.75	1632	29[b]	a
1983	8.90	2659	19[b]	a

[a]Data not available.
[b]Provisional figures.
Adapted from Tobin *et al.* (1985).

age. The incidence of rubella disease declined in all age groups, especially in the children, the primary target group of the programme (Figure 1.1.) (Centers for Disease Control 1986). The programme had successfully prevented epidemic rubella. Serological surveys indicated that the proportion of susceptible individuals among those aged 15 years and more has not been reduced substantially so far. Local outbreaks continued to occur in communities of young adults. A decline in the reported frequency rate of congenital rubella syndrome has been noted especially after the decline in the disease incidence in the post-pubertal population. These results suggest that 'herd immunity' against rubella is not obtained to the extent predicted by simulation models (Bart *et al.* 1985a). An estimation of the costs and savings of the immunization programme for measles, mumps, and rubella for the year 1983 indicated a benefit–cost ratio of 7.7 : 1 for rubella alone (White *et al.* 1985).

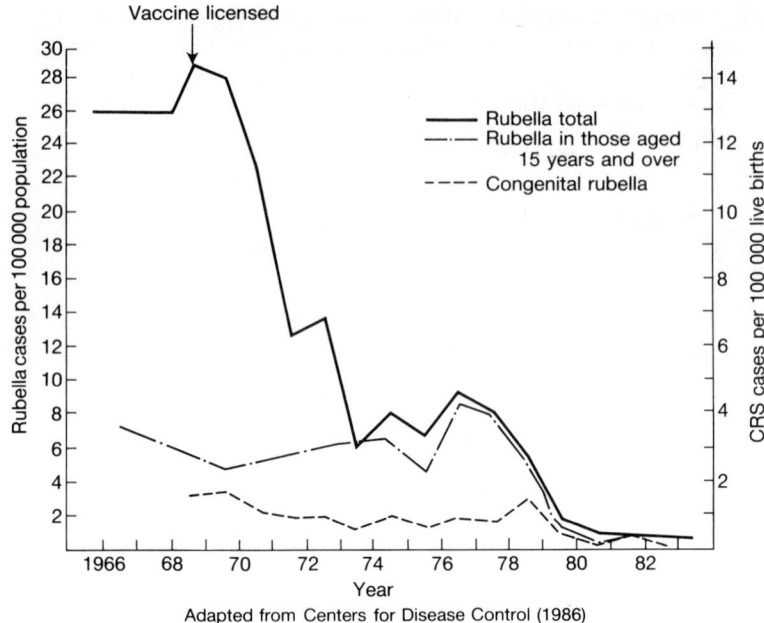

Fig. 1.1 Incidence of reported rubella and of congenital rubella syndrome (CRS) in the United States from 1966 to 1983.

Prospects for achieving elimination of congenital rubella

The experience of rubella control in the United Kingdom and in the United States indicates that both the selective and the mass strategies are effective in reducing the risk of congenital rubella syndrome in the population. However, the programmes currently being carried out reveal limitations, and congenital rubella syndrome has not been eliminated so far.

Whatever the strategy chosen, priority should be given to providing immediate protection to the population currently at risk of infection during pregnancy (Hinman *et al.* 1983). This is needed because immunization of young children or of teenage girls is only effective after a delay of several years, and because the immunization rate achieved is not satisfactory, leaving a significant proportion of susceptible young adults. There are a number of ways in which susceptible females could be identified and immunized. Responsibility for immunization can be given to general practitioners, obstetricians, occupational and school doctors, or community health services. Serological testing before immunization of women of childbearing age is recommended, although, too often, screened women known to be susceptible are lost to follow-up and not immunized (Miller *et al.* 1985).

In countries using the selective immunization of teenage girls, efforts should be made to increase immunization compliance since the long-term effectiveness of the programme is directly proportional to the immunization rate in the target population (Knox 1985). It has been shown in the United Kingdom that levels of immunization of more than 90 per cent can be achieved by motivated general practitioners and community physicians (Andrewes 1983; Jones 1983; Walker *et al.* 1986).

In countries using the systematic immunization of young children, it is essential to achieve high rates of compliance since a low immunization rate could lead to an increasing risk of disease in susceptible pregnant women (Knox 1985). In the United Kingdom, it has been suggested that a change of policy from selective immunization of teenage girls to systematic immunization of young children would not work and would eventually prove dangerous. This is because it seems impossible to achieve a satisfactory immunization rate in the target population as evidenced by the low proportion of infants immunized against measles (50 per cent) in that country (Dudgeon 1985). This situation may, however, change in the future.

Recommendations

There is a safe and effective vaccine against rubella. Although the exact duration of vaccine-induced immunity is not known, it is thought to be lifelong. The benefit of the prevention of congenital rubella syndrome in industrialized countries is beyond doubt. Within each country and within each region, prevention must be handled by an explicit and coordinated choice of strategy. In many European countries, the adopted strategy and the means to implement it are not sufficiently defined and publicized. It is ineffective, inefficient, and even harmful to allow individual clinicians to pursue their own inclinations or different institutions or local authorities to select their own strategy.

In order to reduce the number of cases of congenital rubella syndrome in the short term, it is important to decrease, as soon as possible, the number of susceptible women of childbearing age. Programmes for the control of rubella should be comprehensive and should not ignore this population of adult women currently at risk.

In the long run, the choice of an optimal strategy in European countries depends mainly on the feasibility of achieving an adequate immunization rate in young children and in teenage girls. Both the selective and the mass strategies seem to be effective in reducing the frequency of congenital rubella syndrome. The mass strategy could lead eventually to the eradication of rubella infection.

The key to the success of any programme is to achieve a high level of immunization in the target population. Efforts should be made to improve the awareness of the general population of the dangers of rubella and thus to improve the acceptance of immunization especially in high-risk groups, such as ethnic minorities and less educated social groups. The training and the motivation of health professionals carrying out the immunization programme should be upgraded since it has been demonstrated that this factor affects compliance greatly. Compulsory measures such as those adopted in the United States where, in 36 states, proof of immunization is obligatory for school entry, can certainly lead to an increase in immunization rate, although these kind of measures are not easily accepted in many European countries.

In any case, the implementation of preventive programmes should be properly evaluated. Evaluation requires the availability of a minimum of epidemiological information which is still lacking in most European countries. The establishment of a health information system on rubella, in every country, is a subsidiary but important objective in the fight for the elimination of congenital rubella syndrome.

References

Anderson, R.M. and May, R.M. (1983). Vaccination against rubella and measles: quantitative investigations of different policies. *J. Hyg. Camb.* **90**, 259-325.
—— and Grenfell, B.T. (1985). Control of congenital rubella syndrome by mass vaccination. *Lancet* **2**, 827-8.
Andrewes, D.A. (1983). Rubella immunization: whose baby? *Br. Med. J.* **287**, 1769-71.
Asaad, F. and Ljungars-Esteves, K. (1985). Rubella—world impact. *Rev. Infect. Dis.* **7**, suppl 1, S29-36.
Bart, K.J., Orenstein, W.A., Preblud, S.R., and Hinman, A.R. (1985a). Universal immunization to interrupt rubella. *Rev. Infect. Dis.* **7**, suppl. 1, S177-84.
Bart, S.W., Stetler, H.C., Preblud, S.R., Williams, N.M., Orenstein, W.A., Bart, K.J., Hinman, A.R., and Herrmann, K.L. (1985b). Fetal risk associated with rubella vaccine: an update. *Rev. Infect. Dis.* **7**, suppl. 1, S95-102.
Begg, T., and Noah, N.D. (1985). Immunisation targets in Europe and Britain. *Br. Med. J.* **291**, 1370.
Bisno, A.L., Spence, L.P., Stewart, J.A., and Casey, H.L. (1969). Rubella in Trinidad: sero-epidemiologic studies of an institutional outbreak. *Am. J. Epidemiol.* **89**, 74-81.
Campbell, M. (1965). Causes of malformations of the heart. *Br. Med. J.* **2**, 895-904.
Centers for Disease Control. (1976). Rubella surveillance, July 1973-December 1975. HEW Publication No (CDC) 76-8023, Atlanta, Georgia, 1-15.
—— (1986). Annual summary 1984. *Morbid. Mortal. Wkly Rep.* **33**, 51.

Christenson B., Bottiger, M., and Heller, L. (1983). Mass vaccination programme aimed at eradicating measles, mumps, and rubella in Sweden: first experience. *Br. Med. J.* **287**, 389-91.

Cockburn, W.C. (1969). World aspects of the epidemiology of rubella. *Am. J. Dis. Child.* **118**, 112-22.

Cooper, L.Z.(1985). The history and medical consequences of rubella. *Rev. Infect. Dis.* **7**, suppl. 1, S2-10.

Dudgeon, J.A. (1985). Selective immunization: protection of the individual. *Rev. Infect. Dis.* **7**, suppl. 1, S185-93.

Elo, O. (1974). Health and economic consequences of rubella. *Acta. Univ. Tampere* **60**, 27-47.

Evans, A.S. (1985). The eradication of communicable diseases: myth or reality? *Am. J. Epidemiol.* **122**, 199-207.

Furesz, J., Varughese, P., Acres, S.E., and Davies, J.W. (1985). Rubella immunization strategies in Canada. *Rev. Infect. Dis.* **7**, suppl. 1, S191-3.

Gregg, N.M. (1941). Congenital cataract following german measles in the mother. *Transactions of the Ophthalmological Society of Australia* **3**, 35-46.

Gudnadottir, M. (1985). Cost-effectiveness of different strategies for prevention of congenital rubella infection: a practical example from Iceland. *Rev. Infect. Dis.* **7**, suppl. 1, S200-9.

Heggie, A.D., and Robbins, F.C. (1969). Natural rubella acquired after birth. Clinical features and complications. *Am. J. Dis. Child.* **118**, 12-17.

Hethcote, H.W. (1983). Measles and rubella in the United States. *Am. J. Epidemiol.* **117**, 2-13.

Hinmann, A.R. (1985). Prevention of congenital rubella infection: symposium summary. *Rev. Infect. Dis.* **7**, suppl. 1, S212-15.

——, Bart, K.J., Orenstein, W.A., and Preblud, S.R. (1983). Rational strategy for rubella vaccination. *Lancet* **1**, 39-41.

Holland, W.W. (1983). *Evaluation of health care,* pp. 61-7. Oxford University Press, Oxford.

Hortsmann, D.M. (1982). Rubella. In *Viral infections of humans* (ed. A.S. Evans) pp. 519-39. Plenum Medical Book Company, New York.

Jones, A.E. (1983). Implementation of the rubella vaccination programme in Manchester. *Comm. Med.* **5**, 287-94.

Knox, E.G. (1980). Strategy for rubella vaccination *Int. J. Epidemiol.* **9**, 13-23.

—— (1985). Theoretical aspects of rubella vaccination strategies *Rev. Infect. Dis.* **7**, suppl. 1, S194-7.

—— (1987). Evolution of rubella vaccine policy for the UK. *Int. J. Epidemiol.* **16**, 569-78.

Kono, R., Hiramaya, M., Sugishita, C., and Miyamura, K. (1985). Epidemiology of rubella and congenital rubella infection in Japan. *Rev. Infect. Dis.* **7**, suppl. 1, S56-63.

Menser, M.A., Hudson, J.R., Murphy, A.M., and Upfold, L.J. (1985). Epidemiology of congenital rubella and results of rubella vaccination in Australia. *Rev. Infect. Dis.* **7**, suppl. 1, S37-41.

Miller, E., Cradock-Watson, J.E., and Pollock, T.M. (1982). Consequences of confirmed maternal rubella at successive stages of pregnancy. *Lancet* **2**, 781-4.

Miller, C.L., Miller, E., Sequeira, P.J.L., Cradock-Watson, J.E., Longson, M., and Wiseberg, E.C. (1985). Effect of selective vaccination on rubella susceptibility and infection in pregnancy. *Br. Med. J.* **291**, 1398–401.

Morgan-Capner, P., Hodgson, J., Hambling, M.H., Dulake, C., Coleman, T.J., Boswell, P.A., Watkins, R., Booth, J., Stern, H., Best, J.M., and Banatvala, J.E. (1985). Detection of rubella-specific IgM in subclinical rubella reinfection in pregnancy. *Lancet* **1**, 244–5.

Orenstein, W.A., Preblud, S.R., Bart K.J., and Hinman, A.R. (1985). Methods of assessing the impact of congenital rubella infection. *Rev. Infect. Dis.* **7**, suppl. 1, S22–8.

Parkman, P.D., Buescher, E.L., and Artenstein, M.S. (1962). Recovery of rubella virus from army recruits. *Proc. Soc. Exp. Biol. Med.* **111**, 225–30.

Peckham, C.S., Martin, J.A.M., Marshall, W.C., and Dudgeon, J.A. (1979). Congenital rubella deafness: a preventable disease. *Lancet* **1**, 258–61.

——, Tookey, P., Nelson, D.B., Coleman, J., and Morris, N. (1983). Ethnic minority women and congenital rubella. *Br. Med. J.* **287**, 129–30.

Peltola, H., Karanko, V., Kurki, T., Hukkanen, V., Virtanen, M., Penttinen, K., Nissinen, M., and Heinonen, O.P. (1986). Rapid effect on endemic measles, mumps, and rubella of nationwide vaccination programme in Finland. *Lancet* **1**, 137–8.

Perkins, F.T. (1985). Licensed vaccines. *Rev. Infect. Dis.* **7**, suppl. 1, S73–6.

Preblud, S.R., Serdula, M.K., Frank, J.A., Brandling-Bennet, A.D., and Hinman, A.R. (1980). Rubella vaccination in the United States: a ten-year review. *Epidemiol. Rev.* **2**, 171–94.

Schiff, G.M., Young, B.C., Stefanovic, G.M., Stamler, E.F., Knowlton, D.R., Grundy, B.J., and Dorsett, P.H. (1985). Challenge with rubella virus after loss of detectable vaccine-induced antibody. *Rev. Infect. Dis.* **7**, suppl. 1, S157–63.

Schoenbaum, S.C., Hyde, J.N., Bartoshesky, L., and Crampton, K. (1976). Benefit–cost analysis of rubella vaccination policy. *New Engl. J. Med.* **294**, 306–10.

Sever, J.L., Hardy, J.B., Nelson, K.B., and Gilkeson, M.R. (1969). Rubella in the collaborative perinatal research study. *Am. J. Dis. Child.* **118**, 123–32.

Sheppard, S., Smithells, R.W., Dickson, A., and Holzel, H. (1986). Rubella vaccination and pregnancy: preliminary report of a national survey. *Br. Med. J.* **292**, 727.

Stray-Pedersen, B. (1982). Economic evaluation of different vaccination programmes to prevent congenital rubella. *NIPH Annals* **5**, 69–83.

Swartz, T.A., Hornstein, L., and Epstein, I. (1985). Epidemiology of rubella and congenital rubella infection in Israël, a country with a selective immunization program. *Rev. Infect. Dis.* **7**, suppl. 1, S42–6.

Tobin, J.O'H., Sheppard, S., Smithells, R.W., Milton, A., Noah, N., and Reid, D. (1985). Rubella in the United Kingdom, 1970–1983. *Rev. Infect. Dis.* **7**, suppl. 1, S47–52.

Walker, D., Carter H., and Jones, I.G. (1986). Measles, mumps, and rubella: the need for a change in immunisation policy. *Br. Med. J.* **292**, 1501–2.

Weller, T.H., and Neva, F.H. (1962). Propagation in tissue culture of cytopathic agents from patients with rubella-like illness. *Proc. Soc. Exp. Biol. Med.* **111**, 215–25.

White, C.C., Koplan, J.P., and Orenstein, W.A. (1985). Benefits, risks and costs of immunisation for measles, mumps, and rubella. *Am. J. Publ. Hlth* **75**, 739-44.

White, L.R., Sever, J.L., and Alepa, F.P. (1969). Maternal and congenital rubella before 1964: frequency, clinical features, and search for isoimmune phenomena. *J. Pediat.* **74**, 198-207.

Witte, J.J., Karchmer, A.W., Case, G., Herrmann, K.L., Abrutyn, E., Kassanoff, I., and Neill, J.S. (1969). Epidemiology of rubella. *Am. J. Dis. Child* **118**, 107-11.

2
Whooping cough

Shane Allwright

SUMMARY

Whooping cough (pertussis), although no longer a significant contributor to childhood mortality in Europe, is still a disease which is sufficiently serious, particularly in infants, to warrant protection by immunization. Whole-cell vaccines currently in use are of fairly high efficacy, moderate population effectiveness, and low toxicity. The benefits derived from immunization generally outweigh the risks. In some countries public and medical confidence in immunization has been greatly undermined by fears of serious neurological side-effects. This has led to a lowering of vaccine uptake and subsequent increase in incidence of whooping cough in these countries. The new component vaccines appear promising and are likely to be more acceptable to the general public. It is unlikely that whooping cough will be eliminated in this century, but, with current vaccines, containment can and should be achieved throughout Europe within the next decade.

Defining the problem

Until the end of the nineteenth century, whooping cough caused more deaths than any other infectious disease except measles. It remained a major cause of childhood mortality in Europe until the Second World War. In Europe deaths from whooping cough are now rare.

But whooping cough (pertussis) is still a serious, epidemic, respiratory disease affecting mainly children. The aetiological agent is *Bordetella pertussis*. Typically, whooping cough lasts 4 to 8 weeks and throughout much of this period there are frequent episodes of repetitive paroxysmal coughing, often, but not always, followed by the characteristic whoop sound caused by sudden deep inspiration. The coughing episodes are extremely distressing and frightening, and are often followed by vomiting. Furthermore, exacerbation of symptoms at night means excessive sleep disturbance for both children and parents (Johnston *et al.* 1985). Although antibiotics are effective for treating bacterial complications, they have little effect on the clinical course of the illness. Whooping cough is highly infectious and susceptibility is universal. One attack usually confers lasting immunity. As there is no transfer of passive immunity from the mother to the newborn infant, neonates are susceptible from birth.

A notable feature of the disease is that its severity is greatest in infants. Rates of admission to hospital are inversely related to age and most deaths occur in infants of less than 1 year. Complications include vomiting, cyanosis, bronchitis, pneumonia, apnoea, convulsions, dehydration, and encephalitis, in decreasing order of frequency (Miller and Fletcher 1976; Swansea Research Unit RCGP 1981; Pollock et al. 1984).

A subsequent excess of respiratory morbidity has been found in children who have had whooping cough in the past, but there are conflicting opinions as to whether this was present before their whooping cough or as consequence of it (Johnston et al. 1983; Swansea Research Unit RCGP 1985).

Severe cases in young children are usually readily diagnosed clinically, but in older children and adults laboratory diagnosis is often required. The best method of diagnosis is isolation of the organism with pernasal swabs from the nasopharynx (Preston 1986). Except for demonstration of a rising titre, serological diagnosis is unreliable.

Size of the problem

Occurrence and trends

Whooping cough occurs throughout the world. The death rate from whooping cough has dropped dramatically in Europe since the start of the twentieth century and is currently less than one per million of the population in most countries. This decline in mortality, which preceded the introduction of whooping cough immunization, reflects a sharp fall in case fatality which is believed to result primarily from improved socio-economic conditions and more effective clinical management. Declining fertility, by increasing the median age at infection, may also have contributed to this improvement (Reves 1985).

Widely differing incidence rates are reported in different countries. Trends based on national notifications to the World Health Organization (WHO) are available for most European countries. As the levels of notification to WHO are known to be very incomplete and to differ widely between countries, examination of the trends over time within countries is more valid than a comparison between countries. Differing recent trends (1974–1983) in European countries are illustrated in Figure 2.1. A short (10-year) time period of observation has been selected so as to minimize bias from temporal changes in completeness of notification, case-finding, and diagnostic accuracy.

The first group of countries in Figure 2.1 had rates that were consistently low during this period and had an immunization coverage of over 90 per cent linked with a booster programme—for example, Hungary, Czechoslovakia, and the German Democratic Republic. The second group of countries experienced a fall in notification rates between 1974 and 1983, with immunization coverage between 70 and 90 per cent, and a booster programme—for example, France and Luxembourg. The final group of countries showed a rise in notification rates over this period, with high baseline notification rates and a fall in immunization coverage to less than 60 per cent—for example, the United Kingdom and Ireland.

It is probably correct to infer from the available data (WHO 1985) that in the past 10 years or so there has been a substantial decline in whooping cough incidence in most of the Eastern bloc countries, France, and, possibly, Austria and Greece. Conversely, Norway, Sweden, Iceland, the United Kingdom, and Ireland have experienced large rises in incidence. Incidence in Denmark, after a big rise in the mid-1970s, has decreased.

Detailed and at least partially reliable information on incidence rates is available from the United Kingdom. About 19 per cent of cases are notified (Jenkinson 1983); this is believed to be the highest notification efficiency in Europe (Clarkson and Fine 1985). Figure 2.2. shows annual statutory notifications in England and Wales from 1940 (when whooping cough first became notifiable) to 1985. There was a sharp decline in the 1950s, then a slower decline and levelling-off in the 1960s and early 1970s, and a dramatic upswing in notifications in the late 1970s. Reasons for the different incidence trends seen in the United Kingdom and other countries will be discussed in the section on vaccine effectiveness.

Nature of the intervention

Vaccines made from whole, killed *B. pertussis* cells were developed before the Second World War. Large-scale clinical trials in the late 1940s and 1950s (Medical Research Council 1951, 1956, 1959) demonstrated the safety and potency of three doses of certain of these vaccines. Thus whooping cough vaccines were used with increasing frequency from the early 1950s (Metcalfe Brown 1965). Eventually national immunization programmes were implemented in most European countries.

Vaccine variability

The Medical Research Council trials showed that different vaccines varied greatly in their protective action. Subsequent research has confirmed that

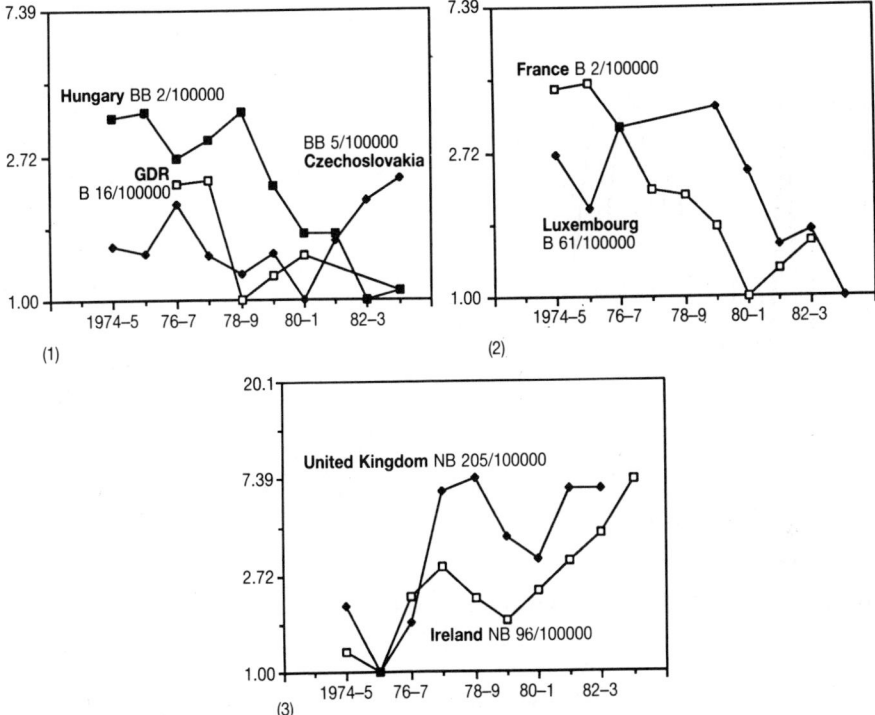

Fig. 2.1 Trends in whooping cough notifications to the World Health Organization and percentage immunization coverage—Europe 1974–84.

(1) Immunization coverage greater than 90 per cent.
(2) Immunization coverage 70–90 per cent.
(3) Immunization coverage fell to less than 60 per cent.

Note:
As less than 10 per cent of whooping cough notifications are in adults, data refer to children under 10 years of age only.

Since whooping cough epidemics usually span more than one year, curves are based on two-year moving averages.

For each country, the biennium with the lowest notification rate per 100 000 children under 10 years has been plotted at base one. This rate is shown beside the country name. All the other biennial rates are displayed relative to this baseline rate on a natural log scale.

Countries are grouped according to recent level of immunization coverage.

B, BB, and NB, shown beside the country name, indicate whether boosters are administered: B—one booster, BB—two boosters, NB—no boosters.

Source: Notifications to WHO 1974–84 (WHO 1985).

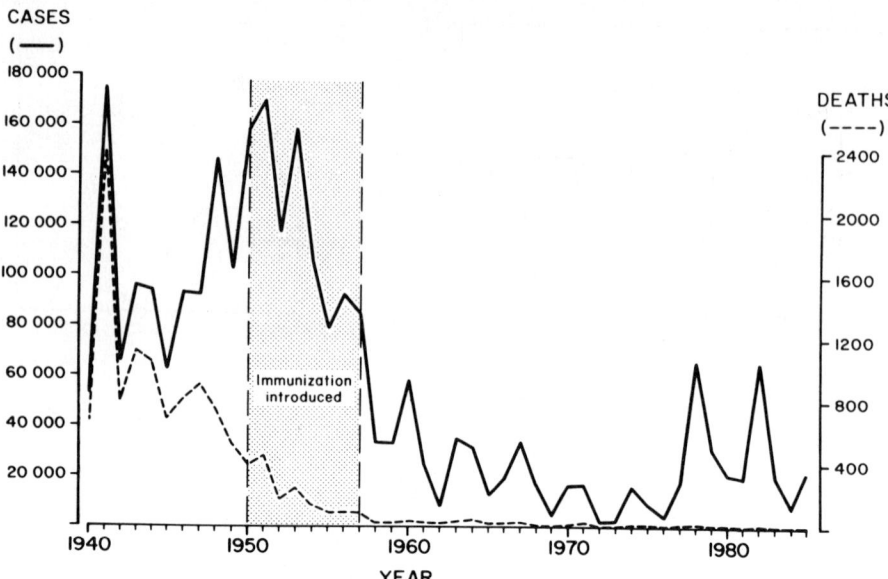

Fig. 2.2 Whooping cough notifications: cases and deaths. England and Wales 1940–85.

whole-cell vaccines vary in efficacy and reactogenicity. The differences relate to many factors including production process and manufacturer (Griffith 1978; Baraff *et al.* 1984), presence or absence of mineral adjuvant (Butler *et al.* 1969; Preston *et al.* 1974), number, size, and timing of doses (Wilkins *et al.* 1971; Baraff *et al.* 1984), differences in injection site (Baraff *et al.* 1984), and combination with other vaccines. Variations in the antigen composition may also contribute to differences between vaccines (Preston 1963, 1976a; PHLS 1973).

Most modern vaccines, which conform to WHO guidelines for adsorption with mineral adjuvant, potency, and antigen content, give adequate protection against whooping cough. Differences in the production process, however, continue to give rise to differences in potency and toxicity. It is therefore essential for surveillance of the vaccines, that not only the fact of immunization, but also the manufacturer and the batch number of vaccine be recorded (Editorial 1978; Griffith 1978). The complexity of batch numbers makes their accurate recording unnecessarily difficult (Rawson *et al.* 1980), and their simplification would aid both manual and computer recording.

Target population

In the early days of immunization the target population for most programmes was not the very young infants (under 6 months) in whom whooping cough is the most lethal, but infants aged 6 to 12 months. This policy was based on concerns about inadequate immune response and toxicity in very young infants. It is now the policy in both Denmark and the United States to start immunization at 6 to 8 weeks and to have the primary course of three doses completed by 6 months of age. This policy narrows the interval during which infants are dependent on herd immunity for their protection. In some countries immunization schedules are still targeted at the 5 to 11 month age group. As inadequate protection is afforded by the first and second doses, this schedule leaves infants unnecessarily vulnerable during their first year, particularly during periods of low immunization uptake when herd immunity is diminished.

High-risk groups

Certain infants—such as those of low birthweight or with conditions such as congenital heart disease, cystic fibrosis, or asthma—are at risk of a particularly severe clinical course of whooping cough. Confusion over contraindications has led to considerable numbers of such infants not being given the benefits of immunization (Hull 1981; Bernbaum et al. 1985; Nicoll 1985). In reality there is a case to be made for more vigorous attempts to achieve for these children both high levels of uptake and an early start to immunization—possibly as early as 2 months in an epidemic. It would probably be necessary to administer a fourth dose of vaccine in the second year of life to children who begin their primary course below the age of 3 months.

Increasing numbers of young infants are now attending day nurseries and are exposed to infection at an earlier age with an increased risk of serious morbidity. These infants constitute another high-risk group for whom both a high uptake and an early start to immunization should be achieved.

Impact of vaccines

The initial impact of the early national immunization programmes was less than dramatic, perhaps as a result both of the low vaccine efficacy and the restriction of immunization to infants. The latter meant that herd immunity could only be built up slowly as successive birth cohorts of infants were immunized.

In the United Kingdom (and probably also in other countries) whooping cough vaccine efficacy appeared to drop further in the early 1960s (PHLS 1969). Preston noted (1963, 1976a) that, whereas in the past the prevalent strains of *B. pertussis* were those possessing antigen 2 (types 1, 2, 3 and 1, 2), by 1963–64 type 1, 3 strains had become common. He suggested that the early vaccines were deficient in antigen 3 which left even fully immunized children susceptible to this newly prevalent serotype and accounted for the decline in efficacy in the 1960s.

The results of current vaccination programmes using whole-cell vaccines which contain all three agglutinogens are still somewhat disappointing. Possible reasons for this are discussed in subsequent sections.

Acellular vaccines

Acellular vaccines have recently been developed and have been used in Japan to immunize 2-year-olds since autumn 1981. These vaccines are still being evaluated. Early results indicate that they are safe and have high protective efficacy (about 80 per cent) (Aoyama *et al.* 1985), but concern has been expressed because they are deficient in pertussis agglutinogens 1, 2, and 3 (Preston 1984; Robinson *et al.* 1985). Continued surveillance is required to reveal whether these vaccines are effective in the long term and whether they are truly devoid of rare, serious side-effects. If the early successes are maintained, it is likely that acellular vaccines will soon replace the whole-cell vaccines currently in use.

Evidence for efficacy

Many clinical trials of pertussis vaccine efficacy were carried out between 1930 and 1960. In Europe the most extensive trials were those organized by the British Medical Research Council. The results (Medical Research Council 1951, 1956, 1959) showed that the vaccine conferred substantial levels of protection (efficacy values of nearly 80 per cent). Different vaccines, however, varied in their protective efficacy, and vaccine potency, as measured in mouse protection tests, correlated well with clinical efficacy.

However, whooping cough vaccines have changed considerably since the 1950s. There are no randomized controlled trials to assess the efficacy of the vaccines currently in use. As serology is not a reliable indicator of protection, serosurveys may not be used to measure efficacy. Assessment and monitoring of vaccines is, therefore, usually based on comparisons of incidence or secondary household attack rates in immunized *versus* non-immunized children. Such assessments are subject to a number of biases, the most important of which is that immunization status is self-selected. Thus, observed differences in attack rate may be the result, at least partially, of confounding variables such as family size and socio-economic status. Other possible sources of bias include errors or bias in diagnosis, changes in completeness of notification over time or between areas, selective under-reporting of disease, differences in criteria for hospital admissions and in proportion of suspected cases sent for laboratory confirmation, and inaccuracies of whooping cough vaccine history.

Nevertheless such studies were sensitive enough to identify the waning efficacy of British vaccines in the 1960s (Preston 1963; Wilson et al. 1965; PHLS 1969, 1973) and to show that the later reformulation of British vaccines had led to restoration of efficacy (Noah 1976; Preston 1976b; Church 1979).

More recently, the results of a large study undertaken by the British Public Health Laboratory Service (PHLS 1982) confirmed the protective efficacy of current whooping cough vaccines. Efficacy estimates varied from over 90 per cent for bacteriologically confirmed whooping cough and cases admitted to hospital, to 64 per cent for cases of cough without paroxysms. Overall protection in the home was only 50 to 60 per cent, although estimates based on bacteriologically proved cases yielded a protective efficacy of 81 per cent for home contacts. The findings of this study are important because of its national coverage and because the survey of home circumstances suggested that notification rates within the two vaccine groups (three doses of diphtheria/tetanus/pertussis *versus* three doses of diptheria/tetanus vaccine) were not materially affected by social class.

Some studies have indicated that vaccine-induced immunity wanes appreciably with time (Lambert 1965), but results of long-term immunity studies are not consistent on this point (Halsey and de Quadros 1983). However, protection does extend, at the very least, through the most dangerous period of early childhood. Additionally, many studies indicate that if the disease does occur in immunized individuals it tends to be less severe (Miller and Fletcher 1976; Grob *et al.* 1981; Swansea Research Unit RCGP 1981; PHLS 1982) and, importantly from a public health perspective, to be less infective (Grob *et al.* 1981; PHLS 1982).

Population effectiveness

Vaccine effectiveness is usually measured in terms of reduction in the incidence of clinical disease; mortality rates are less useful for assessing effectiveness. Effectiveness is best assessed by mass randomized trials, but, because of ethical difficulties, trials of the vaccines currently in use are not available. Recent evidence for effectiveness is indirect and most derives either from demonstrating correlations between incidence estimates and immunization uptake, or from the examination of secular trends. It is therefore inevitable that there should be controversies regarding the effectiveness and reactogenicity of current vaccines.

Correlations

Meaningful correlations between immunization uptake and estimated whooping cough incidence on an international level are precluded by differences in reporting systems. Intra-national correlations have provided some evidence regarding vaccine effectiveness. For example, Bassili and Stewart (1976) showed that for the 36 administrative counties in England, there was an inverse correlation between notification rates and both vaccine acceptance rates and socio-economic factors. Analysis of data from 98 English Area Health Authorities during the 1977–79 epidemic (Pollard 1980) showed that this inverse correlation remained even after elimination of the effects of social class and overcrowding.

Secular trends

The secular trend for whooping cough incidence in England and Wales is shown in Figure 2.2 in terms of annual statutory notifications from 1940 to 1985. This shows that routine use of vaccine started in the early 1950s and was widespread by 1957. The decline in notifications seen from the early 1950s can thus be attributed to the effectiveness of the vaccine rather than used as evidence to the contrary (Bassili and Stewart 1976).

The rapid reversal of the downward trend in incidence which occurred in the latter part of the 1970s is striking. This reversal occurred shortly after the dramatic falls in immunization uptake (Figure 2.3) which were a consequence of widespread publicity, from 1974 onwards, about adverse reactions to immunization. In England and Wales in the 1977–79 epidemic, the greatest

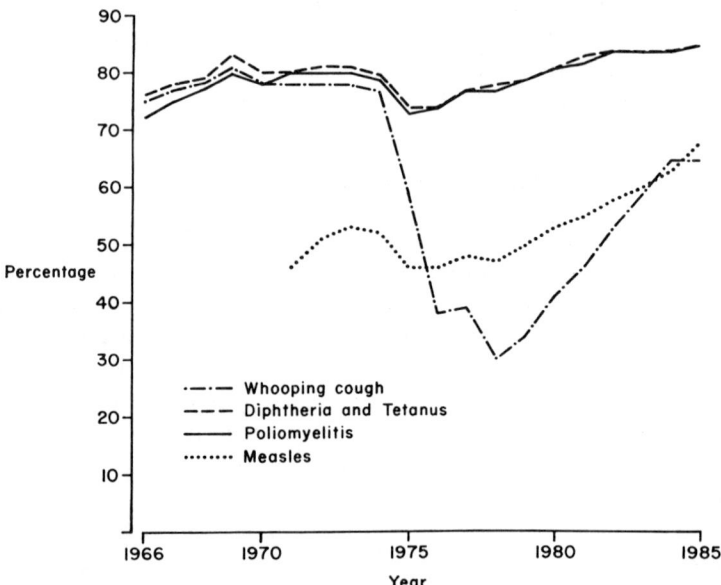

Fig. 2.3 Immunization acceptance rates. Percentage completed immunization by end of second year after birth. England and Wales 1966–85.

increases occurred in children under 5 years of age, the age group most affected by the recent drop in immunization uptake (DHSS 1981).

A significant upswing in notifications was seen only in those countries which experienced drastic falls in vaccine coverage in the mid 1970s—for example, the United Kingdom, Ireland, and Japan. Immunization coverage did not change appreciably in countries such as France, Hungary, the United States, and Canada, and in these countries no upswing in incidence was observed (DHSS 1981; Cherry 1984; WHO 1985). This point is illustrated in Figure 2.1 for some European countries.

The level of disease control, even in periods of high uptake, has been disappointing in comparison, for example, with the impact of immunization programmes against diphtheria and polio. The fact that the efficacy of whooping cough vaccine is not as consistently high as that of other routinely used immunizations may be important.

It has also been suggested that the vaccines have been more efficient in protecting against clinical pertussis than against infection with *B. pertussis* (Fine and Clarkson 1982; Cherry 1984). However, this hypothesis is not widely accepted (Preston 1982; Bass 1987) and evidence against it may be derived from Figure 2.4 which shows that notifications in England and Wales fell from the time immunization was introduced in the 1950s, in children less than 1 year of age, as well as in the older age groups. As whooping cough immunization is generally not complete until well into the latter half of the first year, the declining incidence in children under 1 year of age suggests that herd immunity does exist and that immunization, therefore, does interrupt transmission.

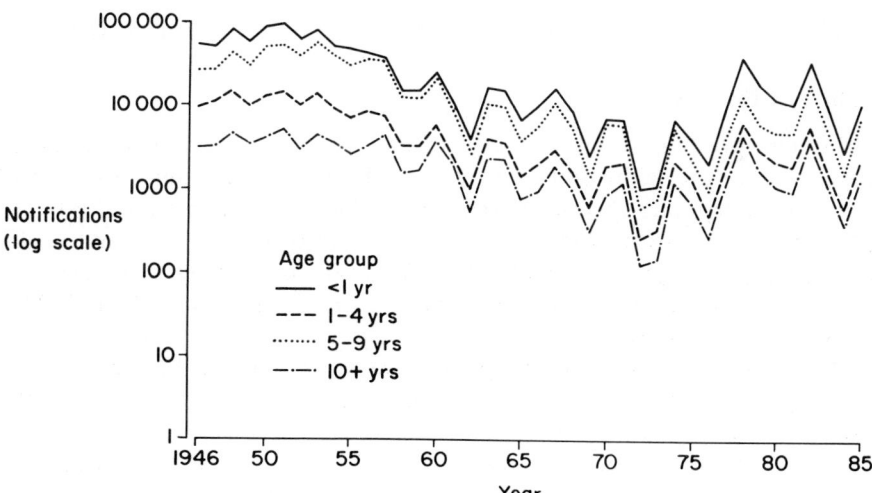

Fig. 2.4 Whooping cough notifications by age group. England and Wales 1946–85.

It is generally agreed that current whooping cough vaccine programmes are at least moderately effective in reducing both disease incidence and transmission. However, if the ultimate goal of immunization programmes is to be the elimination of whooping cough, it is important to confirm that realistically achievable levels of uptake of immunization in a community have the potential to halt transmission completely, and then to determine which schedules are likely to be most effective in achieving this goal.

Boosters

At present, in many European countries, in addition to the primary series of three doses of vaccine, a fourth dose is given to children aged between 1 and 3 years; most of the Eastern European countries also give a fifth dose by the age of 6 (WHO 1985). Comparison of levels of control in countries with and without booster programmes would be of great interest. Unfortunately, reliable data are not generally available to ascertain the levels of immunization uptake and the levels of control achieved. As whooping cough is highly infectious, it may be that boosters are required to prevent transmission totally, particularly if there is significant waning of immunity with time. The recent study by Knox and Shannon (1986) is thus of interest. It showed, by mathematical modelling, that the rate of decay of vaccine immunity had an important effect on programme effectiveness and that a two-course vaccine policy (primary schedule plus booster) would yield an improvement of about 50 per cent in protection against attacks compared to a primary schedule alone.

Problems in maximizing population effectiveness

Nature of the disease

Although whooping cough has some of the 'desirable' features for eradication, such as infection limited to human host, disease transmitted from person-to-person, no chronic carrier state, relatively short period of infectivity, and long-lasting immunity, its highly infectious nature and early average age at infection, deem it an unlikely candidate for eradication.

Even for the lesser goals of elimination or containment (Noah 1983), whooping cough poses special problems. Thirty years ago, because of the relatively high death rate and frequent reappearance of the disease, whooping cough had an important emotional impact which fostered a favourable attitude toward immunization. Today, with the possible exception of the British Isles in recent years, the European public, including younger members of the medical profession, has largely forgotten its fear of the disease. Ironically, immunization programmes themselves have probably contributed to this situation because of the relative rarity of the natural disease in immunized communities and the fact that whooping cough which does occur in previously immunized individuals is likely to be mild.

Nature of the intervention

Although whooping cough vaccines do have some of the characteristics required for a viable control programme—for example, stability, can be combined with other vaccines, only a few injections needed—there are problems relating to effectiveness. In addition there are anxieties about toxicity.

Vaccine toxicity

Except for the acellular vaccines used in Japan, vaccines currently used for mass immunization are made from killed *B. pertussis* organisms containing biologically active endotoxins and exotoxins which can cause febrile and neurotoxic side-effects. Severe systemic reactions which have been attributed to the vaccine include seizures, shock, collapse (with occasional death), and encephalopathic states, some of which result in permanent brain damage.

Assessment of side-effects is difficult for three main reasons. First, different vaccines are believed to vary in toxicity as well as efficacy. Second, there is no characteristic post-immunization syndrome such as lower motor neurone paralysis after oral polio vaccine. Third, whooping cough vaccine is administered at the ages when febrile and non-febrile convulsions and encephalopathies are most common, and when a wide range of unexplained neurological degenerative diseases first appear—a temporal association between such events and whooping cough vaccine is therefore to be expected in some infants.

Most estimates of vaccine toxicity are based on uncontrolled and retrospective observation; some examples are given in Table 2.1. Estimates vary widely with much of the variation caused by differences in case definition and method of ascertainment. These estimates must be compared with the 'natural' occurrence of untoward neurological events in children of a similar age. The incidence rate of first convulsions at ages from 3 to 15 months is of the order of 0.8 to 1.4 per 1000 per month (equivalent to one in 1250 to one in 714 children per month) (DHSS 1981). In the National Child Development Study (Ross *et al.* 1980) in England, Scotland, and Wales, 2 per cent of the 1043 children who had a history of seizures or other episodes of loss of consciousness, were, at 11 years of age, epileptic and mentally subnormal. The background frequency of epilepsy with mental subnormality may be estimated, therefore, to be between one in 63 000 and one in 36 000 children per month for children aged from 3 to 15 months.

Table 2.1 Estimates of the frequency of brain damage after immunization for whooping cough.

Author	Reaction	Frequency
Ström (1960)[a]	Vaccine-induced encephalopathy	1 per 6000 injections
	Vaccine-induced encephalopathy leading to death	1 per 16 500 injections
Malmgren et al. (1960)[a]	Severe reactions	1 per 50 000 immunizations
Ström (1967)[a]	Destructive encephalopathy	1 per 170 000 immunizations
Dick (1974)[a]	Brain damage	1 in 10 000 immunized children
Prensky (1974)[a]	Severe encephalopathies	1 in 180 000 immunizations
Stewart (1977)[a]	Brain damage and mental defect	Between 1 in 10 000 and 1 in 60 000 immunized children
Grist (1977)[a]	Permanent mental retardation	1 in 135 000 immunized children
Stewart (1979)[a]	Brain damage and mental defect	Between 1 in 17 000 and 1 in 52 000 immunized children
Meade et al. (in DHSS 1981)[a]	Brain damage following any neurological event after immunization	1 in 155 000 injections
NCES (in DHSS 1981)[b]	Persistent neurological damage in previously normal children one year after immunization	1 in 310 000 immunizations or 1 per 100 000 children receiving the full course of three injections

Source: Wells (1984).
[a] Uncontrolled studies.
[b] Controlled study.

Based on this and other such estimates (DHSS 1981), the likelihood of a convulsion occurring 'naturally' within a day, a week, or a month of any given immunization, and the likelihood of brain damage occurring in any given child, whether immunized with whooping cough vaccine or not, can be used to counterbalance the frequency estimates given in Table 2.1. The disparity between background incidence and some of these frequencies is not great, and this suggests that many of these events should not be attributed to whooping cough vaccine.

The best currently available estimates of vaccine toxicity, including the only estimate of attributable risk, are provided by the National Childhood

Encephalopathy Study (NCES) (DHSS 1981; Miller *et al.* 1981). This was a case-control study which included all children aged 2 months to the third birthday admitted to hospitals in England, Scotland, and Wales with specified serious acute neurological illnesses, from 1 July 1976 to 30 June 1979. A significant association was shown between serious neurological illness and whooping cough vaccine. As the NCES was a national study, it was possible, subject to certain assumptions, to calculate attributable risk estimates (using an expression derived from the population attributable risk). The estimated attributable risk of serious neurological disorders occurring within seven days of immunization with diphtheria, tetanus, and pertussis vaccine in previously normal children irrespective of outcome is one in 110 000 injections (95 per cent confidence limits, one in 360 000 to one in 44 000). The corresponding rate for previously normal children with neurological sequelae persistent one year later is one in 310 000 injections (95 per cent confidence limits, one in 5 310 000 to one in 54 000).

The authors emphasize that these calculations are not precise measures of risk, but only indicators of the magnitude of risk and they conclude that 'it seems likely that permanent damage as a result of pertussis immunization is a very rare event and attribution of a cause in individual cases is precarious' (DHSS 1981).

Any risk estimates must of course be balanced against the risks of whooping cough itself. Thus in approximately one in 1000 cases, there will be major complications such as encephalitis or death. Theoretically, in a country such as Hungary where the incidence of whooping cough is reported to be extremely low (WHO 1985), the risks of routine immunization, if they are of the order suggested by the NCES, may at present outweigh the risks of disease. But the future upsurge in whooping cough to be expected after withdrawal of the immunization programme, and the inevitable delay in regaining control of the disease, would have to be incorporated into any estimation of the balance between risks and benefits, and would probably weigh the balance in favour of continued immunization. The vaccine also provides community protection through herd immunity, so the benefit side of the equation is given considerable extra weight. But from an individual perspective, one encounters an aspect of Rose's 'prevention paradox' (Rose 1985) whereby for individuals in a low incidence community, the risk of immunization may outweigh the risk of encountering a 'gap' in herd immunity.

Contraindications to immunization

In addition to attempts to minimize the toxicity of vaccines by improvements

For more detailed assessment of vaccine toxicity, please refer to the NCES reports (DHSS 1981; Miller *et al.* 1981; Bellman *et al.* 1983) and other controlled studies (e.g. Harker 1977; Melchior 1977; Pollock and Morris 1983) and to the reviews by Cherry (1984), Miller *et al.* (1982), and Griffith (1978) and the (other) Reports from the Committee on Safety of Medicines and the Joint Committee on Vaccination and Immunization (DHSS 1981).

in production and storage procedures, attempts to identify susceptible infants and situations have led to the empirical formulation of contraindications to immunization. Officially stated contraindications differ between countries and have changed with time. This lack of uniformity has led to considerable confusion among the health care professionals responsible for administering immunizations and a tendency to err in the direction of 'safety' by withholding whooping cough immunization if in doubt. The recent British guidelines (JCVI 1984) have helped to clarify the position by differentiating between the few straightforward absolute contraindications and 'special considerations'.

Population acceptability

The acceptability of whooping cough vaccine to a community depends on whether whooping cough is perceived as a threat and on whether the immunization is seen to provide effective protection against that threat with a level of side-effects that is well below the perceived risk of disease. Acceptability is therefore likely to vary according to changes in the incidence and severity of whooping cough. At a period of low incidence, any occurrence of serious side-effects is likely to reduce public acceptability substantially. When high incidence brings a relatively large proportion of the public into contact with the misery of the actual disease, the occasional occurrence of side-effects will be less likely to deter parents from immunizing their children.

For mass whooping cough immunization to be acceptable, the public must be kept aware of the real risks of the disease itself, be informed of the efficacy and effectiveness of the vaccine, accept that, as with all vaccines, there is a slight risk, and be convinced of the unreliability of statements arising from uncontrolled observations about side-effects. The inadequacy of routine surveillance systems means that the reliable, consistent, and up-to-date information required to inform and reassure the general public is not always available.

Cost

With any immunization programme, the ratio of cost to benefit increases as the incidence of the target disease declines. In developed countries, these diminishing returns, as assessed in monetary terms, are not usually considered grounds for discontinuation of low-risk vaccines that protect against diseases of high case fatality, such as diphtheria, tetanus. The cost of whooping cough immunization may be viewed more critically by governments since the disease carries only a small mortality risk and its vaccine carries a risk that, although still very low, appears to be somewhat greater than the risk carried by other childhood vaccines. Health budgets do not usually allow direct abstraction of the cost of individual programmes. Precise figures for the total cost of national infant immunization programmes are not available, nor are there figures for the cost of whooping cough immunization programmes alone. But since most whooping cough immunizations are integrated in other immunization schedules, the incremental cost of the whooping cough component is not much greater than the cost of the vaccine; this could be estimated from the average number of doses administered per year and the average unit cost of vaccine. For the comparatively wealthy countries of Europe the cost of mass immunization for whooping cough is therefore an insignificant percentage of the total health budget.

The only two formal cost–benefit analyses published to date are from the United States (Koplan *et al.* 1979; Hinman and Koplan 1984) and both show that immunization saves far more money than it costs. Cost–benefit analyses put monetary costs on life, death, and disability, and this adds an extra element of arbitrariness to already crude estimates. For a low cost intervention, such as whooping cough immunization in the European context, assessment of worth is better restricted to computation of risk–benefit ratios such as those presented (again for the United States) by Cherry (1984). In this analysis, although estimates in general under-estimated the risk of disease and over-estimated the risk of immunization, the data suggest that the benefits of the present immunization programme in the United States are considerably greater than the risks of the vaccine. Similar analyses for Europe would be most helpful to decision-makers and health education personnel.

Recommendations

Although the whole-cell whooping cough vaccines currently in use are both safe and efficacious, elimination of whooping cough is most unlikely without extremely high levels of uptake. But public and medical confidence has been so profoundly undermined in some countries that it may well be that nothing short of a 'new' vaccine can restore confidence in immunization against whooping cough. In the meantime there are a number of measures that could help to improve the level of control of whooping cough:

1. Infants should receive a primary course of three doses at 4- to 6-week intervals of adsorbed vaccine containing all three agglutinogens. This course should start at 3 to 4 months of age and be completed by 6 months.
2. To improve confidence (and therefore vaccine uptake) doctors, nurses, and the general public must be given reliable information about the risks of whooping cough itself and the efficacy, safety, and limitations of modern whooping cough vaccines.
3. Thus routine recording of all immunizations (date, dose, manufacturer,

and batch number) and systematic unbiased monitoring of whooping cough incidence by age, and if possible by serotype, are of utmost importance.

4. Simplification of batch numbers of manufacturers would help to improve accuracy of recording of vaccines administered.

5. The special requirement of certain high-risk infants for early and complete immunization should be made known to both health professionals and the general public.

6. Guidelines for contraindications to immunization should be standardized and if necessary clarified.

7. Finally, further research is required. In addition to systematic evaluation of all new vaccines, further research is required to determine how to maximize the impact of immunization programmes on transmission; this should include assessment of the effect of boosters. Since experience in Japan indicates the safety for 2-year-olds of acellular vaccines, the feasibility of the immediate introduction of an acellular vaccine booster deserves consideration.

Acknowledgements

I am grateful to J. Birmingham for typing the manuscript and to F. Sadek and J. Larragy for preparing Figure 2.1. Figures 2.2, 2.3, and 2.4 were prepared by the CDSC. I would also like to thank Dr N. Preston, Professor D. Miller, Dr N. Noah, and members of the Department of Community Health, Trinity College Dublin, for their helpful comments.

References

Aoyama, T., Murase, Y., Kato, T., and Iwata, T. (1985). Efficacy of an acellular pertussis vaccine in Japan. *J. Pediat.* **107**, 180-2.

Baraff, L.J., Cody, C.L., and Cherry, J.D. (1984). DTP-associated reactions: an analysis by injection site, manufacturer, prior reactions and dose. *Pediatrics* **73**, 31-36.

Bass, J.W. (1987). Is there a carrier state in pertussis? *Lancet* **1**, 96.

Bassili, W.R. and Stewart, G.T. (1976). Epidemiological evaluation of immunisation and other factors in the control of whooping-cough. *Lancet* **1**, 471-4.

Bellman, M.H., Ross, E.M., and Miller, D.L. (1983). Infantile spasms and pertussis immunisation. *Lancet* **1**, 1031-4.

Bernbaum, J.C., Daft, A., Anolik, R., Samuelson, J., Barkin, R., Douglas, S., and Polin, R. (1985). Response of preterm infants to diphtheria–tetanus–pertussis immunizations. *J. Pediat.* **107**, 184-8.

Butler, N.R., Voyce, M.A., Burland, W.L., and Hilton, M.L. (1969). Advantages of aluminium hydroxide adsorbed combined diphtheria, tetanus, and pertussis vaccines for the immunization of infants. *Br. Med. J.* **1**, 663–6.

Cherry, J.D. (1984). The epidemiology of pertussis and pertussis immunization in the United Kingdom and the United States: a comparative study. *Curr. Prob. Pediat.* **14**, 1–78.

Church, M.A. (1979). Evidence of whooping-cough-vaccine efficacy from the 1978 whooping-cough epidemic in Hertfordshire. *Lancet* **2**, 188–90.

Clarkson, J.A. and Fine, P.E.M. (1985). The efficiency of measles and pertussis notification in England and Wales. *Int. J. Epidemiol.* **14**, 153–68.

Department of Health and Social Security [DHSS] Committee on Safety of Medicines and the Joint Committee on Vaccination and Immunisation (1981). *Whooping cough. Reports.* Her Majesty's Stationery Office, London.

Dick, G. (1974). Convulsive disorders in young children. *Proc. R. Soc. Med.* **67**, 371–2.

Editorial. (1978). Whooping-cough vaccines. *Br. Med. J.* **1**, 806–7.

Fine, P.E.M. and Clarkson, J.A. (1982). The recurrence of whooping cough: possible implications for assessment of vaccine efficacy. *Lancet* **1**, 666–9.

Griffith, A.H. (1978). Reactions after pertussis vaccine: a manufacturer's experiences and difficulties since 1964. *Br. Med. J.* **1**, 809–15.

Grist, N.R. (1977). Vaccination against whooping-cough. *Lancet* **1**, 358.

Grob, P.R., Crowder, M.J., and Robbins, J.F. (1981). Effect of vaccination on severity and dissemination of whooping cough. *Br. Med. J.* **282**, 1925–8.

Halsey, N.A. and de Quadros, C.A. (1983). Recent advances in immunization. A bibliographic review. *WHO Scientific Publication No. 451*. Pan American Health Organization, Washington D.C.

Harker, P. (1977). Primary immunisation and febrile convulsions in Oxford 1972–5. *Br. Med. J.* **2**, 490–3.

Hinman, A.R. and Koplan, J.P. (1984). Pertussis and pertussis vaccine. Reanalysis of benefits, risks, and costs. *JAMA* **251**, 3109–13.

Hull, D. (1981). Interpretation of the contraindications to whooping cough vaccination. *Br. Med. J.* **283**, 1231–3.

Jenkinson, D. (1983). Whooping cough: what proportion of cases is notified in an epidemic? *Br. Med. J.* **287**, 185–6.

Johnston, I.D.A., Anderson, H.R., Lambert, H.P., and Patel, S. (1983). Respiratory morbidity and lung function after whooping-cough. *Lancet* **2**, 1104–8.

——, Hill, M., Anderson, H.R., and Lambert, H.P. (1985). Impact of whooping cough on patients and their families. *Br. Med. J.* **290**, 1636–8.

Joint Committee on Vaccination and Immunisation [JCVI] for the Secretary of State for Social Services, the Secretary of State for Scotland and the Secretary of State for Wales. (1984). *Immunisation against infectious disease.* 10/83.

Knox, E.G. and Shannon, H.S. (1986). A model basis for the control of whooping cough. *Int. J. Epidemiol.* **15**, 544–52.

Koplan, J.P., Schoenbaum, S.C., Weinstein, M.C., and Fraser, D.W. (1979). Pertussis vaccine—an analysis of benefits, risks and costs. *New Engl. J. Med.* **301**, 906–11.

Lambert, H.J. (1965). Epidemiology of a small pertussis outbreak in Kent County, Michigan. *Publ. Hlth. Reps.* **80**, 365–9.

Malmgren, B., Vahlquist, B., and Zetterstrom, R. (1960). Complications of immunization. *Br. Med. J.* **2**, 1800-1.
Medical Research Council. (1951). The prevention of whooping-cough by vaccination. *Br. Med. J.* **1**, 1463-71.
—— (1956). Vaccination against whooping-cough. Relation between protection in children and results of laboratory tests. *Br. Med. J.* **2**, 454-62.
—— (1959). Vaccination against whooping-cough. *Br. Med. J.* **1**, 994-1000.
Melchior, J.C. (1977). Infantile spasms and early immunization against whooping cough. Danish survey from 1970 to 1975. *Arch. Dis. Child.* **52**, 134-7.
Metcalfe Brown, C. (1965). Pertussis immunization. *Practitioner* **195**, 292-5.
Miller, C.L. and Fletcher, W.B. (1976). Severity of notified whooping cough. *Br. Med. J.* **1**, 117-9.
Miller, D.L., Alderslade, R., and Ross, E.M. (1982). Whooping cough and whooping cough vaccine: the risks and benefits debate. *Epidemiol. Rev.* **4**, 1-24.
——, Ross, E.M., Alderslade, R., Bellman, M.H., and Rawson, N.S.B. (1981). Pertussis immunisation and serious acute neurological illness in children. *Br. Med. J.* **282**, 1595-9.
Nicoll, A. (1985). Contraindications to whooping-cough immunisation—myths or realities? *Lancet* **1**, 679-81.
Noah, N.D. (1976). Attack rates of notified whooping cough in immunised and unimmunised children. *Br. Med. J.* **1**, 128-9.
—— (1983). The strategy of immunization. *Comm. Med.* **5**, 140-7.
Pollard, R. (1980). Relation between vaccination and notification rates for whooping cough in England and Wales. *Lancet* **1**, 1180-2.
Pollock, T.M. and Morris, J. (1983). A 7-year survey of disorders attributed to vaccination in North West Thames region. *Lancet* **1**, 753-7.
——, Miller, E., and Lobb, J. (1984). Severity of whooping cough in England before and after the decline in pertussis immunisation. *Arch. Dis. Child.* **59**, 162-5.
Prensky, A.L. (1974). Pertussis vaccination. *Dev. Med. Child. Neurol.* **16**, 539-43.
Preston, N.W. (1963). Type-specific immunity against whooping-cough. *Br. Med. J.* **2**, 724-6.
—— (1976a). Prevalent serotypes of *Bordetella pertussis* in non-vaccinated communities. *J. Hyg. Camb.* **77**, 85-91.
—— (1976b). Protection by pertussis vaccine. Little cause for concern. *Lancet* **1**, 1065-7.
—— (1982). Whooping cough vaccine efficacy *Lancet* **1**, 860.
—— (1984). Pertussis component vaccine in Japan. *Lancet* **1**, 456.
—— (1986). Recognising whooping cough. *Br. Med. J.* **292**, 901-2.
——, Mackay, R.I., Bamford, F.N., Crofts, J.E., and Burland, W.L. (1974). Pertussis agglutinins in vaccinated children: better response with adjuvant. *J. Hyg. Camb.* **73**, 119-25.
Public Health Laboratory Service [PHLS] Whooping-Cough Committee and Working Party (1969). Efficacy of whooping-cough vaccines used in the United-Kingdom before 1968. A preliminary report to the Director of the Public Health Laboratory Service. *Br. Med. J.* **4**, 329-33.

—— (1973). Efficacy of whooping-cough vaccines used in the United Kingdom before 1968. Final Report to the Director of the Public Health Laboratory Service. *Br. Med. J.* **1**, 259–62.

Public Health Laboratory Service [PHLS] Epidemiological Research Laboratory and 21 Area Health Authorities (1982). Efficacy of pertussis vaccination in England. Report. *Br. Med. J.* **285**, 357–9.

Rawson, N.S.B., Alderslade, R., and Miller, D.L. (1980). Discrepancies in immunization records. *Comm. Med.* **2**, 202–8.

Reves, R. (1985). Declining fertility in England and Wales as a major cause of the twentieth century decline in mortality. The role of changing family size and age structure in infectious disease mortality in infancy. *Am. J. Epidemiol.* **122**, 112–26.

Robinson, A., Irons, L.I., and Ashworth, L.A.E. (1985). Pertussis vaccine: present status and future prospects. *Vaccine* **3**, 11–22.

Rose, G. (1985). Sick individuals and sick populations. *Int. J. Epidemiol.* **14**, 32–38.

Ross, E.M., Peckham, C.S., West, P.B., and Butler, N.R. (1980). Epilepsy in childhood: findings from the National Child Development Study. *Br. Med. J.* **1**, 207–10.

Stewart, G.T. (1977). Vaccination against whooping-cough: efficacy versus risks. *Lancet* **1**, 234–7.

—— (1979). Toxicity of pertussis vaccine: frequency and probability of reactions. *J. Epidemiol. Comm. Hlth.* **33**, 150–6.

Ström, J. (1960). Is universal vaccination against pertussis always justified? *Br. Med. J.* **2**, 1184–6.

—— (1967). Further experience of reactions, especially of a cerebral nature, in conjunction with triple vaccination: a study based on vaccinations in Sweden 1959–65. *Br. Med. J.* **4**, 320–3.

Swansea Research Unit of the Royal College of General Practitioners [RCGP]. (1981). Effect of a low pertussis vaccination uptake on a large community. Report. *Br. Med. J.* **282**, 23–6.

—— (1985). Respiratory sequelae of whooping cough. *Br. Med. J.* **290**, 1937–40.

Wells, N. (1984). *Childhood vaccination. Current controversies.* No. 76. Office of Health Economics, London.

Wilkins, J., Williams, F.F., Wehrle, P.F., and Portnoy, B. (1971). Agglutinin response to pertussis vaccine. I. Effect of dosage and interval. *J. Pediat* **79**, 197–202.

Wilson, A.T., Henderson, I.R., Moore, E.J.H., and Heywood, S.N. (1965). Whooping-cough: difficulties in diagnosis and ineffectiveness of immunization. *Br. Med. J.* **2**, 623–6.

World Health Organization [WHO]. Regional Committee for Europe. (1985). Expanded programme on immunization and related activities in Europe. Progress report. (EUR/RC35/8.1364G).

3
Measles

Norman Noah

'It's unprecedented in the history of preventive medicine to try to eradicate an entire disease in one year, but there is good reason to believe it can be done'. [On measles. B.H. Dull, Communicable Disease Center, Atlanta, Georgia. *Time* 17.3.67. Vol. 89, p. 38.]

SUMMARY

The high benefit-to-cost ratio of immunizing against measles in developed countries has been established beyond any doubt. The burden of measles in these countries is still great, and the vaccine is reasonably cheap, highly effective, produces long-lasting immunity, and is safe. Nevertheless measles immunization rates within Europe vary widely, and in many countries are still low. The tools and resources for eradication of measles are not yet available, and even measles elimination is probably not yet feasible with available vaccines. These vaccines, even with an efficacy of 95 per cent, require extremely high immunization rates of more than 95 per cent, which are costly to achieve. In general, an aggressive containment policy for measles is recommended, with a target coverage of greater than 90 per cent for the vaccine.

Defining the problem

History

Measles is a widespread and highly contagious viral infection causing a characteristic and easily recognizable illness. It has probably been present since antiquity but the first authentic account of the illness was by Rhazes in AD 910. He clearly differentiated measles from smallpox (Gastel 1973), although he considered that both diseases arose from a common morbid process. In the London Bills of Mortality, in 1629, measles and smallpox were reported separately (Gastel 1973). It thus seems appropriate that smallpox was the first disease to be successfully eradicated by man and that measles is now being considered for eradication.

Burden of measles

Measles is not a mild disease, although it is less severe in affluent societies. In 1670, Sydenham described some complications of measles and noted that the adult disease was more severe; and John Graunt, in 1662, listed it as a major cause of death in children under 6 years of age (Gastel 1973). Even in more modern times measles is noted as a severe disease. Cutting (1983) estimated that in 1981—more than 10 years after the introduction of a safe and effective vaccine against it—measles claimed 1-1.5 million deaths in children throughout the world, and the World Health Organization Expanded Programme on Immunization (EPI) estimate (Bart *et al.* 1983) is towards the higher end of this range.

Diagnosis of measles

As measles produces a highly characteristic illness, the clinical diagnosis is reliable; laboratory confirmation is seldom necessary—the virus is difficult to isolate and the serological tests fairly time-consuming and expensive.

Complications

The complications of measles are many and serious. The gastrointestinal complications of diarrhoea and stomatitis, and the respiratory complications of otitis media, pneumonia, bronchitis, croup, and laryngitis score by their frequency and the burden they impose on health care services. The rarer neurological complications of encephalitis and, especially, subacute sclerosing panencephalitis (SSPE), create an impact by causing permanent severe disability and high mortality. In less developed countries measles produces additional morbidity by causing blindness, and mortality by exacerbating protein-energy malnutrition (from a protein-losing enteropathy). All these complications may lead to developmental retardation, lifelong handicaps, and direct and indirect economic loss.

Estimates of severity in developed countries confirm the considerable burden of uncontained measles. Between 1963 and 1976 (Miller 1964; Miller 1978), there was little change in the various indices of severity of measles in England and Wales: the hospital admission rate for notified cases was 1 per cent, the respiratory complication rate 4 per cent, otitis media 2.5-5.0 per cent, and the neurological complication rate for convulsions and encephalitis remained at 0.7 per cent, with the rate of incidence of encephalitis at about 1 per 1000 cases. The ratio of deaths to notifications did not change appreciably between 1970 and 1983, when measles accounted for an average of 23 deaths annually, about half of them estimated to have been in previously healthy children (Miller 1983). Bronchopneumonia and encephalitis or a combination of both were the most common causes of death. In Denmark (Horwitz *et al.* 1974), the otitis media rate was 9 per cent, other respiratory complications 7 per cent, and other inflammatory conditions 3 per cent. One child in their sample of 612 had encephalitis. In France (Rey 1985), measles caused 30 deaths, 6000 admissions to hospital, 100–200 cases of encephalitis (15 per cent residual neurological disease), 10–20 cases of SSPE, and costs of over 100 million francs a year. There are still about 800 measles deaths each year in European countries. In adults, measles is a serious disease, with a high mortality rate (Centers for Disease Control 1982).

Size of the problem

Measles can be found world-wide; before mass immunization 95 per cent of children in the United States were immune by age 15 years (Langmuir 1962). Pre-school children tend to be most frequently affected in urban areas, primary school-aged children in rural. In less developed countries infection occurs at younger ages than in developed countries.

Any variation in the reported incidence of measles in the EEC and other European countries is likely to be a reflection either of vaccine uptake or adequacy of surveillance. An increase in cases reported by some countries such as Greece, Denmark, Italy, Luxembourg, and Spain can almost certainly be attributed to more efficient surveillance.

In England and Wales, the number of notified cases of measles fell from about 400 000 a year on average, between 1940 and 1967, to 100 000 a year. During this period there was an immunization rate of about 50 per cent. By 1984, the immunization rate had crept up to 64 per cent. In Scotland, the immunization rate and the reduction in measles incidence were similar. In France, the estimated numbers of cases of measles infection increased from 300 000 to 500 000 new cases each year (542–903/100 000) before 1983, when the immunization rate was very low (about 10 per cent) (Rey 1985). In 1985, after the introduction of a national programme to immunize all children at 12–15 months, the incidence had fallen to 470 per 100 000 (260 000 cases), with an immunization rate by the end of the second year of life of 37 per cent (Dr C. Goujon, Personal Communication).

Immunization rates vary widely within the European region—from less than 10 per cent, to 99 per cent in Czechoslovakia where eradication is the declared aim. Measles immunization is only compulsory in the Eastern European countries. In all such countries, except Poland and Yugoslavia, the reported number of cases is low. Vaccine coverage in 1980 was stated to be 98.7 per cent in Greece and 91 per cent in the Netherlands (Velimirovic 1984).

Nature of intervention

Live vaccines have been available since 1963, and widely available since 1968. A killed vaccine is no longer used as it is less effective and is liable to produce serious side-effects. The vaccines used in Western Europe and Yugoslavia are grown in tissue culture, not eggs, and all derive from the Edmonston B strain isolated by Enders in 1954; they differ only in the number of passages. In Eastern Europe the Smorodinstev 1959 strain is the origin of all vaccine strains, and these are grown in chick embryos (Velimirovic 1984).

Live vaccines are about 95 per cent efficacious when used under optimal conditions: these include immunizing no earlier than about 12-13 months of age in developed countries, and ensuring that the vaccine has been kept at the correct temperatures, has not been exposed for long periods to light, and is not out of date. An aerosol vaccine (Whittle *et al.* 1984) may produce high seroconversion and protection rates in much younger infants, about 4 months of age. If these results are confirmed, they will prove a significant advance, as measles vaccine can then be given at the same time as the triple/quadruple vaccine given before 12 months of age.

The incidence of convulsions after measles vaccine is 7-10 times lower than after the disease itself (Miller 1982). For encephalitis it is even less, at 1 per million doses distributed (Landrigan and Witte 1973). In Britain, the National Childhood Encephalopathy Study Research Team (1981) found a significant association between serious neurological illness and measles vaccine 7-14 days after its administration. The relative risk for all these illnesses was assessed at 2.5 or 3.9 depending on whether cases were related to the date of onset or date of admission to hospital. Of the 16 cases in this group, from the 1000 studied, 11 had convulsions and 5 encephalitis.

Target population

In Western countries vaccine cannot be used in infants under 1 year of age. The seroconversion and protection rates are unacceptably low because of persisting maternal antibody (Noah 1983a). By 13-15 months, however, the seroconversion rate is 95 per cent. Measles is uncommon in children under 1 year of age. In England and Wales, for example, only 4-5 per cent of notified cases of measles in the pre-vaccine era were in this age group. Immunization is therefore necessary through the 'narrow window in time when maternal antibody has waned sufficiently to permit vaccination, and before the child's exposure to the virus' (Henderson 1982). Hence 13-15 months appears to be the optimal age for measles immunization, and this is accepted in most developed countries. In developing countries, the epidemiology of measles is different and the optimal age for immunization is somewhat lower, around 9 months. When a measles immunization policy in a country is first implemented, however, for maximum efficiency it may be advisable to include all children up to 10 years of age (by which age about 97 per cent of infections have occurred) or even 15 years (99 per cent).

A selective vaccine policy is sometimes advocated (Smith 1980), but it is likely to prove inefficient. It is not often possible to predict which children will react adversely to measles, and complications are common enough to warrant a mass immunization policy.

Effectiveness of intervention

The effectiveness of an intervention programme is related to the aims of the programme. The aims may be eradication, elimination, or containment, and the relative merits of these strategies are discussed.

Eradication

A case for the global eradication of measles was made by Hopkins and colleagues (1982). The arguments for eradication were that measles was a universal disease affecting large numbers of children, which caused serious complications and more than one million deaths a year in the world, and that its eradication would bring considerable savings in cost. Measles had many similarities to smallpox: recognizable rash, lifelong immunity, and the absence of both an animal reservoir and a chronic carrier state. There was a heat-stable cheap effective vaccine, with, furthermore, the recent availability of a potent freeze-dried preparation. Gambia had already eliminated reported measles for over 2 years, and large areas of the United States were free of indigenous measles. Hopkins *et al.* accepted on the other hand that measles was far more contagious than smallpox, that the average age of measles infection in developed countries was 12–18 months (compared with 4–5 years for smallpox), that measles vaccine could not be used in neonates, and that measles immunity (unlike the scars of smallpox) was visually unrecognizable, making surveillance more difficult. Henderson (1982), however, put forward cogent arguments as to why measles would be ineradicable at present: with methods used for smallpox eradication a certain amount of variation in quality of execution was possible, but with measles and present measles vaccine much more precision was necessary. Compared with smallpox vaccine, the measles vaccine was more heat-labile (although more stable vaccines are now available), the technique was more cumbersome, a high vaccination rate of 90 per cent was required in a target age-group that was more difficult to reach (smallpox vaccine could be administered from birth), and measles was highly communicable. These factors did not suggest that measles eradication was feasible. Indeed with measles, large-scale immunization would be a far more important part of the strategy than it was with smallpox. These arguments, and the failure of the United States to achieve the stated goal of measles eradication 4 years after the target date, strongly suggest that measles is not eradicable at present, possibly even in highly organized and developed countries which have legislated to make measles vaccination compulsory. Moreover, on account of the high contagiousness of measles, it may not be worthwhile for single countries to aim for eradication (Noah 1982), because the constant risk of importation would make it necessary to sustain indefinitely the considerable effort expended in achieving that goal. Yekutiel's six preconditions for the eradication of a disease (Yekutiel 1981) and their applicability to measles are illustrated in Table 3.1.

Elimination

By the World Health Organization definition (WHO 1983), the elimination of measles would be achieved when no case of measles is discovered which

Table 3.1 Feasibility of measles eradication.

Essential preconditions for eradication of a disease	Comment
Availability of effective tool for breaking transmission	Vaccine efficacy not high enough Practical problems in administration
Favourable epidemiological features of the disease	Yes, confined to humans and easy to recognize, *but* highly communicable and no stigmata in immunes
Recognized socio-economic importance of the disease	Yes
Specific reason for eradication rather than control	Only if world-wide
Adequacy of administrative, operational, and financial resources	Too variable at present; condition fulfilled in some developed countries
Favourable socio-economic conditions	Condition fulfilled in few developed countries; major population movements, seasonal migrations, remote populations, cultural habits and beliefs, and politics generally unfavourable in underdeveloped countries

After Yekutiel (1981).

cannot be traced within a few generations of transmission to a foreign source—that is, an imported case. Others define elimination as the disappearance of the disease without extinction of the organism.

Feasibility of elimination

Predictions of vaccine uptake necessary to eliminate measles in a country have varied from 50 per cent in 1967 to 95 per cent in 1982 (Fine and Clarkson 1983). A simple calculation shows that 95 per cent coverage with a 95 per cent effective vaccine leads to 90 per cent immunity rate. Various models (Anderson and May 1983; Hethcote 1983) predict that from 93.5 per cent to 96 per cent of children would need to be immune to eliminate measles transmission. If the lower estimate of 93.5 per cent is correct, then a vaccine of 95 per cent efficacy would need to cover 98 per cent of the population, and even if the vaccine were 98 per cent effective, 95 per cent of the population would need to be vaccinated. Hethcote (1983) calculated that a vaccine efficacy of 100 per cent required vaccine coverage of 93.5 per cent. For more realistic vaccine efficacy rates of 95 per cent at 12 months and 97 per cent at 15 months, the coverage required was 98.4 per cent and 96.8 per cent, respectively. For a two-dose schedule of vaccine given at 15 months and 5 years, the required uptake rates were below 80 per cent for each dose but these calculations were based on a vaccine efficacy rate of 100 per cent and also assume that those who missed the first immunization had a 'normal' chance of being immunized at the second. Anderson and May (1982) found that the average age at which measles was acquired was 4–6 years in Europe and North America, but that this was much lower in underdeveloped countries and generally higher in rural than in urban areas. Presumably because of increasing urbanization and greater mingling of populations, the average age of infection in England changed from 5.5 years in 1944 to 4.4 years in 1968, the year before mass immunization was introduced. Clearly if the average age at immunization is greater than the average age at infection eradication is impossible. At present, the average age at immunization in England and Wales is 2.2 years, and with 100 per cent vaccine efficacy, the immunization rate required for eradication would be 96 per cent. If the average age at immunization was 1 year, the required immunization rate would be 94 per cent, with higher rates in densely populated and lower rates in sparsely populated areas. A low intrinsic reproduction rate (R) for an infection also signified good prospects for control, but measles and whooping cough had high R values of about 13–17, while mumps, rubella, and polio had low values of 4–7. Reproduction rate R is the expected number of secondary cases produced by an infectious individual in a population; the disease will die out if R is less than one, or propagate itself if R is greater than one.

The feasibility of elimination can also be judged by the progress of countries which have attempted it. If elimination is defined as the disappearance of the disease, the United States have not yet succeeded in eliminating measles in spite of a high vaccine uptake rate and a well-organized and aggressive strategy. They have achieved a 99 per cent reduction in the rate of measles from the pre-vaccine era, but since 1981 the number of cases has remained fairly constant at between 1500 and 3000 a year. In a recent outbreak among immunized high-school students in Illinois (*Morbid. Mortal. Wkly Rep.* 1984), a large proportion of non-preventable cases was involved; this was found to be disturbing because it suggested that, even in optimal conditions (that is immunization of 100 per cent of those in whom the vaccine is indicated), measles might not be eliminable. Czechoslovakia had 25 cases of measles in 1982, although most of them were imported (WHO 1983). Finland, Sweden, and Canada began their elimination campaigns more recently.

Strategy of elimination
The three fundamentals of any strategy to eliminate measles, as first propounded in the United States and subsequently endorsed by the World Health Organization, are: (1) the achievement and maintenance of high immunization levels; (2) surveillance; and (3) measures to control outbreaks. Practical details of methods required to attain efficiency in these three elements need not be considered here. Some broad comments will be made. Organization is important in achieving high immunization levels, and it may not be necessary in European countries to introduce school entry immunization laws similar to those in the United States and Canada. The Netherlands, for example (WHO 1981), has achieved a measles vaccine rate of 90 per cent without such laws. A strategy encouraging immunization at school entry for those without a recorded history of previous immunization or measles diagnosed by a physician could, however, be worth considering. For efficient surveillance, measles should be notifiable, and as the incidence of the infection decreases, the completeness and accuracy of notification should increase. Outbreak control requires prompt reporting of outbreaks and the efficient identification and immunization of those who are susceptible.

The failure to eliminate measles transmission in the United States has been analysed in detail (Frank *et al.* 1985). The main reason for failure appears to be non-immunization of some persons for whom the vaccine is indicated. Both vaccine and implementation failures continue to play a role in transmission, and sustained transmission in a totally immunized community has not been demonstrated. The essential role in transmission of non-preventable cases implies a failure in the adequacy of the strategy. Nevertheless major changes in strategy are not contemplated. Most of the preventable cases were in pre-school children, and greater coverage of this most accessible of the age groups is important. Young adult transmission, mostly on college or high school campuses, occurs regularly (*Morbid. Mortal. Wkly Rep.* 1985), and immunization of this age group before entry is now (since May 1983) being encouraged by the American College Health Association.

Two-dose regimes

The extremely high immunization rates required for measles elimination, apparent both theoretically and from practical experience, have stimulated some enthusiasm for a two-dose regime for measles vaccine (Rabo and Taranger 1984). This means that, theoretically, an uptake rate of 90 per cent for the first dose of measles vaccine, if repeated for the second, will result in a final coverage of 99 per cent. This assumes that the 10 per cent who do not have the first dose will have a 90 per cent chance of receiving the second, an assumption that cannot be made (Thornton 1985). Moreover the 5 per cent or so who do not respond serologically to the first dose of vaccine are unlikely to respond to the second. A second, theoretical, advantage of a two-dose regime is that outbreaks of measles in older children and adults will be prevented if the second dose is given fairly late in childhood—that is, at about 12 years of age. The cost-effectiveness of a two-dose regime, which in effect sets out a second mass immunization programme to achieve a small percentage of gain, is bound to be low, and the cost high. Many countries may not afford it.

Information systems

Any organized programme for the elimination of measles needs reliable data to monitor progress. First, information is needed on the incidence of the disease. Measles, fortunately, is easily recognizable clinically and sub-clinical infections are unusual, so that laboratory tests are not often necessary. A notification system should cover the whole country, and completeness of notification becomes more important as the incidence of the disease diminishes. Also, as cases become less frequent, a notification system allied to an outbreak control plan, as in the USA, will be necessary. Equally important is a reliable estimate of vaccine coverage by district or region. Efficiency is required all along the chain from the vaccinator recording the immunization to the event being noted centrally. Errors in calculating vaccine coverage can occur in estimating both denominator and numerator, especially in areas where there are large numbers of transfers in and out. Computerization of records generally improves efficiency.

Containment

Containment of measles can be defined as the point at which the disease, although still occurring, is no longer a public health problem (Noah 1983b). The definition is deliberately vague because the point at which a country is satisfied with its measles programme will depend on its own priorities, and would take into account various factors, such as opportunity costs. An important consideration in choosing a containment policy is the greatly increased marginal costs of immunizing the last small percentage of the target population. A policy of containment for measles should not automatically be considered a second-best alternative—it may be a natural choice for that country. On the other hand it should not be used as an excuse for sloppy management of a vaccine programme, and motivation and efficiency are as important with a containment policy as with any other. Other aspects of a containment policy have been discussed by Noah (1983b).

The second World Health Organization Conference on Immunization Policies in Europe (held in Karlovy Vary, Czechoslovakia, in 1984), set a goal of elimination of measles by 1995 by reaching a 95 per cent uptake of vaccine in children by 1990 (Begg and Noah 1985). This may, in effect, be a policy of containment, because in those countries that have set out to eliminate measles, a 95 per cent vaccine uptake rate has not yet proved to be high enough. This has more or less been acknowledged by the British who, in spite of the Karlovy Vary recommendations, set a target for measles immunization of 90 per cent by 1990.

Epidemiological side-effects of mass immunization

Mass immunization is ecological interference, and unless elimination is achieved some change in the epidemiological features of measles is inevitable. The striking biennial pattern of measles in England and Wales in the pre-vaccine era disappeared shortly after mass immunization was introduced, and the seasonal pattern almost disappeared too. Fine and Clarkson (1983) suggested that this was almost entirely accounted for by obliteration of the major biennial and seasonal epidemics, leaving the minor epidemics almost as before. They suggest that this lack of impact on the 'minimum period' of measles is an important sign of the failure of measles to 'fade out' from a community.

Mass immunization has also had an effect on the age distribution of measles cases in populations. In England and Wales the total number of susceptibles is said to have remained fairly constant at 4–4.5 million individuals, in spite of the vaccine programme (Fine and Clarkson 1982), while the number of susceptibles over 10 years of age may be increasing.

In Czechoslovakia (Sejda 1983), a successful immunization programme reduced measles incidence to less than 2 per cent of its pre-vaccine level, but there was a gradual shift in the age distribution of cases to older non-immunized children. In the United States (Hinman et al. 1980) the age-specific incidence of the disease has also changed. In no age group did the incidence of measles actually increase (Table 3.2) but the fall in incidence was considerably less in the older than in the younger age groups and the

Table 3.2 Age distribution and average annual age-specific incidence of reported measles cases in the United States, 1960–64, 1976–78.

Age group (years)	1960–64[a]		1976–78[b]	
	% of total	Cases per 100 000	% of total	Cases per 100 000
< 5	37.2	766.0	15.5	40.2
5–9	52.8	1236.9	26.4	64.1
10–14	6.5	168.1	35.5	74.6
15 +	3.4	10.0	23.7	6.0

[a]Data from 5 reporting areas.
[b]Data from at least 45 reporting areas.
Source: Hinman *et al.* (1980).

10–14-year age group is now the most susceptible, having been less susceptible not only than the 5–9-year olds but also than the 0–4-year olds. A computer model simulation by Levy (1984) suggested that, although the proportion of susceptibles in the United States has fallen from 10.6 per cent to 3.1 per cent since immunization was introduced, this proportion has begun to rise by 0.1 per cent a year, so that it should reach 10.9 per cent, higher than the pre-vaccine level (and older in age) by the year 2050!

Numerous recent outbreaks of measles on American campuses have supported these theoretical, but worrying, considerations. Since January 1985 at least three such outbreaks have occurred (Centers for Disease Control 1985) involving respectively 12, 82, and 128 cases. In two the index case contracted measles abroad, in the third the immunization level of the students was low. In 1983, 296 (19.8 per cent) of 1497 cases of measles reported in the United States were college cases, and a further 274 were college-associated cases (Centers for Disease Control 1984). In 1984 the proportion was somewhat lower, but in 1985 this increased again to 18.5 per cent (334/1802). Outbreaks in pockets of unimmunized religious anti-immunization groups have also been recorded (*Morbid. Mortal. Wkly Rep.* 1980).

Cost–benefits of measles vaccine

One problem of cost–benefit analysis of immunization procedures is that the costs are health costs while the benefits are often social (Patrick and Woolley 1981); hence the arguments may not be as convincing to health managers as one would wish. Benefit calculations usually entail savings on treatment costs, mortality, and morbidity, the avoidance of intangibles such as pain and grief, and external benefits (Creese and Henderson 1980). The benefits from 10 years of measles immunization were clearly shown both in terms of costs and social benefits more than 10 years ago in the United States (Witte and Axnick 1975). Since then, other studies, quoted in Creese and Henderson (1980), have indicated that in developed countries the estimated ratio of benefit to cost is about 10 to 1; a more recent study suggests 15 to 1 (Koplan 1985). The prevention of SSPE by measles vaccine means a further 10 per cent increase in benefit (Elo 1979). In the United States the cost of measles without immunization was estimated to be $1.4 billion. The vaccine costs were $96 million plus $14.5 million for residual measles cases (White *et al.* 1985). In the USSR the measles vaccine programme was stated to be justified as economical by part of the treatment savings alone (Burgasov 1973). A study in one general practice in England revealed that over 20 years measles immunization had not only brought financial reward to the practice but had reduced the number of measles-related consultations by 40 per cent, even though a home visit was often required to immunize a patient (Binnie 1984).

Recommendation

Elimination or containment?

What should be the goal of a measles control programme in a developed country, more specifically one in the EEC? A selective immunization policy for measles cannot be seriously considered. For reasons given, eradication also should probably not be considered—except on a world-wide basis, a target not likely to be attempted for many years. The goal of elimination has its own problems, as stated, not the least of which is the high cost in manpower spent on the surveillance, control, and investigation of outbreaks. The marginal costs of a vaccine programme will rise steeply when attempting complete immunization coverage (Noah 1983b). Moreover, until a concerted attempt can be made world-wide to control measles, the risks of the importation of measles leading to spread will always be present. Given finite resources therefore, containment may be the best policy for much of Europe at present. A shift in the age distribution of measles with all its consequences may, however, occur more rapidly than with a policy of elimination, and careful and strict surveillance will be necessary if such a policy is chosen.

Nevertheless, the efficiency and enthusiasm with which the countries, particularly the United States, that have aimed to eradicate measles have set about their goal is to be admired. They have shown what can be achieved, and the extremely low incidence of measles in most of these countries would be a more than adequate result of an elimination policy, even if measles has not been eliminated. Whatever the goals of the immunization strategy, a more aggressive attitude to improving measles vaccine uptake is certainly required.

References

Anderson, R.M. and May, R.M. (1982). Directly-transmitted infectious diseases: control by vaccination. *Science* **215**, 1053–60.

—— (1983). Vaccination against rubella and measles: quantitative investigations of different policies. *J. Hyg.* **90**, 259–325.

Bart, K.J., Orenstein, W.A., Hinman, A.R., and Amler, R.W. (1983). Measles and models. *Int. J. Epidemiol.* **12**, 263–5.

Begg, N.T. and Noah, N.D. (1985). Immunization targets in Europe and Britain. *Br. Med. J.* **291**, 1370–1.

Binnie, G.A.C. (1984). Measles immunization—profit and loss in a general practice. *Br. Med. J.* **289**, 1275–6.

Burgasov, P.N. (1973). The status of measles after 5 years of mass vaccination in the USSR. *Bull. WHO* **49**, 571.

Centers for Disease Control. (1982). Measles Surveillance Report No. 11, 1977–81. Atlanta.

—— (1984). Measles—New Hampshire. *Morbid. Mortal. Wkly Rep.* **33**, 549–59.

—— (1985). Multiple measles outbreaks on college campus—Ohio, Massachusetts, Illinois. *Morbid. Mortal. Wkly Rep.* **34**, 129–30.

Creese, A.L. and Henderson, R.H. (1980). Cost–benefit analysis and immunization programmes in developing countries. *Bull. WHO* **58**, 491–7.

Cutting, W.A.M. (1983). Measles immunization. A review. *J. Trop. Pediat.* **29**, 246–7.

Elo, O. (1979). Cost benefit studies of vaccination in Finland. *Dev. Biol. Stand.* **43**, 419–28.

Fine, P.E.M. and Clarkson, J.A. (1982). Measles in England and Wales—II: the impact of the measles vaccine programme on the distribution of immunization in the population. *Int. J. Epidemiol.* **11**, 15–25.

—— —— (1983). Measles in England and Wales—III: assessing published predictions of the impact of vaccination on incidence. *Int. J. Epidemiol.* **12**, 332–9.

Frank, J.A., Orenstein, W.A., Bart, K.J., Bart, S.W., El-Tantawy, N., Davis, R.M., and Hinman, A.R. (1985). Major impediments to measles elimination. *Am. J. Dis. Child.* **139**, 881–8.

Gastel, B. (1973). Measles: a potentially finite history. *J. Hist. Med.* **28**, 34–44.

Henderson, D.A. (1982). Global measles eradication. *Lancet* **2**, 208.

Hethcote, H.W. (1983). Measles and rubella in the US. *Am. J. Epidemiol.* **117**, 2–13.

Hinman, A.R., Brandling-Bennett, A.D., Bernier, R., Kirby, C.D., and Eddins, D.L. (1980). Current features of measles in the United States: feasibility of measles elimination. *Epidemiol. Rev.* **2**, 153–70.

Hopkins, D.R., Hinman, A.R., Koplan, J.P., and Lane, J.M. (1982). The case for global measles eradication. *Lancet* **2**, 1396–98.

Horwitz, O., Grünfeld, K., Lysgaard-Hansen, B., and Kjeldsen, K. (1974). The epidemiology and natural history of measles in Denmark. *Am. J. Epidemiol.* **100**, 136–49.

Koplan, J.P. (1985). *The value of preventive medicine*, pp. 55–68. Pitman,

London (Ciba Foundation Symposium 110).
Landrigan, P.J. and Witte, J.J. (1973). Neurologic disorders following live measles vaccination. *JAMA* **223**, 1459.
Langmuir, A.D. (1962). Medical importance of measles. *Am. J. Dis. Child.* **103**, 224-6.
Levy, D.L. (1984). The future of measles in highly immune populations. A modelling approach. *Am. J. Epidemiol.* **120**, 39-48.
Miller, C.L. (1978). Severity of notified measles. *Br. Med. J.* **1**, 1253.
—— (1982). Surveillance after measles vaccination in children. *Practitioner* **226**, 535-7.
—— (1983). Current impact of measles in the U.K. *Rev. Infect. Dis.* **5**, 427-32.
Miller, D.L. (1964). Frequency of complications of measles 1963. *Br. Med. J.* **2**, 75-8.
Morbid. Mortal. Wkly Rep. (1980). Measles—New York. **29**, 452.
—— (1984). Measles outbreak among vaccinated high school students. Illinois. **33**, 349-51.
—— (1985). Measles on college campuses. U.S. **34**, 445-9.
National Childhood Encephalopathy Study Research Team. (1981). The National Childhood Encephalopathy Study. In *Whooping cough.* pp. 79-154. Her Majesty's Stationery Office, London.
Noah, N.D. (1982). Measles eradiction policies. *Br. Med. J.* **284**, 997-8.
—— (1983a). Epidemiological aspects of viral vaccines. In *Recent advances in clinical virology* (ed. A.P. Waterson). Churchill Livingstone, Edinburgh.
—— (1983b). The strategy of immunization. *Comm. Med.* **5**, 140-47.
Patrick, K.M. and Woolley, F.R. (1981). A cost-benefit analysis of immunization for pneumococcal pneumonia. *JAMA* **245**, 473-7.
Rabo, E. and Taranger, J. (1984). Scandinavian model for eliminating measles, mumps and rubella. *Br. Med. J.* **289**, 1402-4.
Rey, M. (1985). Eradication of measles by widespread vaccination is beneficial and feasible. *Sem. Hop. Paris* **61**, 21-5.
Sejda, J. (1983). Control of measles in Czechoslovakia (CSSR). *Rev. Infect. Dis.* **5**, 564-7.
Smith, H. (1980). Measles again. *Br. Med. J.* **280**, 766-7.
Thornton, A.S. (1985). Scandinavian model for eliminating measles, mumps, and rubella. *Br. Med. J.* **290**, 242.
Velimirovic, B (1984). *Infectious diseases in Europe—a fresh look.* World Health Organization, Copenhagen.
White, C.C., Koplan, J.P., and Orenstein, W.A. (1985). Benefits, risks and costs of immunization for measles, mumps and rubella. *Am. J. Publ. Hlth* **75**, 739-44.
Whittle, H.C., Rowland, M.G.M., Mann, G.F., Lamb, W.H., and Lewis, R.A. (1984). Immunization of 4-6-month-old Gambian infants with Edmonston-Zagreb measles vaccine. *Lancet* **2**, 834-7.
Witte, J.J. and Axnick, N.W. (1975). The benefits from 10 years of measles immunization in the U.S. *Publ. Hlth Rep.* **90**, 205.
World Health Organization (WHO) (1981). Incidence of 5 vaccine preventable diseases and immunization coverage. *Wkly Epidemiol. Record* **56**, 369-72.
—— (1983). Measles surveillance: feasibility of measles elimination in Europe. *Wkly Epidemiol. Record* **58**, 229-30.
Yekutiel, P. (1981). Lessons from the big eradication campaigns. *World Hlth Forum* **2**, 465-81.

4
Mumps
Norman Noah

SUMMARY

The case for the elimination of mumps, either on humanitarian or monetary grounds, is not strong. The disease itself is unpleasant, but not severe, and the complications of mumps, on the whole, are self-limiting. Economic studies suggest marginal benefit for a mass immunization programme for mumps vaccine alone, but the cost–benefit ratio increases greatly when mumps vaccine is given together with measles and rubella vaccines as MMR vaccine. Thus mumps vaccine is in the curious and probably unique position of being scarcely justifiable on its own, but is beneficial when used 'as a passenger' with two other vaccines of proven value.

Defining the problem

History

Mumps, like measles, is a widespread and highly infectious viral infection which causes a characteristic and easily recognizable illness. Hippocrates described an outbreak of what could have been mumps in the fifth century BC, but there is little else in the literature until the eighteenth century when several outbreaks were described.

The burden of mumps

Like measles, mumps is universal, with 95 per cent of adults immune. Neither the disease nor its complications, however, are as severe as measles. A complication rate of 24 per 1000 cases has been estimated (Research Unit 1974). It is one of the two most commonly diagnosed causes of viral meningitis (Noah and Urquhart 1980; Rey 1985), but this complication, together with orchitis and pancreatitis, does not usually leave permanent sequelae (Research Unit 1974). The much feared risk of sterility in men has little evidence to support it (Beard *et al.* 1979), although bilateral testicular atrophy may undoubtedly result from orchitis. Deafness is a serious complication as it is of the nerve type, and is often complete and permanent. Fortunately it is rare, and occurs in less than five cases per 100 000 (Westmore *et al.* 1979) or one case per 20 000 of deafness (Rey 1985). Juvenile onset diabetes may possibly follow mumps. This association, if real, would account for less than 1 per cent of this type of diabetes (Gamble 1980).

Death, usually a complication of encephalitis, is also rare, with a case-fatality rate estimated to vary between 1.0 and 3.4 per 10 000 (Hayden *et al.* 1978; Centers for Disease Control 1984). As 30–40 per cent of mumps infections are asymptomatic, a better indicator of the rarity of fatal mumps is the average of 5 certified deaths a year in England and Wales between 1962 and 1981 (a rate of about 1 per 10 million population), more than half of which, on closer inspection, were probably not caused by mumps (Galbraith *et al.* 1984).

Pregnant women who develop mumps in the first trimester are more likely than control women to lose their baby (Siegel *et al.* 1966), and the virus has been isolated from a fetus aborted spontaneously at 10 weeks (Kurtz *et al.* 1982).

Thus the rarity of severe complications, and the facts that one attack of mumps leads to permanent immunity and that attack rates are highest at a time of life when illness is not economically important, collectively make the control or eradication of mumps a less urgent problem than, for example, measles. Nevertheless, it is still cost-effective to control the infection, and the cost–benefit is greatly enhanced by the availability of mumps vaccine in a combined formulation with measles and rubella vaccines (MMR) with little extra cost.

Nature of intervention

Although the transmissibility of mumps by a filtrable agent in saliva (from man to monkey) was demonstrated experimentally in 1934 (Johnson and Goodpasture), mumps virus was isolated in 1948. Some early vaccines were prepared, but it was not until 1963 that a live attenuated vaccine from virus grown in chick embryo cell cultures was developed. A live vaccine is now commercially available in most European countries, although in only a few is it used widely.

Target population

As with measles vaccine, mumps vaccine should be given after 12 months of age, and mass immunization is the accepted strategy. Selective immunization is not generally indicated as the complications of mumps cannot be predicted.

The vaccine is not effective in the control of outbreaks in those in whom exposure has already occurred.

Evidence for efficacy, effectiveness, and safety

The vaccine appears to be safe, the attenuated virus is not communicable, and seroconversion rates of 94–99 per cent have been achieved after one dose (Hillemann et al. 1968). No significant waning of antibody has been reported almost 20 years after the vaccine came into regular use. Like measles vaccine, mumps vaccine should be given after 12 months of age to ensure reasonable seroconversion rates. An important characteristic of mumps vaccine virus is its ability to be combined with measles and rubella vaccine viruses to produce one vaccine (MMR).

The United States has probably had more experience of mumps vaccine than any other country. During the period 1968–82, 59.3 million doses of mumps vaccine were distributed in that country. In 1968, 152 209 cases of mumps were reported, with under-reporting clearly at a high level. By 1981–82 when surveillance had almost certainly improved, only 5000 cases a year were being reported. The immunization rate was 95 per cent in those entering school. States without a compulsory mumps immunization law, but with a mumps vaccine policy, had an overall rate of 34.7 cases/million population/year, about twice that of 17.5 cases/million/year in states with such laws (Centers for Disease Control 1984). When mumps vaccine is used in the combined vaccine, mumps antibodies are stimulated as efficiently as with a single vaccine (Weibel et al. 1980a) without an increase in side-effects (Lerman et al. 1981), and persist for at least 10 years (Weibel et al. 1980b), and probably much longer.

Administration of the mumps vaccine has been followed by some conditions known to be complications of mumps, such as nerve deafness, but a causal association has not been proved. The attenuated virus has been recovered from the placenta, but not the fetus, when given to volunteers.

Cost–benefit considerations

Koplan and Preblud (1982) estimated that mumps immunization would prevent 540 000 cases of mumps and 23 deaths for a 'model cohort' of 1 million people followed up for 30 years. The estimated benefit–cost ratio was 3.3:1 for single mumps immunization, and 39:1 for MMR (Koplan and Preblud 1982; Centers for Disease Control 1984). These estimates include indirect costs of mumps infection: for single mumps vaccine the ratio falls to 1:1 if only direct costs of mumps are taken into account, thereby reducing the apparent gain from immunization (Koplan and Preblud 1982; Koplan 1985).

Others (White *et al.* 1985) estimated the benefit–cost ratio as 6.7:1 for mumps only, and 14:1 for MMR.

Yorke *et al.* (1979) on the other hand, felt that it was debatable whether the costs of mumps eradication were justified by the potential benefits, and the few studies in Europe show only a marginal benefit. In Austria (Weidermann and Ambrosch 1979) the estimated benefit–cost ratio was 3.6:1, though unusually high vaccine costs were used of US$20.50 for measles and mumps (including administration). In Switzerland (Just 1978) a benefit–cost without consideration of indirect costs of mumps was 2.1:1.

Conclusion

The case for mumps elimination is clearly not as strong as it is for measles, even though a safe, efficient, and inexpensive vaccine is available. Nevertheless, most economic studies show some benefit, and the ability to combine mumps with measles and rubella vaccines enhances its claims for consideration. The Scandinavians, like the North Americans, firmly believe that 'both the individual and society should be protected against measles, mumps, and rubella' (Rabo and Taranger 1984). Nevertheless, the same theoretical misgivings about mass immunization against measles apply to mumps, in that a susceptible population may accumulate in the older age groups, when the disease is more severe. In Sweden, this possible alteration of the natural ecology of the disease is considered sufficiently seriously to warrant their immunizing as many children as possible twice, once at 18 months and once at 12 years. A similar programme has also been implemented in Finland and Norway.

It is important not to assume, however, that those who do not attend or do not seroconvert after the first injection will necessarily do so after the second, and the elimination of mumps, like measles, has not yet proved to be a feasible proposition in most countries of the world. It can certainly be stated that elimination of these diseases will be impossible without considerable motivation and organization on the part of health authorities.

References

Beard, C.M., Benson, R.C., Kelalis, P.P., Elveback, L., and Kurland, L.I. (1977). The incidence and outcome of mumps orchititis in Rochester, Minnesota, 1935-1974. *Mayo Clin. Proc.* **52**, 3-7.

Centers for Disease Control. (1984). Mumps Surveillance. January 1977–December 1982. Issued Sept. 1984. US Department Health and Human Services.

Galbraith, N.S., Pusey, J.J., Young, S.E.J., Crombie, D.L., and Sparks, J.P. (1984). Mumps surveillance in England and Wales. 1962-1981. *Lancet* **1**, 91-4.

Gamble, D.R. (1980). Relationship of antecedent illness to development of diabetes in children. *Br. Med. J.* **12**, 99-101.

Hayden, G.F., Preblud, S.R., Orenstein, W.A., and Conrad, J.L. (1978). Current status of mumps and mumps vaccine in the United States. *Pediatrics* **62**, 965-9.

Hilleman, M.R., Buynak, E.B., Weibel, R.E., and Stokes, J. Jr. (1968). Live attenuated mumps-virus vaccine. *New Engl. J. Med.* **278**, 227-32.

Johnson, C.D. and Goodpasture, E.W. (1934). An investigation of the etiology of mumps. *J. Exp. Med.* **59**, 1-19.

Just, M. (1978). Rentiert die Masem—und/oder mumps: impfung fur Schweizerische verhaltnisse? *Schweiz Med. Wochenschr.* **108**, 1763-8.

Koplan, J.P. (1985). Benefits, risks and costs of immunization programmes. In *The value of preventive medicine*, pp. 55-68. Pitman, London (Ciba Foundation Symposium 110).

—— and Preblud, S.R. (1982). A benefit-cost analysis of mumps vaccine. *Am. J. Dis. Child.* **136**, 362-4.

Kurtz, J.B., Tomlinson, A.H., and Pearson, J. (1982). Mumps virus isolated from a foetus. *Br. Med. J.* **1**, 471.

Lerman, S.J., Bollinger, M., and Brunkan, J.M. (1981). Clinical and serologic evaluation of measles, mumps and rubella virus vaccines, singly and in combination. *Pediatrics* **68**, 18-22.

Noah, N.D. and Urquhart, A.M. (1980). Virus meningitis and encephalitis in 1979. *J. Infect.* **2**, 379-83.

Rabo, E. and Taranger, J. (1984). Scandinavian model for eliminating measles, mumps and rubella. *Br. Med. J.* **289**, 1402-4.

Research Unit, Royal College of General Practitioners. (1974). The incidence and complications of mumps. *J. R. Coll. Gen. Pract.* **24**, 545-51.

Rey, M. (1985). Le vaccination contre les oreillons. *Rev. Prat. (Paris)* **35**, 410-12.

Siegel, M., Fuerst, H.T., and Peress, N.S. (1966). Comparative foetal mortality in maternal virus disease. *New Engl. J. Med.* **274**, 768-71.

Weibel, R.E., Buynak, E.B., McLean, A.A., Roehm, R.R., and Hillerman, M.R. (1980a). Persistence of antibody in human subjects for 7-10 years following administration of combined live attenuated measles, mumps, and rubella virus vaccines. *Proc. Soc. Exp. Biol. Med.* **165**, 260-3.

——, Carlson, A.J. Jr., Villarejos, J.M., Buynak, E.B., McLean, A.A., and Hilleman, M.R. (1980b). Clinical and laboratory studies of combined live measles, mumps and rubella vaccine using the RA27/3 rubella virus (40979). *Proc. Soc. Exp. Biol. Med.* **165**, 323-6.

Westmore, G.A., Pickard, B.H., and Stern, H. (1979). Isolation of mumps from the inner ear after sudden deafness. *Br. Med. J.* **1**, 14-15.

White, C.C., Koplan, J.P., and Orenstein, W.A. (1985). Benefits, risks and costs of immunization for measles, mumps and rubella. *Am. J. Publ. Hlth* **75**, 739-44.

Wiedermann, G. and Ambrosch, F. (1979). Costs and benefits of measles and mumps immunization in Austria. *Bull. WHO* **57**, 625-9.

Yorke, J.A., Nathanson, N., Piangiani, G., and Martin, J. (1979). Seasonality and the requirements for perpetuation and eradication of viruses in populations. *Am. J. Epidemiol.* **109**, 102-23.

5
Hepatitis B
Jens Ole Nielsen

SUMMARY

The hepatitis B virus (HBV) represents a major health problem to the vast majority of the world's population, both as a major cause of chronic liver disease and as a possible aetiological agent of hepatocellular carcinoma. Serological studies have confirmed that the predominant feature of hepatitis B epidemiology is a continuous cycle of sub-clinical infections resulting in an appreciable percentage of overtly healthy hepatitis B surface antigen carriers. The incidence and prevalence of hepatitis B show considerable geographical variations in Europe. In addition, a number of social and professional activities are associated with an increased risk of contracting hepatitis B. Sexual transmission and transmission among drug abusers are probably the most important routes of transmission in Europe today. Because some of these activities are illegal or discriminated against (intravenous drug abuse, homosexuality) the target groups for control measures are difficult to identify or recognize before they contract hepatitis B. Defining the risk groups in the individual countries and promoting an appropriate immunization strategy may to some extent reduce the incidence of hepatitis B in Europe during the next decades. However, the presence of a virus carrier state in combination with social and financial constraints militate against elimination of the disease in Europe.

Definiting the problem

Although a number of viral and bacterial infections may induce hepatitis in man, most clinical hepatitis in Europe can be characterized as hepatitis type A, B, or non-A, non-B. In most cases it is not possible to distinguish between these three forms on the basis of the past history or clinical or histological findings. The evidence for hepatitis non-A and non-B is primarily epidemiological and, as yet, agents have not been characterized unequivocally. Hepatitis A is characterized either by seroconversion or by the presence of IgM antibodies against hepatitis A virus (IgM anti-HAV). The disease is self-limiting, and chronic liver disease or a chronic HAV carrier state has never been demonstrated. There are a few reports of fulminant hepatitis A with a fatal outcome. The presence of anti-HAV is a sign of immunity and reinfection does not seem to occur.

Hepatitis B virus (HBV) is a DNA virus. It is a complex virus with a number of antigens (surface antigen, core antigen, e-antigen) with the capacity to induce an antibody response in a susceptible host. In addition the complete HBV particle contains a protein kinase and a DNA polymerase.

The result of individual contact between hepatitis B virus and a susceptible person may be a variety of clinical conditions as indicated in Figure 5.1. However, the infection inevitably produces a serological scar in terms of the presence of either antigen markers (HBsAg, HBeAg) or the corresponding antibodies (anti-HBs, anti-HBc, and anti-HBe). There is considerable geographical variation in the relative numerical importance of the different clinical courses of acute type B hepatitis throughout the world and even within Europe. In general, fulminating hepatitis B is seen in less than 1 per cent of patients and the development of a chronic carriership of HBV and chronic liver disease is seen in 5–10 per cent of the patients in Europe. Very little is known about the development of the healthy HBV carrier state found in blood donors. From an epidemiological point of view, the healthy carrier state is characterized by the presence of anti-HBe, indicating that this group, in general, is less contagious than the group of carriers with chronic liver disease and HBeAg.

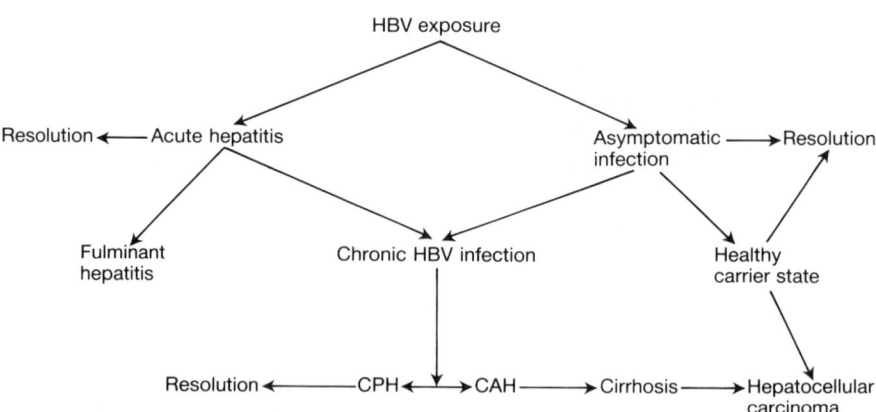

Key: HBV = hepatitis B virus
CAH = chronic active hepatitis
CPH = chronic persistent hepatitis

Fig. 5.1 Possible outcomes of hepatitis B virus infection.

Size of the problem

Epidemiological data on the occurrence of hepatitis B may be based on national notification systems or on serological surveys in different well-defined populations—for example, blood donors, drug addicts, homosexual men, dentists, surgeons.

Routine separate notification for hepatitis A and B was introduced in a number of European countries in the late 1970s, and recently a few countries have also introduced separate notification of non-A, non-B hepatitis. The development of cheap and reliable serological tests for hepatitis A and B has improved the assessment of the respective diagnostic types. The official notified numbers of all three types of hepatitis indicate that it is possible to divide Europe into three hepatitis regions (Velimirovic 1984).

1. *Central and North-West Europe* with an annual incidence of 10 notified cases per 100 000 population and with a constant decrease in the last two decades.
2. *East Europe* with annual incidences around 100 notified cases per 100 000 population and a slight increase in the last two decades.
3. *Mediterranean* with a high incidence until the mid 1970s, when the trend seemed to level off and reach a plateau.

The remarkable difference between Eastern Europe and the rest of Europe can be explained to some extent by a stricter notification of hepatitis in Eastern European countries.

Official figures are hampered by a reporting rate of no more than 5–10 per cent in most countries. Thus these figures can only give an impression of the changing pattern of disease and do not reflect its total impact on the population. Table 5.1 gives some data on the occurrence of hepatitis B in a number of EEC countries at a time when immunoprophylaxis was not possible. The Table shows the considerable difference between the low incidence areas in North and North-West Europe and the regions with high incidence in Southern Europe (WHO 1978).

During the last decade there have only been minor changes in the annual reported numbers of hepatitis B cases in the EEC. Most surprisingly, the introduction of the hepatitis B vaccine, in 1982 and 1983, has still not resulted in a significant reduction in the number of cases reported to the health authorities.

From the data in Table 5.1, it can be estimated that a total of 463 000 new hepatitis B infections occurred in 1976 in a population of approximately 266 million people. It has been demonstrated that 10 per cent of patients with clinically overt hepatitis B become HBsAg carriers for years (Nielsen *et al.* 1971). This is probably a minimum figure since patients with sub-clinical

Table 5.1 Hepatitis B in some EEC countries in 1976

Country (population millions)	Prevalence of HBsAg in donors (%)	Notified cases of hepatitis (all types)	Estimated[a] hepatitis B (per 100 000)
Belgium (10)	0.5	876	44
Denmark (5)	0.2	713	56
France (50)	0.2–0.5	3 656	70
Greece (10)	2.6–4.1	2 897	150
Italy (60)	1–4.1	48 000	320–500
Netherlands (14)	0.2	1 195	43
Spain (38)	1.9–2.2	?	?
UK (56)	0.1–0.2	7 581	45
FRG (62)	0.2–0.3	21 355	221

[a]Estimated on a reporting rate between 5 and 10 per cent, on the basis of the information on the percentage of hepatitis B cases among the total number of cases of hepatitis reported to the World Health Organization.

infections are believed to have a greater risk of becoming carriers. Thus, approximately 46 000 new HBsAg carriers emerged in 1976. Other studies from Europe have shown a spontaneous clearance rate of 1 per cent per year of HBsAg carriers (Dormeyer et al. 1981). This would suggest a steady state would exist when the existing carrier pool equals 100 times the annual number of new carriers. Based on 1976 rates, therefore, this would occur if there were 4.6 million carriers—that is, 1.7 per cent of the total regional population. This figure is probably too high for the EEC countries and as a result it is reasonable to assume, given the new carrier rates above, that the HBV reservoir has increased in the past decade. There is thus a considerable HBV reservoir of chronic carriers in the EEC countries, but it is not equally distributed throughout Europe.

Hepatitis B risk groups

The frequency of hepatitis B infection is a function of several known risk factors (Table 5.2). Additional factors determine the risk of developing a chronic virus carrier state, and, finally, there are circumstances which reflect both an increased risk of infection and persistent carriage of the virus (Lewellys et al. 1983). As can be seen from Table 5.2, the factors which increase the risk of contracting hepatitis B are predominantly related to environment and life-style. From a global point of view, perinatal transmission is an important and self-perpetuating factor. However, in Europe horizontal spread seems to be by far the most important route of hepatitis B transmission. Overall exposure to hepatitis B (HBsAg and anti-HBs) varies

Table 5.2 Risk factors for hepatitis B

Increased risk of exposure
Blood and blood-product transfusion
Percutaneous exposure to blood or serum for example, via contaminated needles, tattooing, narcotics abuse
Sexual contact with an infected person
Household contact with an infected person
Health care workers

Increased risk of persistence
Inherited or acquired immunodeficiency
Exposure in infancy or childhood
Male sex
Ethnic and genetic factors

Increased risk of exposure and persistence
Infants of infected mothers
Residents of custodial institutions for retarded children

from 5 to 30 per cent in the general population. There is, however, considerable variation not only from one country to another, but also between the different age and risk groups within a particular geographical region. In Denmark the total exposure to hepatitis B among blood donors varies with the age of the donor from 5 to 15 per cent. In contrast, the exposure among homosexual men is 70 per cent (Kryger *et al.* 1984).

Hepatitis B transmission by the transfusion of blood and blood products has been an important risk factor for transfusion recipients, but of rather limited importance for the overall epidemiology of the disease. The introduction of routine screening of all blood donations for HBsAg has almost completely eliminated transfusion-associated hepatitis B in the EEC.

Percutaneous exposure to the virus by contaminated needles is an important risk factor in drug abusers. There are no valid figures for the number of intravenous drug abusers in the individual countries, but the impression is that this problem is greater in the North and North-West of Europe than in Southern Europe. Intravenous drug abusers represent one of the most important reservoirs of hepatitis B virus in Europe. In general, drug abusers represent a risk to other drug abusers but not to the entire population, with the exception that prostitutes with an intravenous drug abuse problem are a risk to their clients.

Sexual contact is of major importance for the continuous transmission of hepatitis B. Sexual promiscuity increases disease transmission (Szmuness *et al.* 1975), as illustrated by the extremely high rate of spread of hepatitis B among male homosexuals. The existence of an apparently healthy carrier state which does not cause any reduction in sexual activity makes this route of transmission probably the most important in Europe today.

Low socio-economic status is associated with an increased risk of infection, perhaps as a result of poor hygiene and crowded living conditions (Cherubin et al. 1972). Under unsatisfactory living conditions horizontal spread to children is seen. This might be the reason for the very high prevalence of HBsAg carriers in certain areas of Southern Italy. Otherwise, hepatitis B is very uncommon in European children, except for those living in large institutions for the mentally retarded.

Much attention has been focused on the occupational hazard for health care workers from hepatitis B. From an epidemiological point of view, hepatitis B among health care workers represents only a minor problem, although it might be very important for the individual person. A number of serological surveys from the Western world have demonstrated an increased risk of hepatitis B among those who are in regular contact with blood or body secretions from hepatitis patients. The risk groups include surgeons, emergency room nurses, technicians, dentists, and so on. Once more there seem to be considerable differences from one country to another. Although American dentists seem to be a high-risk group (Mosley et al. 1975), it was not possible to demonstrate any increased risk among Danish dentists in a similar study (Aldershvile et al. 1978). A strong correlation exists between the number of years spent working in a health care setting and the prevalence of HBV markers in health care workers, supporting the fact that the health care environment is a definite risk factor for hepatitis B virus exposure.

In a population with quite a constant incidence of hepatitis B, the size of the hepatitis reservoir depends on the factors which aid the development of chronic HBsAg carriers (Table 5.2). There is accumulating evidence to suggest that impaired cell mediated immunity is an important factor for the progression from an acute type B hepatitis to a chronic carrier state (Thomas 1980). An identical mechanism may account for the high carrier rate found in babies born to mothers with HBV infection at the time of delivery (Beasley and Stevens 1978). It is likely that persistence of perinatal infection is one of the principal factors responsible for the maintenance of a high prevalence of infection in those parts of the world where HBV infection is most common. In Europe this mechanism is of minor importance numerically, and in high-incidence areas may account for even less than 5 per cent of the carrier population.

The existence of several antigenic sub-types of the hepatitis B virus is well documented. The different sub-types are of epidemiological interest, but they are not correlated with the clinical outcome of the infection (Nielsen and Le Bouvier 1973). In contrast, epidemiological studies indicate that some genetic or racial factors may be associated with the response to HBV infection. For some unknown reason, persistence of HBV infection is more common in males than in females even after identical exposure.

In recent years a large number of South-East Asian refugees have arrived in Europe. The prevalence of HBsAg carriers in this population is up to 20 per cent, even among children. In Denmark it has been estimated that the refugees have increased the carrier population in the country by at least 25 per cent.

Interventions

The elimination or eradication of an infectious disease may, in principle, be based on elimination of the reservoir of the infectious agent, interruption of the routes of transmission, or immunization of the susceptible population at risk.

Elimination of reservoirs

In modern medicine there is no example of eradication of a human infectious disease by primary elimination of the reservoir of infection by treatment. Only in diseases with a natural animal reservoir has it been possible to control the spread by attacking the reservoir. There is some limited evidence that hepatitis can be transmitted by mosquitoes, but there seems to be no natural reservoir for the virus in animals. With hepatitis B there is still no effective treatment of the virus carrier state. In recent years a number of reports have described successful treatment with antiviral chemotherapy in combination with interferon or steroids. Most of the studies have been uncontrolled open studies. It is, however, reasonable to assume that an effective treatment will become available within the next few years.

The treatment is obviously going to be expensive, and can probably be offered only to a limited number of patients with chronic active type B hepatitis. Although important for the individual patient, the treatment will have, therefore, no impact on the epidemiology of hepatitis B which is largely determined by the number of healthy HBsAg carriers.

Interruption of transmission

The interruption of the transmission routes by general hygienic precautions is often neglected, but this is nevertheless of utmost importance in the control of hepatitis B. The elimination of hepatitis B from some dialysis units at the beginning of the 1970s is an excellent example of what can be achieved by improving standards of hygiene. The most important routes of transmission in Europe seem to be by sexual contact and the sharing of needles by drug abusers. There is a considerable social barrier to be crossed in reaching these target groups with sufficient information to change their hazardous lifestyles. Although drug addicts do not, in general, regard hepatitis B as a major problem, they should be encouraged not to share needles or syringes with others. Some societies believe that the restriction of access to needles or syringes is a weapon against drug addiction. It is rather a weapon against the control of AIDS and hepatitis B in this particular risk group. In an attempt to stop the spread of AIDS among drug addicts in Denmark, clean needles and syringes are now provided free of charge. If successful this may also have a beneficial impact on the spread of hepatitis B.

People with many, often anonymous, sexual contacts should be advised to follow the same safe sex guidelines being used in the efforts to control the AIDS epidemic. A considerable proportion of homosexual and bisexual men have regular sex contacts with people belonging to hepatitis B high-risk groups. All those within a particular risk group should be recommended to practise safe sex and to reduce their number of sexual partners because a considerable number of HBsAg carriers do not know that they are carriers of hepatitis B virus.

In order to interrupt the routes of infection in health care settings, personnel should be well educated and encouraged to follow good hygienic practices not only when they care for hepatitis patients but also in their daily routine. This is believed to reduce substantially the risk from healthy HBsAg carriers. All carriers should be informed about their carrier status and about the risk of transmitting the virus by sexual contact, blood donation, and in health care settings. In general there should be no occupational restrictions for carriers. In individual situations, however, where transmission from a carrier has occurred, the health authorities should be able to take specific action in order to prevent further transmission.

It is reasonable to speculate that improvement of the socio-economic condition in some high-incidence areas could have a positive impact by reducing the prevalence of HBsAg carriers. However, there is still only circumstantial evidence to support this.

Immunization

Immunization against hepatitis B can be either passive or active. Passive immunoprophylaxis against hepatitis B is of very limited value (Seef and Hoffnagle 1979). Standard preparation of human immune serum globulin has no documented effect either before or after exposure. The efficacy of specific hepatitis B immune globulin preparation remains controversial, but it is recommended in most countries as a part of post-exposure prophylaxis. The preparation is very expensive and the only well-documented beneficial effect is to prevent the development of a virus carrier state when given at the time of birth to babies of HBsAg carrier mothers (Stevens *et al.* 1982).

A major breakthrough in the prevention of hepatitis B was the introduction of inactivated hepatitis B vaccines with high levels of efficacy and safety—as demonstrated in well-designed controlled clinical trials in high-risk groups (Szmuness *et al.* 1980; Maupas *et al.* 1981). The main limitation in the use of these vaccines is the cost. One immunization course of three doses costs at least US$150. From an international point of view this cost prohibits any large-scale immunization programmes against hepatitis B. It has been estimated that the immunization of all newborn babies in the high-risk areas of Africa and Asia would cost 100 times more than the total World Health Organization expenditure on all other immunization programmes (Arthur *et al.* 1984).

Hepatitis vaccines have been licensed in all EEC countries, and their use can be considered in three groups: newborn babies of carrier mothers, homosexual men, and drug addicts.

It has been demonstrated that the vaccine, in combination with hepatitis B immune globulin, prevents the development of a carrier state in newborn babies of carrier mothers. Pregnant women from hepatitis B risk groups should be tested for HBsAg during pregnancy in order to give immediate prophylaxis to the babies. This is a very important point for individuals, but it has almost no impact on the incidence or prevalence of hepatitis B in Europe.

Hepatitis B infection may occur in children living under poor conditions in large families. The reasonable action in this situation is to improve the hygienic and sanitary conditions rather than to offer an expensive vaccine to a population that is not very well defined (Caporaso *et al.* 1983).

The major routes of hepatitis B transmission in adult life are by sharing needles and by sexual intercourse. The two major risk groups are assumed to be homosexual men and drug addicts. There is a considerable social barrier surrounding both groups. From a medical point of view, susceptible people in both groups should be offered hepatitis B immunization along with information about how to reduce the risk of contracting hepatitis B (and AIDS). However, the extremely high cost of the vaccine make it necessary, even in EEC countries, to consider the indications for its use on the basis of cost-effectiveness. Hepatitis is a heavy financial burden on health care systems. According to a World Health Organization study, the cost varies between US$20 000 and $75 000 per 100 000 population per year (WHO 1982). The considerable difference between countries was to some extent the result of differences in hospitalization practices. Mulley and co-workers (1982) calculated that hepatitis B immunization of susceptible persons would save medical costs in population groups with annual attack rates above 5 per cent in USA. Immunization might even be considered cost-effective for populations with attack rates as low as 1 to 2 per cent. From a similar study in the United Kingdom, Adler and co-workers (1983) concluded that considerable savings could be made to the national economy by offering hepatitis B immunization to homosexual men. It might be difficult to make similar studies in a population of drug addicts, and the problem in both studies is to define and reach the risk groups before they contract hepatitis B.

The development of cheaper recombinant vaccines may change the economic balance in favour of the vaccine in the near future. However, there are fundamental problems in the elimination of hepatitis B by immunization, whichever vaccine is used. The eradication of smallpox is probably the greatest medical success of this century. In smallpox, the recognition of infectious people was simple, those with sub-clinical infections did not transmit the disease, and there was no healthy carrier state. It is estimated that smallpox required between 200 000 and 1 million infected persons for endemicity. The healthy carrier state in hepatitis B is not affected by immunization and perhaps as few as 100 HBsAg carriers may sustain hepatitis B in the population.

Recommendations and conclusions

Continuing and intensified surveillance is required in each country in order to define the risk groups and elaborate control strategies based on cost-effectiveness. Practices found to favour the spread of the virus must also be changed. New and cheaper—and possibly single dose—vaccines are now being investigated. These include synthetic polypeptide vaccines, recombinant antigen vaccines, recombinant vectored vaccines, and anti-idiotypic antibody vaccines. Safe and effective vaccines should be offered to reduce the vertical transmission from infected mothers to their offspring and to reduce the hepatitis B risk in drug addicts and homosexual men. The effect of an immunization offer depends entirely on the co-operation of the population at risk. The reservoir of HBV carriers in Europe—and in the rest of the world—guarantees that hepatitis B will remain a considerable health problem for the foreseeable future.

References

Adler, M.W., Belsey, E.M., McCutchan, J.A., and Mindel, A. (1983). Should homosexuals be vaccinated against hepatitis B? Cost and benefit assessment. *Br. Med. J.* **286**, 1621-4.

Aldershvile, J., Brock, A., Dietrichson, O., Hardt, F., Juhl, E., Madsbad, S., Mathiesen, L., Matzen, P., Nielsen, J.O., Schlichting, P., Sorensen, S., and Tage-Jensen, U. (1978). Hepatitis B virus infection among Danish dentists. *J. Infect. Dis* **137**, 63-6.

Arthur, M.J.P., Hall, A.J., and Wright, R. (1984). Hepatitis B, hepatocellular carcinoma and strategies for prevention. *Lancet* **1**, 607-10.

Beasley, R.P., and Stevens, C.E. (1978). Vertical transmission of HBV and interruption with globulin. In *Viral hepatitis* (eds Vyas, Cohen, and Schmid) pp. 333-45. Franklin Institute Press, Philadelphia.

Caporaso, N., Coltori, M., Del Vecchio-Blanco, C., Mele, A., Ambrogio, G., Stroffolini, T., Aldershvile, J., and Nielsen, J.O. (1983). Acute viral hepatitis in childhool: etiology and evolution. *J. Pediat. Gastroenterol. Nutr.* **2**, 99-104.

Cherubin, C.E., Purcell, R.H., Lander, J.J., McGinn, T.G., and Cone, L.A. (1972). Acquisition of antibody to hepatitis B antigen in three socioeconomically different medical populations. *Lancet* **2**, 149-53.

Dormeyer, H.H., Arnold, W., Schonborn, H., Braun, B., Klinge, O., Pfeifer, U., Knolle, J., Hess, G., Kryger, P., Nielsen, J.O., and Meyer zum Buschenfelde, K.H. (1981). The significance of serologic, histologic and immunohistologic findings in the prognosis of 88 asymptomatic carriers of hepatitis B surface antigen. *J. Infect. Dis.* **144**, 33-7.

Kryger, P., Hofmann, B., Pedersen, N.S., Sprechler, H.H., Tjerk Van den Berg, and Korner, E.A. (1984). Hepatitis among homosexual men in two saunas in Copenhagen. *Ugeskr. Laeger.* **146**, 1276-79.

Lewellys, F., Dodd, R.Y., and Sandler, S.G. (1983). Epidemiology of hepatitis B and of posttransfusion and nosocomial hepatitis. In *Viral hepatitis: laboratory and clinical science* (eds Deinhardt and Deinhardt) pp. 215-30. Marcel Dekker, New York.

Maupas, P., Chiron, J.P., Baring, F., Coursaget, P., Goudeau A., Perrin, J., Denis, F., and Diopmar, I. (1981). Efficacy of hepatitis B vaccine in prevention of early HBsAg carrier state in children. *Lancet* **1**, 289-92.

Mosley, J.W., Edwards, V.M., Casey, G., Redecker, A.G., and White, E. (1975). Hepatitis B virus infections in dentists. *New Engl. J. Med.* **293**, 729-34.

Mulley, A.G., Silverstein, M.D., and Dienstag, J.L. (1982). Indications for use of hepatitis B vaccine, based on cost-effectiveness analysis. *New Engl. J. Med.* **293**, 644-52.

Nielson, J.O. and Le Bouvier, G.L. (1973). Subtypes of Australia antigen among patients and healthy carriers in Copenhagen. *New Engl. J. Med.* **288**, 1257-61.

——, Dietrichson, O., Elling, P., and Christoffersen, P. (1971). Incidence and meaning of persistence of Australia antigen in patients with acute viral hepatitis: development of chronic hepatitis. *New Engl. J. Med.* **285**, 1157-60.

Report of World Health Organization Working Group: Economic aspects of communicable disease. *WHO Euro Reports and Studies* No. 68, Copenhagen, 1982.

Seef, L.B., and Hoffnagle, J.H. (1979). Immunoprophylaxis of viral hepatitis. *Gastroenterology* **77**, 161-82.

Stevens, C.E., Beasley, R.P., Lin, C.D., Hwang, L.Y., Sun, T.S., Hsieh, F.J., Wang, K.Y., and Szmuness, W. (1982). In *Viral hepatitis* (eds Szmuness, Alter and Maynard) p. 527. Franklin Institute Press, Philadelphia.

Szmuness, W., Much, M.I., Prince, A.M., Hoffnagle, J.H., Cherubin, L.E., Harley, E.J., and Block, G.H. (1975). On the role of sexual behaviour in the spread of hepatitis B infection. *Ann. Intern. Med.* **83**, 489-95.

—— Stevens, C., Harley, E.J., Zang, E.A., Olesko, W.R., William, D.C., Sudovsky, R., Morrison, J.N., and Kellner, A (1980). Hepatitis B vaccine. Demonstration of efficacy in a controlled clinical trial in a high-risk population in the United States. *New Engl. J. Med.* **303**, 833–41.

Thomas, H.C. (1980). Cellular immunity to the hepatitis B virus. In *Virus and liver* (eds Bianchi, Gerok, Sickinger and Stradler) pp. 161–68. MPT Press Limited, Lancaster.

Velimirovic, B. (1984). *Infectious diseases in Europe*. World Health Organization, Regional Office for Europe, Copenhagen.

World Health Organization (WHO) (1978). *World Hlth Stat. Rep.* **31**, 84–108.

6
Tuberculosis

Matthijs A. Bleiker and Karel Styblo

SUMMARY

The incidence of tuberculosis has been decreasing since the end of the nineteenth century. Improving socio-economic conditions and the practice of isolating infectious cases in sanatoria made important contributions to this decline in the pre-chemotherapy era. Today in Western Europe primary infection in children and young adults is rare, and the prevalence of infection among them is very low. Almost all cases of bacillary tuberculosis are now caused by endogenous exacerbation of the remote infection. Such cases will continue to occur for many years until the prevalence of infection has become very low in all age groups. It is expected that tuberculosis will be eliminated from most of Western Europe by the first half of the twenty-first century. The most important interventions against tuberculosis will remain case-finding and treatment; BCG vaccination and chemoprophylaxis will have limited scope in future.

Defining the problem

Tuberculosis continues to be a major problem in developing countries, but will be virtually eliminated in developed countries within a few decades. Many factors can influence the level of tuberculosis prevalence in a community and these include density of population, extent of overcrowding (very intensive during the Industrial Revolution), socio-economic conditions and standards of housing, cultural background, general health care, malnutrition, and associated diseases. Another factor, after the emergence of the tubercle bacillus in 1882 and before the discovery of chemotherapy, was the isolation in sanatoria of an increasing number of patients with infectious tuberculosis. Since a larger proportion of these highly infectious cases was isolated and treated for many months in sanatoria, the risk of infection in the community must have been, to some extent, curtailed.

Limitations of anti-tuberculosis therapy

Deaths from bacillary tuberculosis continue to occur in spite of the so-called '100 per cent successful chemotherapy' available in all European countries from the late 1950s or early 1960s. Nowadays there is evidence that the results of chemotherapy, under routine conditions, in many countries are nearly as good as those obtained in controlled clinical trials (Heffernan et al. 1976; van Geuns et al. 1984; Blaha et al. 1988).

Much research into modern short-course chemotherapy for pulmonary bacillary tuberculosis has been conducted since the late 1960s and was reviewed by Fox (1980). There are now a number of short-course regimens of 6–9 months' duration that are highly effective, of low toxicity, and well tolerated (Fox 1981). These potent regimens are based on an initial intensive phase of isoniazid, rifampicin, and pyrazinamide supplemented by a fourth drug (streptomycin or ethambutol). There is a choice between 6-month regimens with rifampicin throughout or cheaper regimens lasting 8–9 months with the four drugs given in an initial phase, followed by a less costly continuation phase. In spite of these comparatively short regimens, compliance can be a problem, particularly when the disease occurs among disaffected groups within the population.

Unfortunately, death from tuberculosis is not a rare event, even in newly diagnosed cases. Heffernan et al. (1976) reported 15 (2 per cent) deaths from tuberculosis among 770 patients with pulmonary tuberculosis within 2 years of the start of chemotherapy. The number of deaths from tuberculosis among the 372 patients with bacillary pulmonary tuberculosis and the 398 patients with culture-negative tuberculosis are not given in the report, making comparisons with other studies difficult. Humphries et al. (1984) have analysed Medical Research Council data on notifications in England and Wales covering 6 months (from October 1978 to March 1979) and noted that 12 per cent of 1312 adult patients died before chemotherapy was completed, approximately half of them from tuberculosis. In Bavaria (Blaha et al. 1988), 197 (3.7 per cent) of 5157 diagnosed bacillary pulmonary tuberculosis cases in 1975–76 were reported as having died from tuberculosis during the first 2 years after diagnosis. In a further 73 (1.4 per cent) patients who died during the first 2 years after diagnosis, 'sequelae of tuberculosis' were given on death certificates as the cause of death. It is probable that this group included a number of patients who died from tuberculosis rather than tuberculosis sequelae. In the Netherlands in 1975–81 (van Geuns et al. 1984), the death rate from tuberculosis during the first 2 years after diagnosis was low, namely 1.5 per cent. However, it cannot be excluded that a small number of newly detected patients who died within the first few days after diagnosis were registered under 'death from tuberculosis', but not under 'incidence'. In some patients the cause of death was unknown and it is possible that a few of them died from tuberculosis. The fatality rate increased to 3.8 per cent in 1981–84 (data not yet published).

Primary and post-primary tuberculosis

It is known that the risk of developing clinical tuberculosis as a result of tuberculous infection is greater for subjects recently infected than for those infected in the past. Primary tuberculosis describes disease occurring soon after infection with the bacillus. Post-primary tuberculosis describes the occurrence of clinical disease in individuals whose primary infection was some time in the past.

Primary tuberculosis

When the risk of infection is high—as it was in Europe before the Second World War and still is in many developing countries—primary tuberculosis occurs mostly among children. When the risk of infection is low, primary tuberculosis also occurs, at a low rate, among young persons and adults. When the risk of infection becomes very low, as is the case now in many countries of Western Europe, an increasing number of old people remain uninfected earlier in life and primary infection will also occur at a very low rate in the elderly.

Post-primary tuberculosis

There are two possible explanations for the development of this stage of the disease. The first is that it results from tubercle bacilli acquired by primary infection, which remained viable but dormant in diseased areas (foci) produced shortly after primary infection. The acquired immune response will inhibit the multiplication of the tubercle bacilli, but will not confer on the cells the capacity for destruction of all the tubercle bacilli (Youmans 1979). Therefore, tubercle bacilli within macrophages located in small tubercles in a lymph node, for example, or in the lung, may be held in check for long periods, but are perfectly capable of metabolizing and dividing again if local immunity is lowered (*endogenous reactivation*). The present very low risk of primary tuberculous infection in a number of developed countries enables us to measure the rate of endogenous exacerbation, provided that the tuberculin status of the population is known before the development of bacillary tuberculosis (Styblo 1984). It is probable that approximately 10–15 subjects per 100 000 persons with a remote tuberculous infection will continue to develop bacillary pulmonary tuberculosis per year as a result of endogenous exacerbation.

The second explanation is that it develops because of reinfection with virulent tubercle bacilli in subjects who had primary infection several years before (*exogenous reinfection*). Since reinfection with virulent tubercle bacilli in Europe is low or very low and has been decreasing constantly, its role can be virtually disregarded in the elimination and eradication phases of tuberculosis.

Transmission characteristics

Several studies (Shaw and Wynn-Williams 1954; Hertzberg 1957; Grzybowski and Allen 1964; Grzybowski et al. 1975; van Geuns et al. 1975a; Rouillon et al. 1976) among close contacts of tuberculous patients show that patients in whom bacilli can be found by microscopic examination of the sputum (smear-positive) play the greatest role in the spread of infection. In contrast, those patients in whom the presence of tubercle bacilli in the sputum can be demonstrated by culture only, or who are culture-negative, play a lesser role in the transmission of infection. In the Netherlands (van Geuns et al. 1975a), the prevalence of positive infection, defined as reaction to the tuberculin test, was high among household contacts of smear-positive index cases: 50 per cent of such contacts aged 0–14 years were found to be infected, as compared with 1 per cent of the same age group among the general population. Notably, the prevalence of infection was about 6 per cent in child contacts of culture-positive and culture-negative index cases.

Since few children with primary tuberculosis develop bacillary tuberculosis before the age of puberty and even fewer children develop smear-positive tuberculosis, the infectivity of tuberculosis is also related to the age at which primary infection occurs. The proportion of smear-positive primary tuberculosis cases increases sharply (to about 25 per cent) in those who contracted primary infection at 15–29 years of age, but, even in this age group, smear-negative cases form three-quarters of all clinical tuberculosis cases (Barnett and Styblo 1977). The chest X-ray appearance of primary tuberculosis in adults differs from the primary complex seen in children (Malmros and Hedvall 1938; Barnett and Styblo 1977). Very little is known about symptoms, X-ray appearance, and bacteriological status in those who contract primary infection after about 50 years of age, but one can assume that a proportion of cases with primary disease is smear-positive.

It is estimated that one unknown smear-positive case of pulmonary tuberculosis infects, on average, 10 persons with tubercle bacilli during a year (Styblo 1980). Since the patient's[1] and doctor's delay[2] in diagnosing smear-positive cases in the Netherlands is about 2.5 months (Baas et al. 1982), one open case may infect 2–3 people before being identified. This agrees with the observation made in the United States (Johnston and Wildrik 1974) where it

---

[1] Patient's delay:interval (in months) between the appearance of the first symptoms referable to tuberculous disease and the first visit of the patient to a health service.

[2] Doctor's delay:interval (in months) between the first visit of the patient to a health service and diagnosis of tuberculosis.

was estimated that an open case infects, on average, 2–3 people. One of the major aims of the study of transmission of tubercle bacilli is to estimate the annual risk of tuberculous infection and its trend in the community.

Annual risk of tuberculosis infection and its trend

The annual average risk of tuberculosis infection (referred to hereafter as risk of infection) indicates what proportion of the population will be infected (whether primarily infected or reinfected) with tubercle bacilli in the course of 1 year. It is usually expressed as a rate.

The risk or rate of infection is derived from the results of tuberculin testing. Techniques for converting information on prevalence of infection into a smooth series of annual rates of incidence of infection have been described by Styblo *et al.* (1969), Sutherland (1976), and Sutherland *et al.* (1984a). To obtain a reliable estimate of the risk of infection and its changes over a given period of time, several tuberculin surveys are required at certain intervals. Provided that non-BCG-vaccinated subjects are representative of the general population, each survey should take a representative sample of non-BCG-vaccinated subjects of the same age, and test them by the same technique. For routine evaluation of a tuberculosis control programme, a simple method of estimating the risk of infection and its trend has been described by Bleiker (1974).

Size of the problem and trends

There is reliable evidence that, irrespective of its magnitude, the tuberculosis problem in Europe and other developed countries has been decreasing since at least the turn of this century. Between the two World Wars, tuberculosis mortality in most developed countries showed an annual decrease ranging from 3 to 5 per cent.

In some developed countries tuberculosis probably started to decline in the nineteenth century or even earlier. Figure 6.1 shows tuberculosis mortality rates in children aged 0–4 years in England and Wales between 1851 and 1940. Nearly 600 per 100 000 children of that age died annually from tuberculosis in the 1850s. It took some 55 years to reduce this mortality by 50 per cent. The decrease was much steeper between 1905 and 1940, in spite of the First World War and the serious economic depression in the late 1920s and early 1930s.

It is therefore likely that tuberculosis would eventually be eliminated in Europe even without the introduction of anti-tuberculous chemotherapy, provided that control measures applied at that time continued and that socioeconomic conditions did not deteriorate. The total elimination of tuberculosis would, however, take longer.

The secular trend for incidence of and mortality from tuberculosis, and

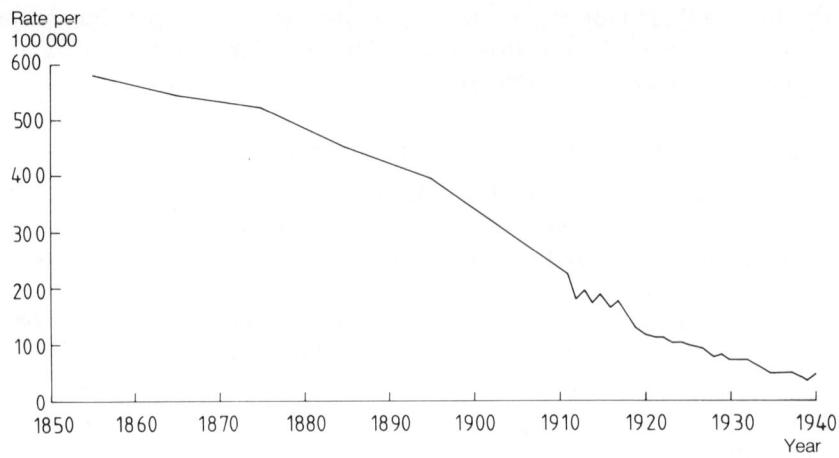

Fig. 6.1 Rates (per 100 000) of mortality from tuberculosis in England and Wales in children aged 0–4 years, 1851–1940. (From Styblo 1986.)

changes in the pattern of risk of infection are described below in some detail for the Netherlands. Similar patterns and trends may be forecast in all other European countries.

Figure 6.2 shows that there was a close relationship, in the pre-chemotherapy era, between the risk of infection and mortality from tuberculosis. This Figure suggests that there was no interruption in the steady decrease in the risk of infection, at least since 1910, not even during the Second World War, in spite of the steep increase in tuberculosis mortality and morbidity during that period (for possible reasons see Styblo *et al.* 1969). There was no close relationship between the risk of infection and the incidence of tuberculosis in all forms reported from 1959 to 1983. The levelling of the incidence curve from the 1950s onwards is predominantly the result of the endogenous exacerbation of tuberculosis, particularly among the elderly. On the other hand, there was a correlation between the risk of infection and the incidence of tuberculosis in children and young adults which was caused by primary infection (Figure 6.3).

The tremendous fall in the risk of infection in the Netherlands during the last 75 years is seen in Table 6.1. This table shows that the proportion of the population infected annually decreased from 11 310 per 100 000 in 1910 to 3920 in 1930, to 530 in 1950, to 12 in 1985, or by 99.9 per cent during the last 75 years.

It is obvious that such a momentous decrease resulted in profound changes in the prevalence of infection in the population. The estimates of prevalence of tuberculous infection in the cohorts born in the year 1910 and, subsequently at 10-year intervals, for those aged 5, 10, 20. . .80 years are given in

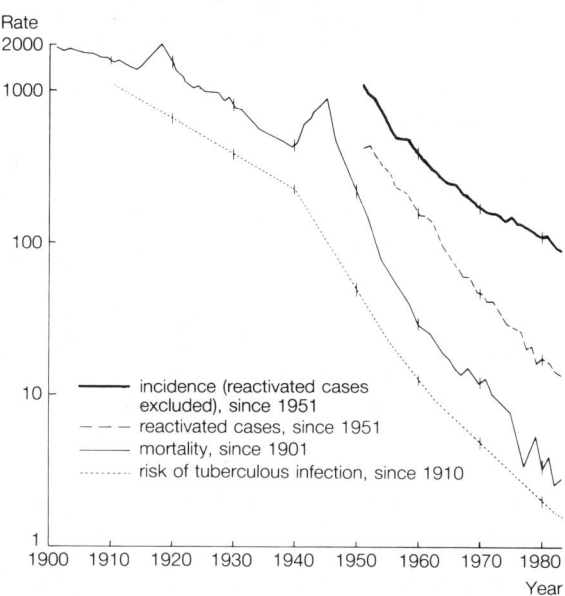

Fig. 6.2 Tuberculosis incidence, reactivation, and death rates (per 1 000 000), and the average annual risk of tuberculous infection (per 10 000) in the Netherlands 1901–83. (From Styblo 1986.)

Figure 6.4. For the individual cohorts each curve follows a similar pattern in that it rises steeply during childhood, continues to rise—though less markedly—during adolescence, and after about 25 years of age becomes nearly level. (It should be noted that a log scale is used for this Figure.) However, prevalence at individual ages has changed dramatically during the last 75 years. For example, the prevalence of infection at age 20 years, nearing 77 per cent for the cohort born in 1910, had already fallen to 1 per cent in 1980 for the cohort born in 1960 and has recently decreased to about 0.7 per cent for the 1965 cohort.

Figure 6.4 also shows estimated prevalence rates of tuberculous infection and their trends for those aged 5, 10, 20, 30. . .80 years for the period 1910 to 2005. At present, the prevalence of infection is very low in children, in subjects aged 20 years (about 0.7 per cent), and in those aged 30 years (about 2.4 per cent), and is also quite low for those aged 40 years (approximately 7.5 per cent) and 50 years (about 24 per cent). However, for those aged 60 years the rate remained unchanged at about 99 per cent until approximately 1970, when the turning point for this age group was reached; the present proportion of infected is about 49 per cent. For those aged 70 years, the turning point was reached in 1978 when their prevalence rates began to decrease from about 99

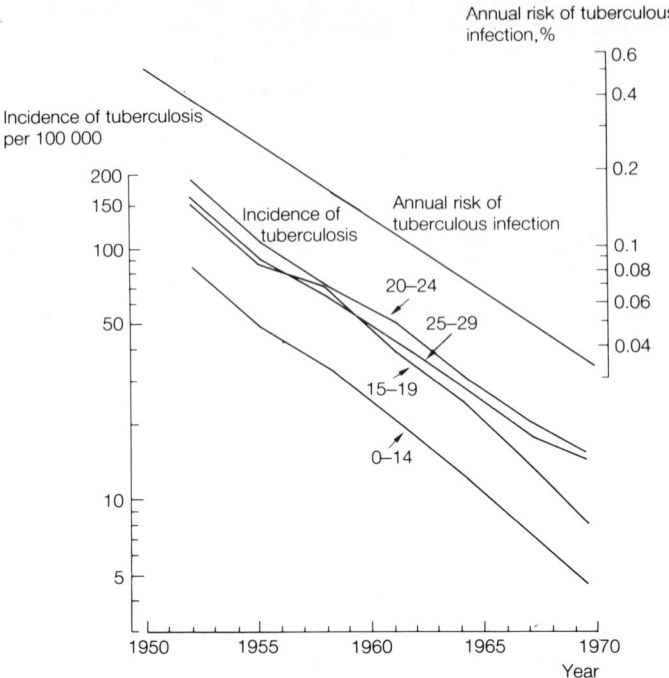

Fig. 6.3 Annual risks of tuberculous infection and incidence of new, active tuberculosis in subjects aged 0–14, 15–19, 20–24, and 25–29 years of age in the Netherlands, 1952–70. (From Styblo 1986.)

Table 6.1 Estimated number of persons infected annually with tubercle bacilli in the Netherlands 1910–85.

Year	Estimated number of persons infected annually (per 100 000)
1910	11 310
1920	6 690
1930	3 920
1940	2 080
1950	530
1960	171
1970	58
1980	21
1985	12

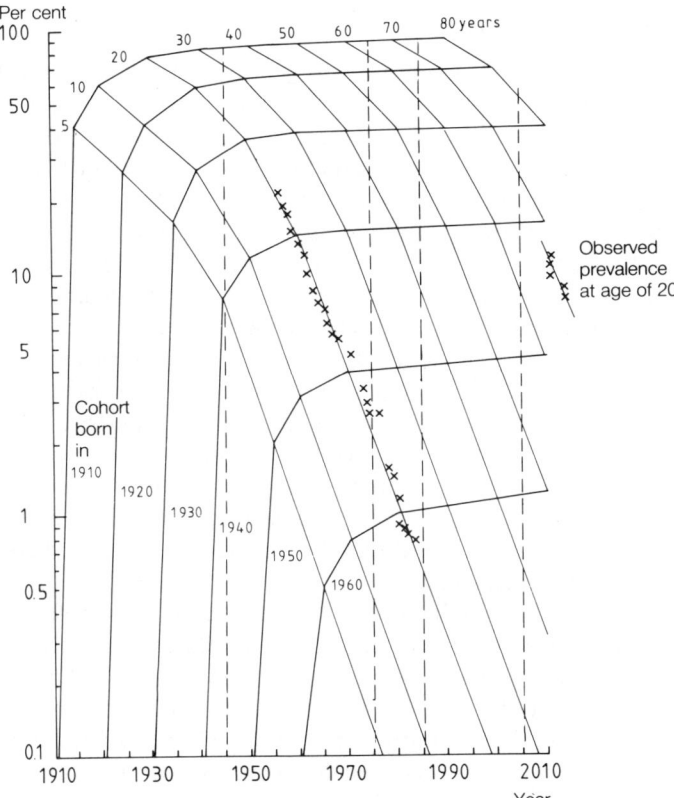

Fig. 6.4 Estimated percentage prevalence of tuberculous infection in cohorts born from 1910 to 1960 in 1945, 1975, 1985, and 2005 in the Netherlands. (From Styblo 1986.)

per cent (the present rate is about 74 per cent). It will take another 20 years for it to fall to about 24 per cent. Finally, in those aged 80 years the prevalence rate will remain high (more than 90 per cent) until about 1990.

It is thus clear that there will still be patients with bacillary tuberculosis resulting from endogenous exacerbation for many years to come and deaths may occasionally occur. Nevertheless the disease will be eliminated from most of Europe in the first half of the next century.

Nature and efficacy of interventions

There are two distinct approaches in the fight against tuberculosis, namely the complex of case-finding and treatment, and the preventive measures (BCG vaccination and chemoprophylaxis).

Case-finding and chemotherapy

Styblo (1984) suggests that, in developed countries, the 8 per cent difference between the present decrease in the risk of infection (12–13 per cent annually), and the natural downward trend for the disease in those countries before chemotherapy (4–5 per cent annually) is a result of intensive case-finding and adequate chemotherapy of all diagnosed bacillary cases. It must be stressed, however, that the magnitude of the decrease of the annual risk of tuberculous infection has a very limited effect on the elimination and eradication of tuberculosis in Europe. The decisive factor in these phases is the proportion of the population infected in the past who continue to give rise to most bacillary cases at present and in future. Therefore the prime aim of early diagnosis of tuberculosis in Europe is to reduce human suffering in patients and their contacts. Unfortunately, we do not succeed in performing this task in all patients who develop tuberculosis, even in countries with the most sophisticated health service structures. In a proportion of those who suffer from tuberculosis, the disease is not diagnosed until after death. The figure varies in developed countries and may be on average 3 to 5 per cent of the total incidence of tuberculosis.

It is useful for differential diagnosis to introduce the Mantoux test into the daily work of some hospital departments and other health services. The testing and reading techniques should conform to those described by the World Health Organization (1963). In the few developed countries not using mass BCG vaccination, nearly all children, more than 98 per cent of young adults, more than 90 per cent of subjects aged 40 years, 75 per cent of those aged 50 years, and more than 50 per cent of those aged 60 years are at present tuberculin-negative (non-infected). As shown in Table 6.2, the proportion of non-infected subjects in the Netherlands will rapidly increase in the near future and will soon extend to old people. The prevalence of tuberculin reactors may be higher in countries which use BCG effectively and widely, but a similar overall decline in the proportion of reactors is to be expected.

It is obvious that indiscriminate mass miniature radiography has no place in any tuberculosis control programme and surveillance must be applied selectively to groups considered to be at high risk. There are three main high-risk categories. The first consists of contacts, and contact examination will remain an important measure in all countries until tuberculosis is eradicated. The second group includes newly arrived immigrants and refugees from high-prevalence countries. Newly arrived immigrants from high-prevalence countries continue to have a high incidence of tuberculosis for the first 5 years or so. Afterwards there is a decrease in tuberculosis incidence in the host country, the result of a substantial decrease in the risk of infection. Many European countries, therefore, keep newly arrived immigrants under public health surveillance for tuberculosis for about 5 years. The third high-risk

Table 6.2 Estimated prevalence of tuberculous infection, by age group, in the Netherlands.

Age	1945			1985			2005			2025		
	1	2	3	1[a]	2	3	1[b]	2	3	1[c]	2	3
0–14	27.8	11.0	3.0	20.9	0.1	—	18	0.0	—	18	—	—
15–24	17.4	44.7	7.8	17.4	0.8	0.1	14	0.1	—	12	—	—
25–34	15.1	72.0	10.9	16.3	2.4	0.4	12	0.3	—	13	—	—
35–44	13.3	90.8	12.1	13.6	7.5	1.0	14	0.9	0.1	12	0.1	—
45–54	10.8	97.2	10.5	10.6	24.2	2.6	15	2.5	0.4	14	0.3	—
55–64	8.0	99.2	7.9	9.4	48.9	4.6	13	7.6	1.0	14	0.9	0.1
65–74	5.4	99.5	5.3	7.0	74.1	5.2	8	24.2	1.9	11	2.5	0.3
75	2.2	99.7	2.2	4.8	91.5	4.4	6	48.9	2.9	6	7.6	0.5
Total	100		59.7	100		18.3	100		6.3	100		0.9

1 = percentages of the general population in the given age groups.
2 = estimated per cent prevalence of tuberculous infection in age groups 0–14 years, 15–24 years, 25–34 years . . .
3 = estimated percentage of the total population infected with tubercle bacilli, by age group.
[a]based on 1983 census.
[b]based on estimated population for 2010.
[c]based on estimated population for 2020.

group includes people with inactive tuberculosis (ex-patients) and those with fibrotic lesions who in many developed countries had and continue to have repeated routine chest X-ray and culture examinations. However, Styblo *et al.* (1984) showed that in tuberculosis clinics in Holland the yield of these control examinations was not of sufficient clinical value to justify the cost and the inconvenience to the patient. This conclusion may not apply to other populations.

Other high-risk groups include deprived inner city populations in overcrowded housing, homeless indigents, alcoholics, drug addicts, and gypsies. These exist to varying extent in different countries.

There should be no major problems connected with tuberculosis chemotherapy in developed countries in the future. However, as the disease becomes progressively more rare, so too will the medical expertise required to prescribe appropriate treatment. Hence case-finding and diagnosis of the continuously falling number of new cases of tuberculosis will remain the most difficult problems until the disease has been eradicated.

Preventive measures

In European countries, anti-tuberculosis preventive measures (BCG vaccination and chemoprophylaxis) will have limited scope in future.

Mass BCG vaccination

BCG protects against the consequences of primary infection rather than preventing infection *per se*. It has been shown that mass BCG vaccination cannot therefore, substantially influence the chain of transmission (Styblo and Meijer 1976). It has, however, considerably reduced the incidence of clinical tuberculosis in children and young adults in those European countries where it was adequately applied.

Waaler and Rouillon (1974) have dealt in detail with the problem of the present and future place of BCG vaccination in low-prevalence countries. They have analysed the three aspects of a BCG programme: epidemiological, economic, and psychological (the worry created by immunization or by the consequence of the absence of immunization). It goes without saying that they could not give a conclusive answer to the question of when to stop systematic BCG vaccination in countries where it is now applied. In European countries, the suffering and psychological aspects are most relevant to the decision as to when to stop. There is no doubt that the final decision on when to discontinue mass BCG vaccination is political, but as Waaler and Rouillon stress, decision-making should be based on the three essential elements mentioned above.

In Europe, Sweden abandoned BCG vaccination at birth in 1975; it had been introduced there in the 1940s and covered at least 95 per cent of all newborn infants. The main reason for stopping routine BCG immunization was the high incidence of BCG osteitis observed in children born and immunized in or after 1972. It is suggested that its reintroduction would not be appropriate (Romanus 1983). It is inevitable that, in Europe, the time will come when mass BCG immunization will have to cease because, quite apart from economic considerations, the complications it causes (suppurative lymphadenitis, osteitis, lupus vulgaris, 'BCG-itis') will outweigh the benefits obtained. Instead, selective BCG vaccination should be applied in community groups with a high risk of tuberculous infection—for instance, in foreign residents coming from high-prevalence countries. In most European countries with no mass BCG vaccination policy, BCG is given to tuberculin-negative health service employees.

Chemoprophylaxis

Chemoprophylaxis is applied either to freshly infected, so-called tuberculin converters, or to those who have been infected with virulent tubercle bacilli in the past with or without radiological abnormalities in the lungs.

The tuberculin converters undoubtedly represent a very rewarding group in terms of chemoprophylaxis results, and the chemoprophylaxis policy has been adopted as a routine procedure in a number of low-prevalence countries. However, mass chemoprophylaxis of converters is impossible since their identification depends on repeated tuberculin testing. It would be unrealistic to attempt to find converters among the general population of a European country where as many as three-quarters or more are, at present, tuberculin-negative and risks of infection are so small. Through annual school tuberculin surveys, only 22 per cent of all tuberculin-converters in the population could be identified (van Geuns et al. 1975b). On the other hand, a selective search for converters in high-risk groups, such as close family contacts of smear-positive sources, remains fully justified.

Chemoprophylaxis in tuberculin-positive subjects in a developed country would reduce, theoretically, the number of sources of infection. But this reduced incidence would have little, if any, impact on the time needed for eliminating tuberculosis in the population, because the present risk of tuberculous infection is extremely low. It would, however, still alleviate human suffering.

Chemoprophylaxis has never been extensively practised in Europe (Horne 1985). On the other hand, it is considered an important tool in tuberculosis control and surveillance in the United States and Canada (National Consensus Conference on Tuberculosis 1985).

Feasibility of tuberculosis elimination

The conventional definition of tuberculosis elimination is when the number of new sputum-positive cases drops to 1 per million population per year. Reliable information on two specific conditions is necessary to estimate when the elimination of tuberculosis will be achieved in a country—(1) the prevalence of tuberculous infection, by age groups, in the past and in several decades to come; (2) the rate of breakdown to smear-positive tuberculosis in subjects infected in the remote past with tubercle bacilli. With this information, it is easy to estimate when the target of one new case of sputum-positive tuberculosis per million population per year will be reached. Moreover, information on the first condition will also indicate when the proportion of the general population infected with tubercle bacillus will fall to less than 1 per cent.

Estimates of prevalence of tuberculosis infection in the Netherlands

These estimates are based on the risks of tuberculous infection in the Netherlands for the period 1910–79 (Styblo et al. 1969; Sutherland et al. 1984a). The

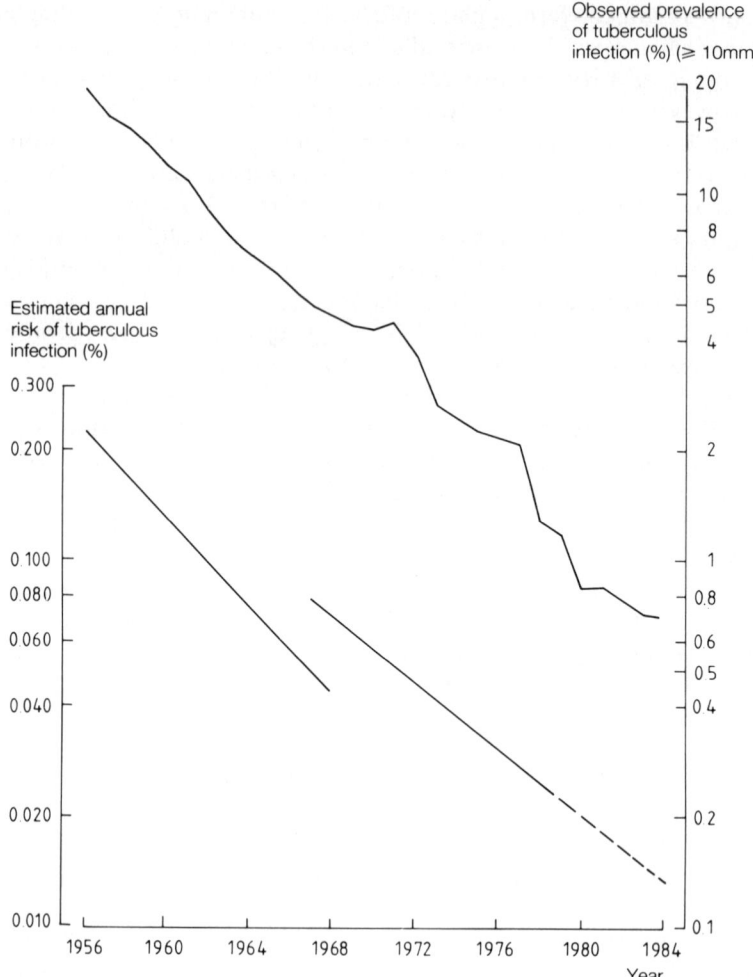

Fig. 6.5 Prevalence of tuberculosis in unimmunized recruits aged 20 years, and the estimated annual risk of infection in the Netherlands 1956–84. (From Styblo 1986.) Number of recruits tested annually: 37 376–45 896.

prevalence data on recruits and the risk of tuberculous infection for the period 1956–84 are given in Figure 6.5. The estimated and observed prevalence rates of tuberculous infection for recruits during 1956–79 are very similar (Figure 6.4).

Table 6.2 shows estimates of the proportions of infected subjects in the Netherlands, by age groups, for the years 1945, 1985, 2005, and 2025. In 1945, 59.7 per cent of the Dutch population (total population 8.1 million) were infected with tubercle bacilli. By 1985 (total population 14.5 million) there had been a very marked decrease in the prevalence of infection in subjects below 45 years, and a distinct decrease in those aged 45 to 64 years. It is projected that the proportion of infected will decrease to 6.3 per cent in 2005 and to 0.9 per cent in 2025.

Rate of endogenous exacerbation

The present very low risk of tuberculous infection in a number of developed countries enables us to measure the effect of endogenous exacerbation, provided that the tuberculin status of the population is known before the development of bacillary pulmonary tuberculosis. Since development of disease caused by reinfection can be practically excluded, most of the cases observed must be the result of endogenous exacerbation.

The annual rate of breakdown resulting from endogenous exacerbation is approximately 12 to 15 cases of bacillary pulmonary tuberculosis per 100 000 previously infected, about half of whom are sputum-positive (Styblo 1986).

In the Netherlands, the estimated prevalence of tuberculosis infection will be 0.9 per cent in the year 2025 (Table 6.2). Thus, given the breakdown rate above, by the year 2025 the expected incidence of smear-positive pulmonary tuberculosis will be less than 1 per million—the conventional limit proposed for tuberculosis elimination.

Problems in maximizing population effectiveness

Horne (1985) has recently pointed out that 'forecasts that tuberculosis would disappear within a generation have been made for nearly a century, but it seems likely that several more generations will come and go before eradication is achieved'. He adhered to the conventional limit suggested for eradication, namely less than one new case of sputum-positive tuberculosis per million population per year. In this context, he also arrived at an estimate according to which some countries would reach this target in 40–50 years—that is, during the period 2025–35.

The most formidable obstacle to eliminating tuberculosis in low-prevalence countries is the population previously infected with the tubercle bacillus, particularly among the elderly. They continue to be the main source of the infectious disease caused by endogenous exacerbation, even if the community is virtually cleared of tuberculous infection. Preventive therapy may seem the obvious solution, but there are serious problems with this. First, the difficulty and cost of identification of reactors will greatly increase as their prevalence further decreases. Second, isoniazid prophylaxis can pose problems in general usage among older adults. In spite of recent improvements in therapy for this group, routine treatment of all reactors may not be acceptable.

Figures 6.4 and 6.6 and Table 6.1 show that the spectacular change in the risk of infection in the Netherlands during the last 75 years (particularly during the last four decades) resulted in profound changes in the prevalence of infection not only in children and adolescents but also in adults. However, the level and trend of the risk of tuberculous infection, even if observed for several decades, cannot in themselves give an answer as to when tuberculosis will be eliminated in a given country. In very low-prevalence countries, it is observed already that the incidence rate of infectious tuberculous disease in the elderly is higher than the annual rate of tuberculous infection.

Other causes of delay in elimination

There are two other main factors which could delay the elimination of tuberculosis in Europe. These are continued immigration from high-incidence areas and delay in diagnosis.

Immigration from high incidence areas

In a number of developed countries, continued migration from high-incidence areas has had a substantial effect on slowing the downward trend in national tuberculosis notification rates (Sutherland *et al.* 1984b). Since immigrants were mostly young labourers or young couples, the rates in the host country were particularly inflated in young adults and children (Baas *et al.* 1982; Nunn *et al.* 1984).

The effects of immigration from high-incidence areas are mainly dependent on the extent of the immigration, whether or not it continues, the age and sex of immigrants, and the environment in the country of origin. In several Western European countries with recent immigration from high-prevalence countries, the proportion of immigrants is at present around 3 per cent. Most immigrants are young male labourers who came in the 1960s and 1970s. With the economic recession in the late 1970s, immigration of foreign workers was considerably restricted, but wives and children have joined their husbands and fathers over the last 10 years.

On the other hand the trend of the risk of tuberculous infection was little influenced by the wave of immigrants in the Netherlands and Britain (Nunn *et al.* 1984; Sutherland *et al.* 1984a, b). The prevalence of infection referred to in Table 6.2 would be slightly increased by the infection prevalence that the foreign population acquired in their native countries before immigration.

Fig. 6.6 Estimated prevalence per 100 000 of tuberculous infection at ages 3, 23, 43, 63, and 83 years, and estimated incidence per 100 000 of primary infection and reinfection in the Netherlands 1910–2000. (From Styblo 1986.)

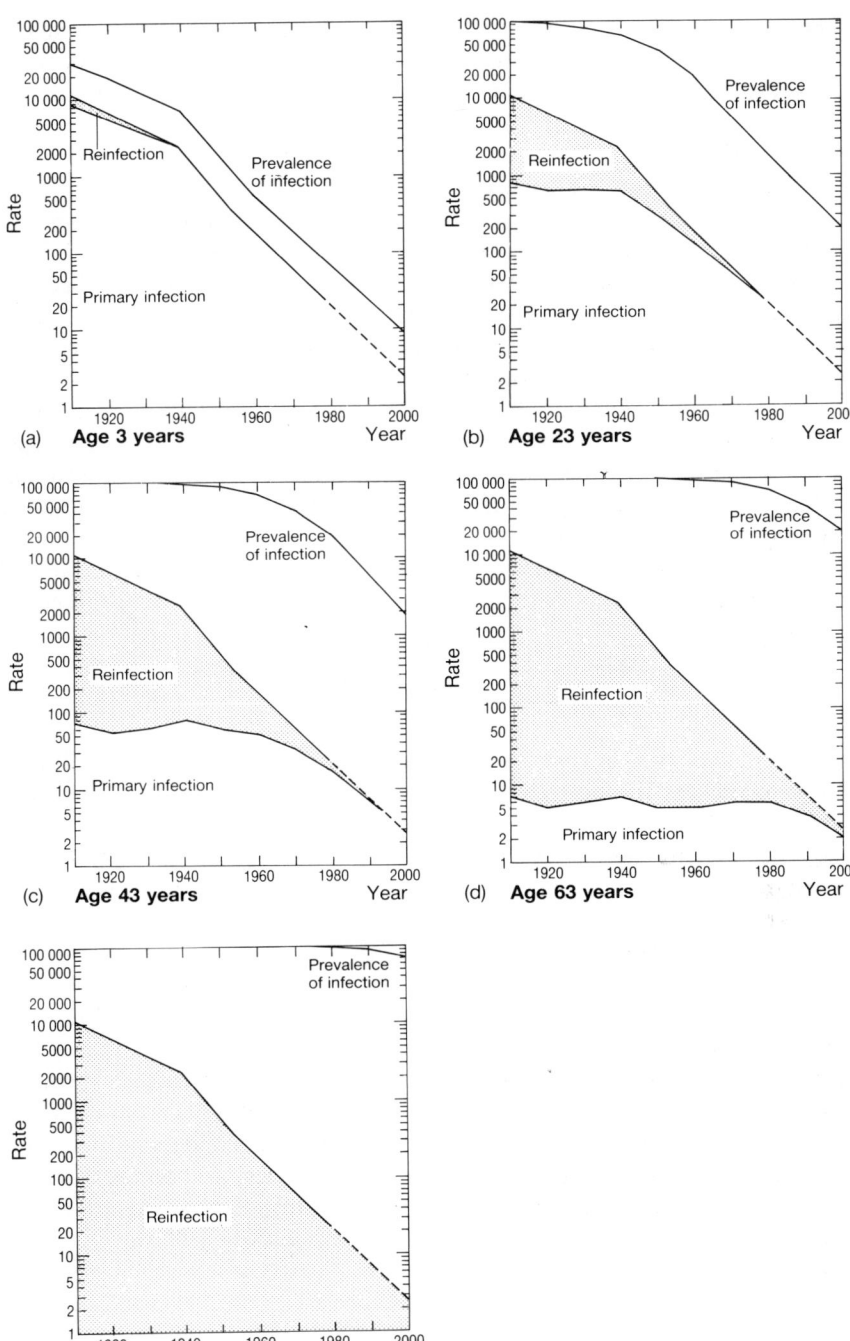

Tuberculosis elimination might thus be delayed, but only for a few years.

If extensive immigration from high-prevalence countries were to continue for several years, this might delay tuberculosis elimination for longer.

Diagnostic delay

As the prevalence of the tubercle bacillus in our environment has been diminishing and will continue to do so in future, tuberculous infection and disease will become distinctly localized. Patients will remain the focal point from which to start case-finding. They will not 'forget' their disease because most serious forms of tuberculosis cause distressing symptoms. Some patients who will have developed tuberculosis may for various reasons postpone a visit to the doctor, but the progressing disease will soon force most of them to seek medical advice. There is no reason to assume that the proportion of persons suffering from symptoms caused by tuberculosis, and who seek medical advice too late (or not at all), will substantially increase in future as the disease becomes infrequent and ultimately rare. However, it cannot be excluded that, because the disease will become increasingly unfamiliar to doctors themselves, the proportion of cases diagnosed late or not at all will increase in future.

Recommendations

It is evident that even in very low-prevalence countries tuberculosis will continue to occur for the next three to four decades. The disease is now seen infrequently by general practitioners in Europe, and will soon become rare. A steady decrease in tuberculosis will result in a readjustment of tuberculosis control programmes in Europe during the elimination and eradication phases of the disease.

Preventive measures, particularly BCG vaccination, will be greatly reduced in countries where they are still carried out on a mass scale. In countries with a mass BCG programme of newborn children or school-leavers, BCG vaccination will be limited to high-risk groups in the 1990s since there will be no justification for its indiscriminate use, with very few exceptions.

In some countries surveillance of immigrants and refugees from high-prevalence countries might be necessary for several decades, depending on the success of tuberculosis control in developing countries, and on the influx of immigrants from high-prevalence countries to Europe.

Future control programmes among native populations will mostly consist of diagnosis of tuberculosis (and notification of active disease to the Ministry of Health), contact examination around index cases, and chemotherapy of active cases of tuberculosis. Chemoprophylaxis will be given to a small number of identified converters.

There is no doubt that diagnosis of the decreasing number of new cases of tuberculosis in developed countries is and will remain the most difficult problem in the future, in spite of the sophisticated health facilities available to the whole population. One reason is that the public has lost interest in tuberculosis and another is that physicians are 'forgetting' the disease in daily practice because they so seldom see it. Furthermore, in some patients, early symptoms are neither serious enough to make the physician think of tuberculosis, nor typical of tuberculosis, particularly among the elderly.

On the other hand, no major problems are to be expected with tuberculosis chemotherapy in developed countries in the elimination phase of the disease. It is improbable that the elimination of tuberculosis in Europe will be delayed by AIDS. The reason is that the European population up to the age of about 40–45 years are or will very soon become virtually free of tuberculous infection and therefore few future AIDS patients should be at risk of developing the endogenous type of tuberculosis.

Appendix

Glossary

Case-finding is an essential component of the control of tuberculosis and most other communicable diseases. Its object is to identify the sources of infection in a community—for example, in the case of tuberculosis, to find persons who are discharging tubercle bacilli. By rendering them non-infectious through chemotherapy, the chain of transmission of tubercle bacilli from man-to-man is cut.

Chronic excretor of tubercle bacilli—a patient who has been excreting tubercle bacilli for more than 2 years.

Incidence—indicates the number of new cases of tuberculosis which develop within a specified period of time, usually 1 year. It is usually expressed as a rate per 100 000 general population. The incidence should be given separately for patients excreting tubercle bacilli demonstrable by direct smear examination; those excreting tubercle bacilli demonstrable by culture only; culture-negative cases of pulmonary tuberculosis, and extra-pulmonary tuberculosis.

Prevalence—tuberculosis prevalence gives the number of cases of tuberculosis present in a defined population at a particular date per 100 000 general population ('point prevalence').

Reactivation (relapse)—tuberculosis reactivation indicates recurrence of the disease after it has been considered cured. Bacteriologically confirmed reactivations belong to the influx of 'new' sources of infection and should be reported separately among the 'newly reported' cases.

Tuberculin survey—a study in which a group of individuals is tested with tuberculin with a view to measuring the prevalence (see above) of infection with *Mycobacterium tuberculosis* or *Mycobacterium bovis*. To perform the tuberculin test, an intradermal injection of 0.1 ml tuberculin (purified protein derivative = PPD) is given in the forearm. Three days later, the reaction (an induration at the injection site), if present, is measured. A person is considered to have been infected in the past when the diameter of the induration measures 10 mm or more. Non-BCG-vaccinated children, usually of school age, are studied in a tuberculin survey. Based on the prevalence of infection the risk of infection with *Mycobacterium tuberculosis* can thus be estimated.

References

Baas, M.A., Geuns, H.A. van, Hellinga, H.S., Meijer, J., and Styblo, K. (1982). Surveillance of diagnostic and treatment measures of bacillary pulmonary tuberculosis reported in the Netherlands from 1973 to 1976. *Selected Papers* 21, 41–80 (K.N.C.V., P.O. Box 146, The Hague, Netherlands).

Barnett, G.D. and Styblo, K. (1977). Bacteriological and X-ray status of tuberculosis following primary infection acquired during adolescence or later. *Bull. Int. Un. Tuberc.* 52, 5–16.

Blaha, H., Heilig, B., Schreiber, M.A., and Styblo, K. (1988). Surveillance of diagnostic and treatment measures, Bavaria, 1974–1976. Results 2 and 5 years after the start of chemotherapy. *Tubercle*. In press.

Bleiker, M.A. (1974). Epidemiological trends in low prevalence countries. *Bull. Int. Un. Tuberc.* 49, 128–135.

Fox, W. (1980). Short-course chemotherapy for tuberculosis. In *Recent advances in respiratory medicine* (ed. Flenley). Churchill Livingstone, Edinburgh, London, Melbourne, and New York.

—— (1981). Whither short-course chemotherapy? *Br. J. Dis. Chest* 75, 331–357.

Geuns, H.A. van, Meijer, J., and Styblo, K. (1975a). Results of contact examination in Rotterdam, 1967–1969. *Bull. Int. Un. Tuberc.* 50, 107–121.

——, ——, —— (1975b). The yield from tuberculin testing on unvaccinated children and adolescents. *Bull. Intl. Un. Tuberc.* 50, 82–89.

——, Bleiker, M.A., Hellinga, H.S., and Styblo, K. (1984). Surveillance of diagnostic and treatment measures in the Netherlands. Comparison between the periods 1973–1976, 1977–1980 and 1981. *Bull. Intl. Un. Tuberc.* 59, 134–137.

Grzybowski, S. and Allen, E.A. (1964). The challenge of tuberculosis in decline. A study based on the epidemiology of tuberculosis in Ontario, Canada. *Am. Rev. Resp. Dis.* 90, 707–720.

——, Barnett, G.D., and Styblo, K. (1975). Contacts of cases of active pulmonary tuberculosis. *Bull. Int. Un. Tuberc.* 50, 90–196.

Heffernan, J.F., Nunn, A.J., Peto, J., and Fox, F. (1976). Tuberculosis in Scotland: a national sample survey (1968-1970). 2. A two-year follow-up of newly diagnosed respiratory tuberculosis notified in 1968. *Tubercle* **57**, 161-175.

Hertzberg, G. (1957). *The infectiousness of human tuberculosis* pp. 57-89. Munksgaard, Copenhagen.

Horne, N.W. (1985) Eradication of tuberculosis in Europe—so near and yet so far. *Bull. Int. Un. Tuberc.* **59**, 107-209.

Humphries, M.J., Byfield, S.P., Darbyshire, Janet, H., Davies, P.D.O., Nunn, A.J., Citron, K.M., and Fox, W. (1984). Deaths occurring in newly notified patients with pulmonary tuberculosis in England and Wales. *Br. J. Dis. Chest* **78**, 149-158.

Johnston, R.F. and Wildrik, H.K. (1974). "State of Art" Review. The impact of chemotherapy on the care of patients with tuberculosis. *Am. Rev. Resp. Dis.* **109**, 636-664.

Malmros, H. and Hedvall, E. (1938). *Studien uber die Entstehung und Entwicklung der Lungentuberkulose.* Joh. Ambrosius Barth, Leipzig.

National Consensus Conference on Tuberculosis (1985). *Chest* **87**, Vol. 2/Supplement.

Nunn, A.J., Springett, V.H., and Sutherland, I. (1984). Changes in tuberculosis notification rates in the white ethnic group in England between 1971 and 1978/79. *Br. J. Dis. Chest* **78**, 159-162.

Romanus, V. (1983). Childhood tuberculosis in Sweden. An epidemiological study made six years after the cessation of general BCG vaccination of the newborn. *Tubercle* **64**, 101-110.

Rouillon, A., Perdrizet, S., and Parrot, R. (1976). Transmission of tubercle bacilli: the effects of chemotherapy. *Tubercle* **57**, 257-299.

Shaw, J.B. and Wynn-Williams, N. (1954). Infectivity of pulmonary tuberculosis in relation to sputum status. *Am. Rev. Tuberc.* **69**, 724-732.

Styblo, K. (1980). Recent advances in epidemiological research in tuberculosis. *Adv. Tuberc. Res.* **20**, 1-63.

—— (1984). Epidemiology of tuberculosis. In *Infektionskrankheiten und ihre Erreger, Band 4/VI. Mykobakteria und mykobakteriellen Krankheiten* (ed. G. Meissner *et al.*). VEB Gustav Fischer Verlag, Jena.

—— (1986). Tuberculosis control and surveillance. In *Recent advances of respiratory medicine*, No. 4 (eds D.C. Flenley and T.L. Petty) pp. 77-108. Churchill Livingstone, Edinburgh, London, Melbourne and New York.

—— and Meijer, J. (1976). Impact of BCG vaccination programmes in children and young adults on the tuberculosis problem. *Tubercle* **57**, 17-43.

——, —— and Sutherland, I. (1969). The transmission of tubercle bacilli. Its trend in a human population. Tuberculosis Surveillance Research Unit Report No. 1. *Bull. Int. Un. Tuberc.* **42**, 5-104.

——, Geuns, H.A. van, and Meijer, J. (1984). The yield of active case-finding in persons with inactive pulmonary tuberculosis or fibrotic lesions. A 5-year study in Tuberculosis Clinics in Amsterdam, Rotterdam and Utrecht. *Tubercle* **65**, 237-251.

Sutherland, I., Bleiker, M.A., Meijer, J., and Styblo, K. (1984a). The risk of tuberculous infection in the Netherlands from 1967 to 1979. *Tubercle* **64**, 241-53.

——, Springett, V.H., and Nunn, A.J. (1984b). Changes in tuberculosis notification rates in ethnic groups in England between 1971 and 1978/79. *Tubercle* **65**, 83-91.

Waaler, H.T. and Rouillon, A. (1974). BCG-vaccination policy according to the epidemiological situation. *Bull. Int. Un. Tuberc.* **49**, 166–189.

World Health Organization (WHO) (1963). *The WHO Standard Tuberculin Test.* WHO/TB Tech. Guide/3.

Youmans, G.P. (1979). *Tuberculosis.* W.B. Saunders Company, Philadelphia, London, Toronto.

B Non-infectious disorders

7
Vitamin D deficiency

Mark Baker

SUMMARY

Vitamin D deficiency is a relatively frequent finding in people of Asian origin living in temperate regions, in vegetarians, and in the elderly housebound. The condition is responsible for impairment of the functioning of the musculo-skeletal system, but severe clinical manifestations are uncommon. Elimination of vitamin D deficiency may be achieved in infants by breast feeding and in others by fortification of foodstuffs and by oral supplementation. These could result in reduced morbidity and, perhaps, mortality.

Vitamin D is a steroid-like molecule which is produced at one site—the skin (Huldschinsky 1919; Beadle 1977)—and acts metabolically at other sites (bone, gut, and kidney); it is therefore a hormone. Uniquely, vitamin D is also found in a slightly different but metabolically equivalent form as a natural component of certain foods, and it has been artificially added to others (Preece *et al.* 1975).

In most communities the endogenous source is the most important (Haddad and Hahn 1973), but prevention of vitamin D deficiency is achieved mainly by enhancing the exogenous component (Anon 1974; Pietrek *et al.* 1976; Conely *et al.* 1977; MacLennan and Hamilton 1977; Singleton and Tucker 1978; Robertson *et al.* 1981).

Profound deficiency of vitamin D can produce early and serious effects on the bone and muscle, characterized by weakness and bowing of the long bones (rickets) in children (Halvorsen and Halvorsen 1983) and bone pain and proximal myopathy (osteomalacia) in adults (Ekbom *et al.* 1964). Vitamin D deficiency which is sufficiently severe to result in hypocalcaemia of clinical importance is extremely rare in the absence of major metabolic disturbance. In addition to its unusual sources, the metabolism of vitamin D is also quite complex (Figure 7.1) and there are a large number of pathways by which vitamin D deficiency can arise.

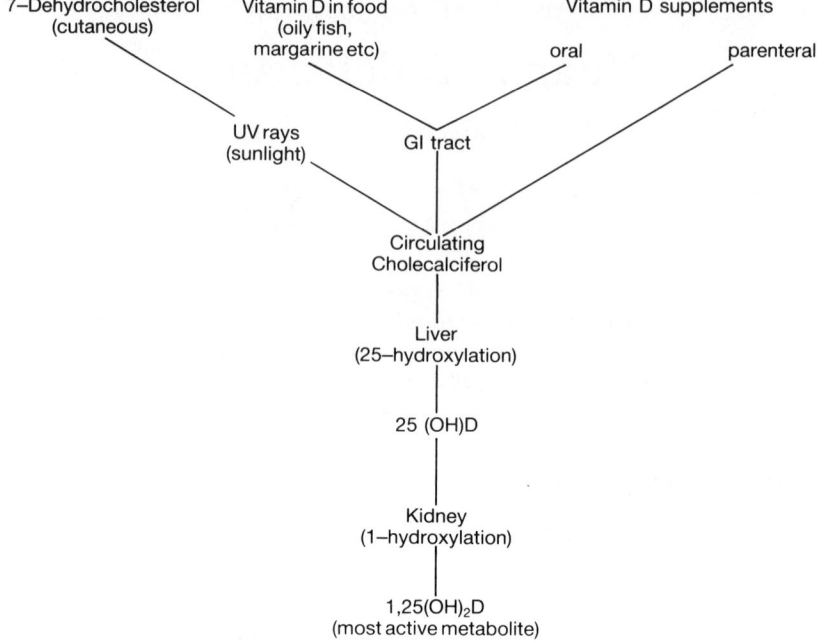

Fig. 7.1 Production and metabolism of vitamin D.

Defining the problem

The complexity of metabolic processes involving vitamin D is reflected in the range of criteria used to define its deficiency (Peach 1984). These include the following: histological evidence of osteomalacia or rickets (bone biopsy); clinical or radiological disease or both; low circulating blood concentrations of metabolites of vitamin D, usually 25-hydroxy vitamin D (25(OH)D); serum biochemical markers (hypocalcaemia, low calcium X phosphate product, raised serum alkaline phosphatase); raised incidence of alleged associated conditions (femoral neck fracture).

The availability of reproducible assays for 25(OH)D offers the best option for comparing groups and for monitoring trends. Healing of diseased bone, however, follows some weeks after an improvement in the blood concentrations of metabolites, so that current plasma vitamin D status may not correspond directly with current bone status (Aaron et al. 1974a).

Does vitamin D deficiency cause femoral neck fracture?

For the last 15 years debate has raged over the relationship, causal or otherwise, between vitamin D deficiency and fracture of the femoral neck in the elderly (Hodkinson 1974; Wootton et al. 1978; Baker et al. 1979a). A large amount of circumstantial evidence has been collected, but the crucial question of causation has not yet been answered.

There are two separate, if related, hypotheses in relation to this controversy. First, that vitamin D deficiency of moderate degree and long duration contributes to the development of osteoporosis which in turn leads to femoral fracture (Nordin et al. 1985); second, that severe vitamin D deficiency with osteomalacia leads to spontaneous non-traumatic fracture or fracture on falling caused by a proximal myopathy, or both (Baker et al. 1979b). These hypotheses are both plausible and, to some extent, supported by research.

Calcium absorption declines after the menopause (Bullamore et al. 1970) and may be raised by vitamin D in moderate doses, thus reducing or removing the negative calcium balance associated with postmenopausal osteoporosis (Nordin et al. 1972). Similarly, metacarpal bone loss in the elderly can be reduced by vitamin D supplements (Nordin et al. 1985). However, the relationship between osteoporosis and fractured neck of femur is by no means absolute and other factors are clearly involved.

A number of studies have shown a high prevalence of osteomalacia or biochemical vitamin D deficiency in series of patients with fractured neck of femur (Aaron et al. 1974a, b; Lund et al. 1975; Pettifer et al. 1978; Baker et al. 1979a; Hoikka et al. 1982; Lund et al. 1982). However, vitamin D status is no better in elderly housebound people without recent fractures (Rapin et al. 1979) or in patients with osteoarthrosis (Bird et al. 1980), a disease with which femoral neck fracture rarely coincides. It is highly probable that frailty and immobility resulting in diminished sunlight exposure and reduced nutrition is responsible for the vitamin D deficiency in elderly housebound people; there is no direct evidence that the resulting vitamin D deficiency causes the fracture. It could be, therefore, that it is the frail elderly who are at risk of fractured neck of femur, vitamin D deficiency being merely a marker of that fraility. Alternatively, end-organ resistance to the active metabolite of vitamin D $(1,25 (OH)_2D)$ has been suggested as a cause (Lund et al. 1982).

Size of the problem

Prevalence

Major factors influencing the prevalence of vitamin D deficiency include latitude, race, age, disability, and, historically, atmospheric pollution.

During the present century, rickets has declined in prevalence while osteomalacia has probably become more common, at least in some groups. More recently, rickets has reappeared in some high-risk populations (Goel *et al.* 1976; Schulpen 1982). Furthermore, international migration has introduced high-risk groups into high-risk locations and has resulted in a dramatic change in the local epidemiology of vitamin D deficiency syndromes (Hodgkin *et al.* 1973; Goel *et al.* 1976; Bachrach *et al.* 1979; Stamp *et al.* 1980; Schulpen 1982; Halvorsen and Halvorsen 1983; Rashid *et al.* 1983).

With ultraviolet radiation being a major feature in the production of cholecalciferol, vitamin D deficiency syndromes increase in prevalence with latitude (Cave and Nordin 1973; Bachrach *et al.* 1979), and are relatively uncommon in warmer climates, including much of Southern Europe.

Although small series of rachitic children have been reported from many countries (Goel *et al.* 1976; Robertson *et al.* 1981; Schulpen 1982), rickets is a significant community problem only in dark-skinned Muslims living in temperate zones (Goel *et al.* 1976; Schulpen 1982). Before anti-pollution legislation, rickets occurred in many northern cities (McLaren 1981), most notably Glasgow (Dunnigan *et al.* 1981), and in children of all races. However, rickets is extremely uncommon in white children in the 1980s except in those with metabolic disturbance—for example, severe renal disease. Dark-skinned ethnic minorities, particularly Asian Muslims (McLaren 1981), living in the United Kingdom and West Germany, do suffer a seasonal biochemical deficiency of vitamin D, up to 40 per cent of the community being affected by late spring, but, in most cases, healing spontaneously during the summer months (Gupta *et al.* 1974; Ford *et al.* 1976).

Even in those high-risk groups, cases of clinical rickets remain uncommon, approximate incidence rates for Bradford's Asian community being 2/1000 per annum for girls aged under 12 years and 0.4/1000 per annum for boys. Slightly higher rates have been recorded in Glasgow (Dunnigan *et al.* 1981). Rickets is relatively uncommon in Afro-caribbeans although biochemical vitamin D deficiency occurs more commonly than in whites (Ford *et al.* 1976). However, the vegetarian Rastafarian community appears to be at greater risk (Ward *et al.* 1982), regardless of their country of domicile, and cases have been reported in other vegetarian and Afro-caribbean groups (Bachrach *et al.* 1979; Schulpen 1982; Curtis *et al.* 1983).

Osteomalacia, characterized by a proximal myopathy and bone pain, is a common finding in pregnant Asian women in the United Kingdom and among housebound elderly people (Exton-Smith *et al.* 1972; Hodkinson *et al.* 1973). Biochemical vitamin D deficiency has been recorded in about 40 per cent of housebound women regardless of age (Baker *et al.* 1979a), and has been considered as a risk factor for fractured neck of femur in this group (Baker *et al.* 1980). The prevalence of histological osteomalacia in patients with a recent fracture of the proximal femur has been assessed at 5 per cent to

37 per cent (Hodkinson 1971; Aaron *et al.* 1974b; Hoikka *et al.* 1982), depending on the definition of thresholds, the former being concomitant with the clinical syndrome, the latter supported by biochemical deficiency.

The prevalence of biochemical vitamin D deficiency in both the housebound and in fracture patients is remarkably consistent and irrespective of latitude. It may be assumed, therefore, that, even in the sunniest and warmest climates, such a prevalence may be observed in the housebound elderly.

The prevalence of biochemical vitamin D deficiency may be as high as 50 per cent in pregnant Asian women (Heckmatt *et al.* 1979). The clinical syndrome is frequently misdiagnosed in this group because of communication difficulties, the classic waddling gait being confused with postural changes associated with pregnancy. The children born to osteomalacic mothers rarely suffer from neonatal hypocalcaemia and early childhood rickets (Congdon *et al.* 1983). Breast-feeding is uncommon in this group and would not protect the child unless the mother's skeleton was fully healed.

In this section I have described those at particular risk from vitamin D deficiency, but no European country is free from the condition since the housebound elderly exist throughout Western Europe.

Current trends

Vitamin D deficiency comprises a range of syndromes, each with its own epidemiology and aetiology. Secular trends in incidence also vary substantially between the different syndromes and between high-risk groups.

First, there are those with an increasing prevalence of vitamin D deficiency. These include people with renal or hepatic disease, the former because of prolonged survival, the latter because of the increasing abuse of alcohol. The elderly housebound with osteomalacia are also increasing in number, mainly for demographic reasons. Rickets is increasing in incidence in migrants from the Equator (Schulpen 1982).

Second, groups with a decreasing prevalence include Asian communities in parts of the United Kingdom where successful intervention programmes have been launched (Dunnigan *et al.* 1985). In addition, as the use of barbiturates declines, so the number of epileptics with osteomalacia may also diminish (Haddad and Hendin 1972), although the most significant reduction in barbiturate use has been as a hypnotic.

Third, adequately nourished and active white populations continue to experience a very low incidence of vitamin D deficiency, as has been the case for most of the twentieth century. An exception was during and after the Second World War when the production and availability of foodstuffs was seriously affected even in non-aligned countries (Robertson *et al.* 1981).

Risk factors

As stated above, the clinical syndromes of rickets and osteomalacia are relatively uncommon whereas less severe degrees of vitamin D deficiency occur not infrequently. The high-risk groups defined below are based mostly on studies of biochemical vitamin D deficiency, but the continuum with clinical significance is constant to all. Vitamin D deficiency can occur at any age, although it is more common in the elderly. In adults vitamin D status declines with age (Baker *et al.* 1980), even in those who are active and taking a good diet (Barragry *et al.* 1978). In all groups and at all ages females are more likely to be affected than males (Dunnigan *et al.* 1981).

At all ages, vitamin D deficiency syndromes are more common in the disabled (Anderson *et al.* 1971) because of both diminished nutrition (Exton-Smith 1975) and low sunlight exposure (Corless *et al.* 1975; Offerman and Biehle 1978). There is no evidence that, in a given location, social class is a feature of vitamin D deficiency (Dandona *et al.* 1985).

Skin pigment reduces the penetration of ultraviolet radiation (Beadle 1977; Clemens *et al.* 1982). Dark-skinned children living in temperate zones are thus at increased risk (Hodgkin *et al.* 1973; Stephens *et al.* 1982). Further, dark-skinned Asians and Afro-caribbeans whose vitamin D status is compromised in any other way are at significantly increased risk of vitamin D deficiency (Ford *et al.* 1976; Bachrach *et al.* 1979), especially, for example, Muslims during pregnancy (Heckmatt *et al.* 1979). Major additional factors may include vegetarianism (Bachrach *et al.* 1979; Schulpen 1982; Curtis *et al.* 1983), adherence to the customs of Islam (Bachrach *et al.* 1979), particularly for women (McLaren 1981), and residence at high latitudes. The dietary vitamin D of Asian schoolchildren in Bradford has been reported as only 38 per cent of that of their white classmates.

The prevalence of vitamin D deficiency increases with distance from the Equator because of the reduced availability of ultraviolet radiation (Bachrach *et al.* 1970; Rush 1977). It has been said that the global distribution of the human race is determined by the effect of latitude, together with skin pigment (Clemens *et al.* 1982), on the anatomical soundness of the bony pelvis in childbearing women. Even within the United Kingdom deficiency is more common at the more northerly latitudes, such as Scotland (Dunnigan *et al.* 1981).

In temperate zones, the angle of the earth prevents the penetration of ultraviolet radiation during the winter months. This, together with the shorter day and lower temperatures, leads to a maximum prevalence of vitamin D deficiency in late spring (Gupta *et al.* 1974; Stamp and Round 1974; Pettifer *et al.* 1978).

Diet

Where exposure to ultraviolet radiation is adequate, diet is relatively unimportant as a source of vitamin D. However, diet can become the critical variable when endogenous production of cholecalciferol is restricted for any reason (Lawson *et al.* 1979).

On its own, the average diet in countries with few fortified foods provides insufficient vitamin D (MacLeod *et al.* 1974; Lonergan *et al.* 1975). In Great Britain, the Ministry of Agriculture, Fisheries and Food recommends 2.5 mcg daily with 10 mcg for children and pregnant and nursing women. These minimum levels are infrequently achieved except with the aid of supplements. In countries where all dairy products are fortified with vitamin D, these minimum levels can be achieved with relative ease and there is some evidence that vitamin D deficiency syndromes may be less common (Lund *et al.* 1975).

Vegetarian, especially vegan, diets are usually deficient in vitamin D. Asians who consume large quantities of chappatti flour probably raise their requirement for vitamin D, perhaps by interfering with calcium absorption from the gut (Dunnigan *et al.* 1981). Similarly, increases in the consumption of wholemeal flour and cereals may interfere with vitamin D metabolism and have been associated with outbreaks of rickets in white children (Robertson *et al.* 1981). In addition, some Asian communities favour the use of butter, which is not fortified with vitamin D in the United Kingdom, to margarine, which is fortified.

Breast-feeding may protect against rickets for a variety of reasons (Novak 1980), not all of which are explained by our current knowledge of vitamin D metabolism. However, the mother's vitamin D status must be adequate and the duration of nursing should not be prolonged (Bachrach *et al.* 1979; O'Connor 1980; Robertson *et al.* 1982).

Given the combination of factors described in this section on those at risk, it is perhaps surprising that vitamin D deficiency is not universal among Asians in the United Kingdom. However, it is not and this serves to demonstrate the relative resistance of humans to vitamin D deficiency.

Intervention and its efficacy

The evidence cited here is based mostly on clinical studies and their extrapolations and not on community intervention programmes. This clinical evidence, supported by circumstantial epidemiological observations, can be assembled into a strong case for the feasibility and probable success of intervention.

With the exception of metabolic and iatrogenic disorders, the principal factor in the aetiology of vitamin D deficiency is disruption to the endogenous production of cholecalciferol in the skin caused mainly by the lack or non-penetration of ultraviolet radiation (Haddad and Hahn 1973; Clemens *et al.* 1982).

Attempts have been made to overcome this deficiency by the provision, in institutions, of fluorescent light sources which emit ultraviolet radiation (Conely *et al.* 1977; Stamp *et al.* 1977; Snell *et al.* 1978). The results of these efforts have been inconclusive, however, and the method cannot therefore be considered suitable or effective in many of the at-risk situations described above (Devgun *et al.* 1980).

The only route of administration of vitamin D which can be entertained as both acceptable and effective for most of those at risk is the oral route. The options for implementing orally administered prevention include dietary modification, individual supplementation, and the fortification of certain foodstuffs.

Health education aimed at increasing the consumption of foods high in vitamin D is difficult to achieve and to monitor, is unlikely to succeed, and could well conflict with other dietary advice being delivered in order to prevent more lethal disorders—for example, butter and vitamin D-fortified margarine, are major sources of vitamin D, yet increasing their consumption conflicts with dietary advice to prevent heart disease. However, the further encouragement of breast-feeding in high-risk groups would be advantageous, provided that the mother's vitamin D status is sustained and that weaning is not delayed too long (Bachrach *et al.* 1979; Novak 1980; O'Connor 1980; Robertson *et al.* 1982).

Alternative education encouraging individual supplementation and possibly enhanced by the provision of supplements without charge might be preferable. But there are difficulties. First, experience of human behaviour causes one to question the effectiveness of such programmes although, when led by motivated practitioners, they can achieve notable success (Dunnigan *et al.* 1985). Second, vitamin D supplements are potentially toxic when taken to excess and their distribution to almost every domestic drug cabinet in the continent must be regarded as less than desirable.

The fortification of a range of foodstuffs, sufficient to reach all but the most faddish, is the least expensive and probably the most effective measure that could be adopted (Pietrek *et al.* 1976). In particular, the fortification of chappatti flour (Hunt *et al.* 1976), milk, and butter (Anon 1974; Exton-Smith 1975) would enable all those with an intact gastrointestinal tract to avoid severe deficiency of vitamin D without presenting any risk of intoxication from dietary sources. The single most effective measure would be the fortification of milk, with additional local measures where the risks were unusually high (Singleton and Tucker 1978). It is notable that the fortification of milk with vitamin D appears to influence the incidence of fractured neck of femur (Eddy 1973; Lund *et al.* 1975).

There is evidence that daily doses as low as 2000 iu (50 mcg) may be associated with hypercalcaemia (Johnson et al. 1980); most people can accept daily doses of up to 15 000 iu without harm, but individual hypersensitivity does occur, especially in people suffering from sarcoidosis or primary hyperparathyroidism. The ideal target range for prevention should therefore be 500–1500 iu/day (12.5–37.5 mcg) (Nordin et al. 1972; Corless et al. 1975; Conely et al. 1977; MacLennan and Hamilton 1977). The addition of 400 iu (10 mcg) per litre of milk, with proportionate quantities in other dairy products, and up to 2000 iu (50 mcg) per kilogram of chappatti flour could eliminate vitamin D deficiency as a community nutritional problem.

Population effectiveness

There are no data on the effectiveness of vitamin D supplementation and the reason for this may be difficulties inherent in mounting suitable trials. Studies to test these causal hypotheses would have to be very large indeed. For the first hypothesis (prevention of osteoporosis), assuming that age-related bone loss can be reduced by vitamin D supplements and that the increase in fracture incidence with age can be reduced by 25 per cent, it would require a cohort of 60 000 women aged about 70 years and followed up for 15 years with continuous recruitment to replace losses in order to demonstrate a significant difference in fracture incidence at the 5 per cent level. It would be difficult to justify the expense of such a study and its feasibility must be open to question.

The second hypothesis (prevention of osteomalacia) is more approachable. On the assumption that vitamin D deficiency doubles the risk of fracture, a cohort of 12 000 women aged 80 years or more and followed up for 4 years, with continuous recruitment to replace losses, would enable a significant difference in incidence at the 5 per cent level to be demonstrated. Further, limiting the study to housebound subjects would significantly reduce the size of the cohort to be followed up, but would require a larger initial sampling frame. This is still a massive undertaking, but the benefits of eliminating vitamin D deficiency would be magnified manyfold were a causal relationship with fractured neck of femur to be confirmed.

Constraints on implementation

Clinical importance

The clinical syndromes associated with vitamin D deficiency are relatively uncommon; vitamin D deficiency is often latent and asymptomatic and is of uncertain importance. In particular, if the apparent association with fractured neck of femur is shown to be spurious, the clinical relevance of vitamin D deficiency will be greatly reduced. Seasonal variation in the prevalence of vitamin D deficiency, with spontaneous healing during the summer months and spontaneous cure of mild rickets when children reach school age, diminish the importance of active intervention which has yet to be shown to positively influence human health. There is, also, some disagreement among clinicians as to what constitutes abnormality; in some communities vitamin D status is a continuum from zero upwards.

Feasibility of intervention

Individual supplementation is always subject to the vagaries of compliance while education programmes tend to be relatively ineffective for those most in need. Fortification of foodstuffs for uncommon health problems rarely attracts widespread popular and political favour, especially when some of those at greatest risk are unpopular minorities.

A relatively narrow therapeutic range and considerable paranoia about potential toxicity hazards also serve as constraining influences.

Nonetheless, fortification can be achieved relatively inexpensively, and precedents exist in almost all countries. Personal liberty may be protected by offering a choice of fortified or non-fortified food as with the fat content of cows' milk. Public health policies should ensure that there should be no price disadvantage for the fortified product.

Recommendations

It should be possible, by nutritional supplements (specifically the fortification of bread and milk), to reduce considerably the prevalence of rickets and osteomalacia, although it is most unlikely that prevalence will fall to zero. The reasons for this include the ubiquity and nature of food faddism and the existence of disease of the gut, liver, and kidney which routine supplements cannot address. A feasible target would be a reduction of 90 per cent for nutritional rickets and of a slightly lower proportion for osteomalacia.

The circumstances necessary to achieve this target include a political will to take action to prevent diseases which affect mainly minority groups, a more receptive public attitude towards beneficial additives, and a mechanism to demonstrate the effectiveness of intervention. This latter requires the value of preventing vitamin D deficiency to be demonstrated by conducting large-scale intervention studies to assess the role of the condition in fracture aetiology. The level of human benefit and cost–benefit will be determined by the extent to which fractured neck of femur is preventable.

References

Aaron, J.E., Gallagher, J.C., and Nordin, B.E.C. (1974a). Seasonal variation of histological osteomalacia in femoral neck fractures. *Lancet* **2**, 84–6.
——, Gallagher, J.C., Anderson, J., Stasiak, L., Loughton, E.B., Nordin, B.E.C., and Nicholson, M. (1974b). Frequency of osteomalacia and osteoporosis in fractures of the proximal femur. *Lancet* **1**, 229–33.
Anderson, W.F., Cohen, C., Hyams, D.E., Millard, P.H., Plowright, N., Woodford-Williams, E., and Barry, W.T.C. (1971). *Clinical and sub-clinical malnutrition in old age. Nutrition in old age.* Swedish Nutrition Foundation, Stockholm.
Anon (1974). Old people's nutrition. *Br. Med. J.* **1**, 212–3.
Bachrach, S., Fisher, J., and Parks, J.S. (1979). An outbreak of vitamin D deficiency rickets in a susceptible population. *Paediatrics* **64**, 871–7.
Baker, M.R., McDonnell, H., Nordin, B.E.C., and Peacock, M. (1979a). Plasma 25-hydroxy vitamin D concentration in patients with fractures of the femoral neck. *Br. Med. J.* **278**, 589.
——, Peacock, M., and Nordin, B.E.C. (1979b). Difference between Leeds fractures and London fractures. *Br. Med. J.* **278**, 1218–9.
——, ——, —— (1980). The decline in vitamin D status with age. *Age and Ageing* **9**, 249–52.
Barragry, J.M., France, M.W., Corless, D., Gupta, S.P., Switala, S., Boucher, B.J., and Cohen, R.D. (1978). Cholecalciferol absorption in the elderly. *Clin. Sci. Mol. Med.* **54**, 28.
Beadle, P.C. (1977). Cholecalciferol production in vitamin D. In *Biochemical, chemical and clinical aspects related to calcium metabolism* (ed. A.W. Norman) pp. 549–51. Walter de Gruter and Co, Berlin.
Bird, H.A., Peacock, M., Storer, J.H., and Wright, V. (1980). Comparison of serum 25-OH vitamin D concentrations in rheumatoid arthritis and osteoarthritis. *Br. Med. J.* **280**, 1416.
Bullamore, J.R., Wilkinson, R., Gallagher, J.C., and Nordin, B.E.C. (1970). Effect of age on calcium absorption. *Lancet* **2**, 535–7.
Cave, W., and Nordin, B.E.C. (1973). *Report on fractures of the proximal femur to International Health Foundation.* (privately published).
Clemens, J.L., Adams, J.S., Henderson, S.L., and Holick, M.F. (1982). Increased skin pigment reduces the capacity of skin to synthesise vitamin D3. *Lancet* **1**, 74–6.
Conely, J., Sumner D., McKinlay, A., McIntosh, W., and Dunnigan, M.G. (1977). Prevention of vitamin D deficiency in the elderly. *Br. Med. J.* **2**, 1668.
Congdon, P., Horsman, A., Kirby, P.A., Dibble, J., and Bashir, T. (1983). Mineral content of the forearms of babies born to asian and white mothers. *Br. Med. J.* **286**, 1233–4.
Corless, D., Beer, M., Boucher, B.J., Gupta, S.P., and Cohen, R.D. (1975). Vitamin D status in long-stay geriatric patients. *Lancet* **1**, 1404–6.
Curtis, J.A., Kooh, S.W., Fraser, D., and Greenberg, M.L. (1983). Nutritional rickets in vegetarian children. *Can. Med. Assoc. J.* **128**, 150–2.

Dandona, P., Okonofua, F., and Clemens, R. (1985). Osteomalacia presenting as pathological fractures during pregnancy in asian women of high socioeconomic class. *Br. Med. J.* **290**, 837.

Devgun, M.S., Paterson, C.R., Cohen, C., and Johnson, B.E. (1980). Possible value of fluorescent lighting in the prevention of vitamin D deficiency in the elderly. *Age and Ageing* **9**, 117-20.

Dunnigan, M.G., Glekin, B.M., Henderson, J.B., McIntosh, W.B., Sumner, D., and Sutherland, G.R. (1985). Prevention of rickets in asian children: assessment of the Glasgow campaign. *Br. Med. J.* **291**, 239-42.

Dunnigan, M.G., McIntosh, W.B., Sutherland, G.R., Gardee, R., Glekin, B., Ford, J.A., and Robertson, I. (1981). Policy for Prevention of Asian rickets in Britain: a preliminary assessment of the Glasgow rickets campaign. *Br. Med. J.* **282**, 357-60.

Eddy, T.P. (1973). Deaths from falls and fractures: comparison of mortality in Scotland and the United States with that in England and Wales. *Br. J. Prev. Soc. Med.* **27**, 247-54.

Ekbom, K., Hed, R., Kirstein, L., and Astrom, K.E. (1964). Weakness of proximal limb muscles, probably due to myopathy after partial gastrectomy. *Acta. Med. Scand.* **176**, 493-6.

Exton-Smith, A.N. (1975). Problems of diet in old age. *J. R. Coll. Phys. Lond.* **9**, 148-60.

——, Windsor, A., and Stanton, B.R. (1972). *Nutrition of housebound old people.* King Edward's Hospital Fund, London.

Ford, J.A., McIntosh, W.B., Butterfield, R., Preece, M.A., Pietrek, J., Arrowsmith, W.A., Arthurton, M.W., Turner, W., O'Riordan, J.L.H., and Dunnigan, M.G. (1976). Clinical and subclinical vitamin D deficiency in Bradford children. *Arch. Dis. Child.* **51**, 939-43.

Goel, K.M., Logan, R.W., Arneil, G.C., Sweet. E.M., Warren, J.M., and Shanks, R.A. (1976). Florid and sub-clinical rickets among immigrant children in Glasgow. *Lancet* **1**, 1141-5.

Gupta, M.M., Round, J.M., and Stamp, T.C.B. (1974). Spontaneous cure of vitamin D deficiency in Asians during summer in Britain. *Lancet* **1**, 586-8.

Haddad, J.G. and Hahn, T.J. (1973). Natural and synthetic sources of circulating 25-hydroxyvitamin D in men. *Nature* **244**, 515-7.

—— and Hendin, B.A. (1972). Effect of chronic anticonvulsant therapy on serum 25 (OH) vitamin D levels. *Clin. Res.* **20**, 238.

Halvorsen, K.S., and Halvorsen, S.R. (1983). En aktuell sykdom. *Tidsskr. Nor. Loegeforen* **103**, 1054-7.

Heckmatt, J.Z., Peacock, M., Davies, A.E.J., McMurray, J., and Isherwood, D.M. (1979). Plasma 25-hydroxy vitamin D in pregnant Asian women and their babies. *Lancet* **2**, 546-9.

Hodgkin, P., Kay, G.H., Hine, P.M., Lumb, G.A., and Stanbury, S.W. (1973). Vitamin D deficiency in Asians at home and in Britain. *Lancet* **2**, 167-71.

Hodkinson, H.M. (1971). Fracture of the femoral neck in the elderly: assessment of the role of osteomalacia. *Gerontol. Clin.* **13**, 153-60.

—— (1974). Seasonal variation of histological osteomalacia in femoral neck fractures. *Lancet* **2**, 463.

——, Round, P., Stanton, B.R., and Morgan, C. (1973). Sunlight, vitamin D and osteomalacia in the elderly. *Lancet* **1**, 910-2.

Hoikka, V., Alhava, E.M., Savolainen, K., and Parviainen (1982). Osteomalacia in fracture of the proximal femur. *Acta. Orthop. Scand.* **53**, 255-60.

Huldschinsky, K. (1919). Heiling con rachitis durch kunsthicke Hohensonne. *Dtsch. Med. Wochenschr.* **45**, 712.

Hunt, S.P., O'Riordan, J.L.H., Windo, and Truswell, A.S. (1976). Vitamin D status in different subgroups of British Asians. *Br. Med. J.* **4**, 1351-4.

Johnson, K.R., Jobber, J., and Stonawski, B.J. (1980). Prophylactic vitamin D in the elderly. *Age and Ageing.* **9**, 121-7.

Lawson, D.E.M., Paul, A.A., Black, A.E., Cole, T.J., Mandal, A.R., and Davie, M. (1979). Relative contributions of diet and sunlight to vitamin D state in the elderly. *Br. Med. J.* **2**, 303-5.

Lonergan, M.E., Milne, J.S., Maule, M.M., and Williamson, J. (1975). A dietary survey of older people in Edinburgh. *Br. J. Nutr.* **34**, 517-27.

Lund, B., Sorenson, O.H., and Christensen, A.B. (1975). 25 (OH)D3 and fractures of the proximal femur. *Lancet* **2**, 300-2.

Lund, B., Sorensen, O.H., Lund, B., Melsen, F., and Mosekilde, L. (1982). Vitamin D metabolism and osteomalacia in patients with fractures of the proximal femur. *Acta. Orthop. Scand.* **54**, 251-4.

McLaren, D.S. (1981). The prevalence and possible causes of fat soluble vitamin deficiencies in the world. *Prog. Clin. Biol. Res.* **77**, 99-107.

MacLennan, W.J. and Hamilton, J.C. (1977). Vitamin D supplements and 25-hydroxy vitamin D concentrations in the elderly. *Br. Med. J.* **2**, 589-61.

MacLeod, C.C., Judge, T.G., and Caird, F.I. (1974). Nutrition of the elderly at home: intakes of vitamins. *Age and Ageing* **3**, 209-20.

Nordin, B.E.C., Aaron, J., Gallagher, J.C., and Horsman, A. (1972). *Calcium and bone metabolism in old age.* Symposia of the Swedish Nutrition Foundation.

——, Baker, R.M., Horsman, A., and Peacock, M. (1985). A prospective trial of the effect of vitamin D supplementation on metacarpal bone loss in elderly women. *Am. J. Clin. Nutr.* **42**, 470-4.

Novak, J. (1980). Profylaxe, vyskyt a diagnostika krivice na venkovskem obvode. *Cesk. Pediatr.* **35**, 686-8.

Offerman, G., and Biehle, G. (1978). Vitamin D deficiency and osteomalacia in old people. *Dtsch Med. Wochenschr.* **193**, 415-19.

O'Connor, P.A. (1980). Clouds, skin colour and rickets. *Pediatrics* **66**, 332.

Peach, H. (1984). A critique of survey methods used to measure the occurrence of osteomalacia and rickets in the UK. *Comm Med.* **6**, 20-8.

Pettifer, J.M., Ross, F.P., and Solomon, L. (1978). Seasonal variation in serum 25-hydroxycholecalciferol concentrations in elderly South African patients with fractures of femoral neck. *Br. Med. J.* **1**, 826-7.

Pietrek, J., Preece, M.A., Windo, J., O'Riordan, J.L.H., Dunnigan, M.G., McIntosh, W.B., and Ford, J.A. (1976). Prevention of vitamin D deficiency in Asians. *Lancet* **1**, 1145-8.

Preece, M.A., Tomlinson, S., Ribot, C.A., Pietrek, J., Korn, H.T., Davies, D.M.,

Ford, J.A., Dunnigan, M.G., and O'Riordan, J.L.H. (1975). Studies of vitamin D deficiency in man. *Quart. J. Med.* **176**, 575-89.

Rapin, C.H., Jung, A., Lagier, R., MacGee, W., Barras, C., Courvoisier, B., Vasey, H., and Junod, J.P. (1979). Y a-t-il une composante osteomalacique dans les fracture due col du femur? *Schweiz Med. Wochenschr.* **109**, 1894-5.

Rashid, A., Mohammed, T., Stephens, W., Warrington, S., Berry J.L., and Mawer, E.B. (1983). Vitamin D state of Asians living in Pakistan. *Br. Med. J.* **286**, 182-3.

Robertson, I., Ford, J.A., McIntosh, W.B., and Dunnigan, M.G. (1981). The role of cereals in the Aetiology of Nutrition Survey 1943-8. *Br. J. Nutr.* **45**, 17-22.

—— Glekin, B.M., Henderson, J.B., McIntosh, W.B., Lakhani, A., and Dunnigan, M.G. (1982). Nutrition deficiencies among ethnic minorities in the United Kingdom. *Proc. Nutr. Soc.* **41**, 243-56.

Rush, J.H. (1977). Osteomalacia in the elderly. *Austr. N.Z. J. Surg.* **47**, 186-8.

Schulpen, T.W.J. (1982). Opnieuw rachitis in Nederland. *Ned. Tijdschr. Geneeskd.* **126**, 610-3.

Singleton, N. and Tucker, S.M. (1978). Vitamin D status of Asian infants. *Br. Med. J.* **1**, 607-10.

Snell, A.P., McLennan, W.J., and Hamilton, J.C. (1978). Ultraviolet irradiation and 25-hydroxy vitamin D levels in sick old people. *Age and Ageing* **7**, 225-8.

Stamp, T.C.B. and Round, J.M. (1974). Seasonal changes in human plasma levels of 25(OH)D3. *Nature* **247**, 563-5.

——, Haddad, J.G., and Twigg, C.A. (1977). Comparison of oral 25-hydroxycholecalciferol, vitamin D and ultraviolet light as determinants of circulating 25-hydroxyvitamin D. *Lancet* **1**, 2341-3.

——, Walker, P.G., Perry, W., and Jenkins, M.V. (1980). Nutritional osteomalacia in Greater London, 1974-79. *Clin. Endocr. Metab.* **9**, 81-105.

Stephens, W.P., Klimuik, P.S., Warrington, S., Taylor J.L., Barry, J.L., and Mawer, E.B. (1982). Observations on the natural history of vitamin D deficiency among Asian immigrants. *Quart. J. Med.* **51**, 171-88.

Ward, P.S., Drakeford, J.P., Milton, J.P., and James, J.A. (1982). Nutritional Rickets in Rastafarian Children. *Br. Med. J.* **285**, 1242-3.

Wootton, R., Brereton, P.J., Clark, M.B., Hesp. R., Hodkinson, H.M., Klenerman, L., Loewi, G., Reeve, J., and Tellez-Yudilevich, M. (1978). A prospective study of some possible aetiological factors in fractured neck of femur. *Clin. Sci. Mol. Med.* **54**, 28.

8
Iodine deficiency and goitre

Claude H Thilly, Beatrice Swennen, and Raphael Lagasse

SUMMARY

Endemic goitre is the result of dietary iodine deficiency and can be classified as mild, intermediate, or severe. Despite many attempts at iodine supplementation and the extremely low cost of this prophylactic measure, endemic goitre remains a health problem of some size, if not a major priority, in many European countries. In addition to the cosmetic problem which mild goitre constitutes, it is also associated with additional avoidable medical costs. Goitre of intermediate severity and pockets of severe goitre, still present in Europe today, raise the question that maternal iodine deficiency might lead to transient hypothyroidism in the neonatal period which could affect brain maturation and subsequent mental and physical development. Iodine supplementation in developed countries is cheap, extremely cost-effective, easy to administer, and virtually without hazard. Changing dietary habits, consumer resistance to food additives, and lack of central direction and political awareness are all factors responsible for the continuing high prevalence of iodine deficiency. Recent awareness of the potential consequences of iodine deficiency on intellectual development, together with the improvement which adequate intake of iodine would have on the yield and the cost of screening for congenital hypothyroidism, bring new impetus to the need to eliminate this health problem from Europe as rapidly as possible.

Defining the problem

The link between goitre (thyroid gland swelling) and iodine deficiency is well established. It is usual to classify endemic goitre as mild, intermediate, or severe, and within Europe there are still many areas where goitre is present in all three degrees of severity (Scriba 1985; Thilly *et al.* 1985). Mild goitre—apart from the obvious and unacceptable cosmetic problem—may lead to additional diagnostic and therapeutic procedures, and thus to supplementary medical costs to differentiate it from other thyroid diseases, mainly thyroid cancer. The true public health burden of intermediate and severe iodine deficiencies includes perinatal and transient neonatal hypothyroidism. It consists of the whole spectrum of iodine deficiency disorders (IDD), such as high rates of stillbirth and perinatal mortality, and severe or sub-clinical mental impairment (Hetzel 1983). These suspected sub-clinical deficits in physical and psychomotor development may affect a small percentage of the children living in iodine-deficient areas, and they are thus a significant public health problem. More recently, the increase in screening for permanent neonatal hypothyroidism which is discussed in Chapter 14 of this book, has added a new dimension to the need for adequate iodine intake, because this type of non-dietary congenital thyroid deficiency is rare (one in 4000 births) and is indistinguishable, at screening, from the transient neonatal hypothyroidism caused by iodine deficiency. The recall rate needed to separate these two types of pathology with very different medical prognoses, may be increased by a factor of three in iodine-deficient areas. This leads to unacceptable medical and psychological costs, especially for those subsequently found to be false-positive (Delange et al. 1986).

Size of the problem

Endemic goitre and iodine deficiency are a health problem of geochemical origin. They arise mainly in areas with soils poor in iodine and they are one of the best examples of a 'place-disease'. Different countries or areas of Europe are either unaffected or affected at the three degrees of severity already mentioned (Scriba 1985).

Several countries such as Denmark, Iceland, the United Kingdom, and Ireland seem always to have had very little goitre. Recent or already well-established programmes of iodine supplementation have altered the occurrence of goitre in other countries. Thus Finland, Switzerland, the Netherlands, and various Eastern European countries have effective and country-wide iodine prophylaxis programmes.

A large proportion of the inhabitants of Europe, however, are still living with an iodine intake which is inadequate. This is the case, for example, in most of the Federal Republic of Germany, as well as in more limited areas of Belgium, France, and Italy. While very few national data are available, a study of 5.4 million military recruits in the Federal Republic of Germany in 1975 showed a relatively high goitre prevalence of 15 per cent, and iodine deficiency has been found in different populations of children and adults (Horster et al. 1975).

Mild or intermediate iodine deficiency has been observed in some of the plains of Europe and even near the sea in countries such as the Netherlands. Figure 8.1 is a map of the iodine intake in different localities of Europe. This

Iodine deficiency and goitre 117

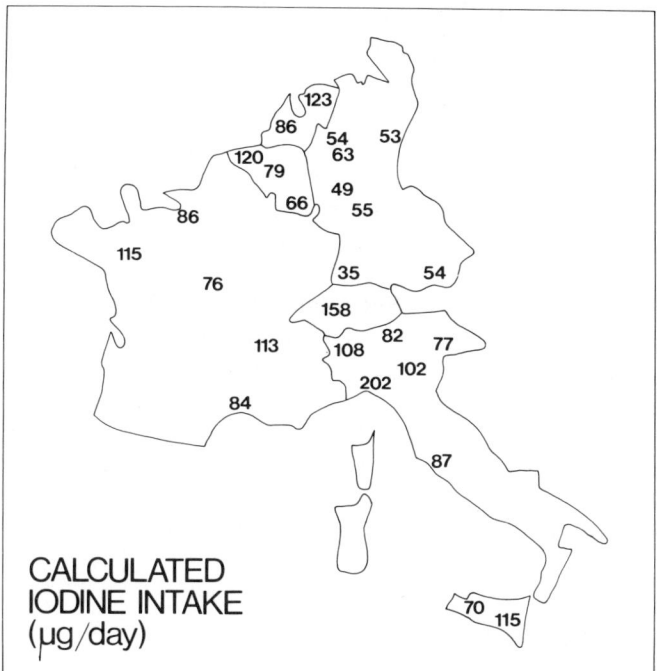

Fig. 8.1 Mean calculated iodine intake in different localities of Europe. Source: Thilly, unpublished data.

represents the results of a survey undertaken in 1972 at the request of the EEC. It can be seen that there are still a few places with a very low daily iodine intake of under 50 µg and quite a number with a borderline intake of between 50 and 100 µg. This work has been extended recently (Scriba et al. 1985), but the main conclusions are that iodine deficiency is still widespread in many areas of Europe and that no major prophylactic interventions, since 1972, have changed this pattern very much.

Historically, severe goitre, accompanied with cretinism, was found in the Alps and in populations that were isolated and largely self-sufficient in the provision of food, especially in areas where communications were poor and the level of health education low. Severe iodine deficiency, in the range 20–40 µg/day, is still observed in areas of Greece and Spain (Beckers et al. 1981; Escobar Del Rey et al. 1981). In an area known as Las Hurdes in Spain, for example, the overall goitre frequency among schoolchildren was 86 per cent. While socio-economic conditions and general nutritional status in the area were also very poor, the physical development and skeletal age of schoolchildren were clearly retarded compared with children from Madrid. High serum TSH levels (above 7.5 µU/ml) were observed in as many as 40 per cent of the children in Las Hurdes and usually coincided with low circulating T4. Therefore it was concluded that these children were probably at a serious developmental disadvantage as a consequence of juvenile hypothyroidism.

The occurrence of neonatal problems caused by thyroid deficiency has also been studied in Europe (Delange *et al.* 1986). The incidence of a low serum thyroxine concentration combined with congenital goitre in the first days of life was observed in almost 1 per cent of newborns from an iodine-deficient area of southern Germany (Heidemann and Stubbe 1978). Figure 8.2 shows the rapid return to normal of the previously low serum T4 (6.3 µg/dl) which occurred after a few days of iodine treatment in these children. In Sicily, a frequency of transient biochemical hypothyroidism of 9.8 per cent (as measured by a cord serum TSH above 50 µU/ml) has been observed in one small endemic area where there were still a few cases of congenital hypothyroidism (Squatrito *et al.* 1981; Sava *et al.* 1984). Interestingly, from a public health point of view, a frequency of 0.67 per cent was also observed in a much larger population from a more moderate endemic goitre area. Although abnormalities of thyroid function were rarely observed in the adult population

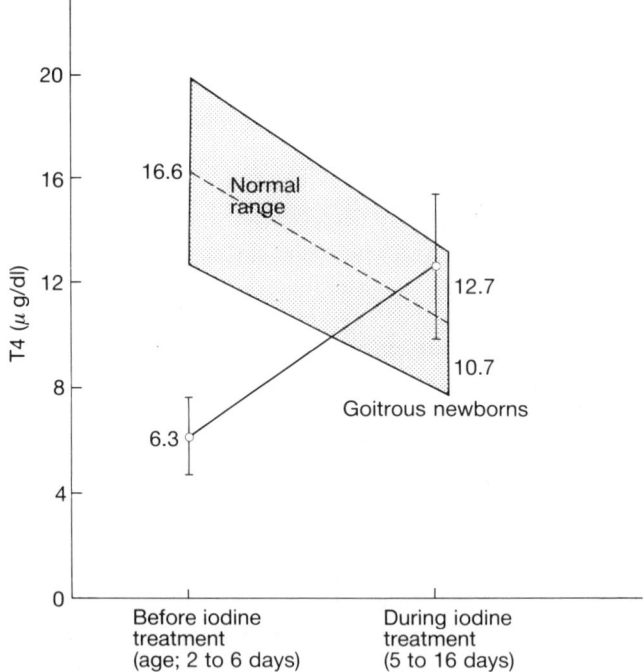

Fig. 8.2 Mean concentration of serum thyroxine in neonates with congenital goitre observed in south Germany just before and a few days after iodine treatment. Source: Heidemann and Stubbe (1978).

from this area, it is not yet known whether this transient biological neonatal hypothyroidism will have deleterious effects on brain maturation. At this moment, data on the possible impairment of intellectual development caused by transient hypothyroidism linked to intermediate iodine deficiency are not conclusive and it is unlikely that stronger data will be available in the near future (Bleichrodt et al. 1986; Muzzo et al. 1986). However, as this disorder can be prevented so easily by iodine supplementation, such 'moderate' endemic populations should be considered at risk and treated as a target for intervention.

Nature of intervention

In the developed countries, endemic goitre and iodine deficiency are among the easiest health problems to control and prevent. One simply adds a minute amount of iodine to table salt. Because this salt is eaten in a relatively constant quantity by almost everyone, it is an ideal vehicle of iodine supplementation. This technique is by far the easiest, cheapest, and most acceptable method of goitre control. The iodine to be added is either potassium iodide (KI) or potassium iodate (KIO_3) at a level of 5–25 mg of iodine per kilo of salt depending on the average salt consumption. For a person eating 10 g of salt per day, the supplement of iodine given would thus be in the physiological range of 50 to 250 µg daily.

Iodization of salt necessitates an understanding of its production. Salt in Europe is mainly of industrial origin, coming from salt mines or as a by-product of other industrial activities. In the south of Europe salt is also obtained from the sea by evaporation. Production, however, lies increasingly in the hands of a few companies and the salt consumed in most of Europe is dry, refined, and vacuum-packed so that the cost of adding iodine to the industrial chain is minimal—on the order of 4 US cents per capita per year (Burgi and Rutishauser 1986).

In order to obtain the active collaboration of the industry, iodine salt prophylaxis has generally been introduced either by making it mandatory by law or on a voluntary basis, mostly by direct discussion between the health authorities and the producers. But, whatever way is chosen, the introduction takes time because it implies change in an industrial procedure or the passage of legislation as well as the understanding and the control of the salt market. The long duration of its introduction is also considered advisable to avoid rare complications such as iodine-induced hyperthyroidism (iod-Basedow). It is appropriate to increase the quantity of iodine in the salt by 5 mg/kg every 5 years until an adequate level is reached. In Switzerland, for example, prophylaxis has been made mandatory progressively, canton after canton, between 1924 and the 1950s, while in Finland it has been introduced on a voluntary basis and its increase in concentration and coverage has extended between the end of the Second World War and the 1970s (Lamberg 1985).

Efficacy and effectiveness of intervention

The correction of dietary deficiency by supplementation is obviously logical, but the population effectiveness of such action must be evaluated. In fact, whenever such an intervention is introduced, a parallel mechanism of surveillance and quality control is also required. In Switzerland a very successful programme was introduced as early as the 1920s. Despite this, significant percentages of both young and old hospital patients were still observed to have goitre in the 1960s—20 per cent and 60 per cent, respectively (Burgi and Rutishauser 1986). This was attributed to the low concentration of 5 mg of potassium iodide (KI) per kilo of salt, to an important decrease in salt consumption in many developed countries, and to the introduction of a non-iodinated luxury salt. As a consequence, the concentration of iodine was increased to 10 mg KI/kg in 1962 and to 20 mg KI/kg in 1977 (Figure 8.3). It is also interesting to note from this figure that sodium fluoride was also added to salt for the prophylaxis of dental caries (Wespi 1982).

The surveillance of iodinated salt prophylaxis has not only to include regular chemical determination of the iodine concentration at both salt producer and consumer levels but also measurements of goitre frequency in schoolchildren, the daily urinary excretion of iodine, and the range of radioiodine concentrations taken up by the thyroid; measured for diagnostic reasons in euthyroid patients (Thilly et al. 1973). New and simpler indices of iodine intake may also be needed (Bourdoux et al. 1985).

In developing countries, however, the cost of introducing iodized salt prophylaxis may have to include rationalization of the production and marketing of salt—which may be expensive or not feasible. The additional cost in the developed countries is only that of adding iodine to an existing industrial chain which is negligible (Thilly et al. 1986). Different authors (Demaeyer et al. 1979; Burgi and Rutishauser 1985) come to very similar cost estimates on the order of 2–5 US cents per capita per year. Thus for a country like the Federal Republic of Germany, the total cost per year would be on the order of 2 million dollars. By contrast, the costs caused by continuous iodine deficiency in Germany have been estimated, in 1981, at 700 million German marks per year (200 million dollars). These costs include the diagnostic expenses for out-patients, the surgical and life-long post-operative therapy, and lost working days (Pfannenstiel 1985). They do not include the economic and psychological costs linked to the large proportion of false-positive results in screening for congenital hypothyroidism at birth. There is thus no question that intervention is extremely cost-effective.

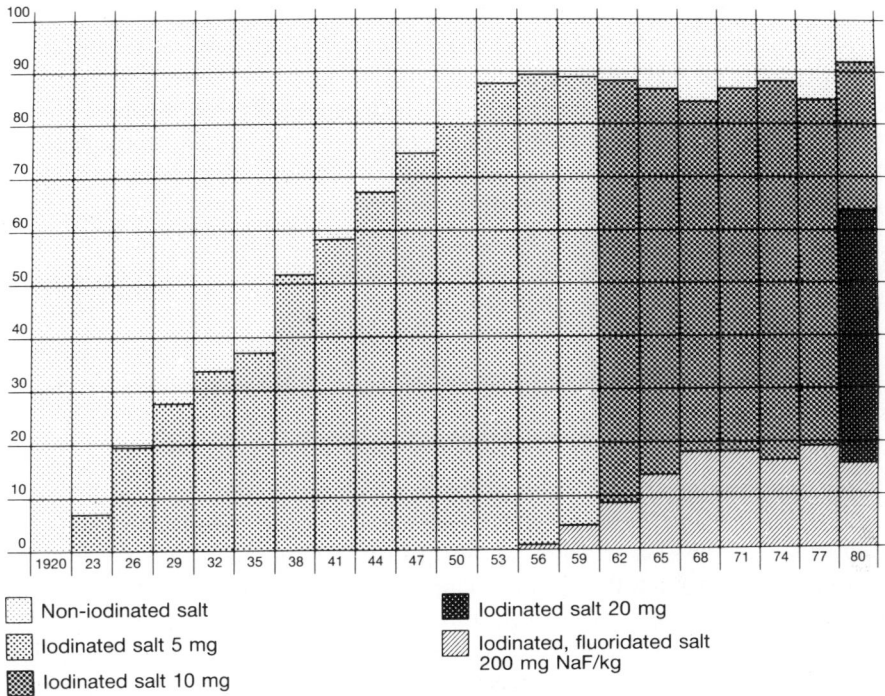

Fig. 8.3 Percentages of non-iodinated salt, of iodinated salt at different concentrations (5, 10 and 15 mg/kg), and of iodinated and fluoridated salt sold by the salines of Rhyn in Switzerland between 1920 and 1980.

Alternatives to iodization of table salt

In less developed areas or where sea salt is produced locally—for example, in many salt marshes in different parts of southern Europe—the introduction of generalized iodine salt prophylaxis may encounter different geographical, administrative, or political obstacles or constraints. As a consequence, alternative methods of supplementing the diet with iodine such as in water, tablets, chocolates, or baby foods have all been proposed as well as the intramuscular injection and oral administration of a supraphysiological dose of slowly resorbable iodinated oil every few years (Thilly *et al.* 1986). The latter method, however, has been restricted to severe goitre which only exists in a few pockets in Europe such as the area of Las Hurdes, where some iodized oil has indeed been used (Escobar del Rey 1981). Previous studies of the supplementation of water with iodine have generally reached the conclusion that it is uneconomical in view of the very small proportion (less than one per cent) of the water used for human drinking in the industrialized countries.

However, in Sicily, where salt iodization faces different obstacles, a very successful programme of iodinated water has been in progress for the last 5 years for the 40 000 inhabitants of Troina. Preliminary assessment of the costs of this programme, undertaken in an area where severe goitre was still present, suggests that they are quite low, on the order of 5 US cents per capita per year (Filetti *et al.* 1985). It is possible that in other special circumstances, other alternative methods of iodine prophylaxis, such as the oral use of iodinated oil, may be of value as complementary measures. For instance, for patients for whom a low salt diet is prescribed for long periods, an alternative source of iodine would be advisable.

Constraints in achieving disease elimination and recommendations

In view of the significant health problem which iodine deficiency still represents in Europe and the ease, effectiveness, and low cost of iodinated salt prophylaxis, it is quite surprising that most of the inhabitants of Europe are still having a sub-normal iodine intake. The reasons are many. Apart from iodine prophylaxis, food diversification and improved nutritional status already increase iodine intake. Goitre is thus perceived as a self-limiting disease, and it does tend to disappear with increasing urbanization and better transportation. However, this may not be a general phenomenon as there are still areas in Europe today where intermediate iodine deficiency is present. The need for supplementation in such populations has not diminished. Indeed the current trend towards reducing salt intake in the developed countries may reduce the effectiveness of salt iodization programmes.

There is also anxiety about possible harmful effects of iodization. In the nineteenth century and more recently in Tasmania (Connolly *et al.* 1970), cases of thyrotoxicosis resulting from iod-Basedow were undoubtedly linked to the introduction of the iodine prophylaxis. However, this syndrome is transient and the number of cases is very small. Cases are also easily diagnosed and treated.

In comparison with the United States, where many additives, vitamin supplements, and iodine have been actively introduced into the diet over the last 30 years, Europe has had a much more ambivalent and conservative attitude, and, perhaps, even hostility against such action. This psychological attitude is difficult to fight which is why recent proposals for the introduction of fluoride into drinking water to combat dental caries have failed (Wespi 1982). In the case of fluoride, however, the margin between deficiency and excess is indeed relatively narrow. With iodine, the prophylactic range is quite large. In the United States, some concern has recently been expressed concerning excessive iodine intake. Higher frequencies of thyrotoxicosis and

Hashimoto thyroiditis (Barsano et al. 1982) have been related to it, although these data have yet to be confirmed. More important is the fact that the average iodine intake in the United States has increased, for non-dietetic reasons, to 0.5 to 2 mg of iodine per day. This is five to twenty times higher than is usual in Europe so there is still a very good case for iodine prophylaxis. It is also known that the exceptional cases of iodide goitre with or without hypothyroidism in neonates, and probably also iod-Basedow and other rare complications of iodine excess, are more common in subjects with previous iodine deficiency. This is again a strong argument in favour of prophylaxis, but, in the developed countries, surveillance of both iodine deficiency and excess must be suggested (Thilly et al. 1986).

The main reasons for the failure to introduce effective iodine prophylaxis in the EEC are largely administrative and political in nature. They are linked to the lack of communication between endocrinologists, who see the diseases in their clinics, and the health authorities, legislators, and salt producers, who have to initiate and direct the preventive action. They are linked to the federal structure of the EEC and some of the countries themselves. The implementation of an efficient control programme implies a multisectorial approach with specialists from different disciplines grouped in a sufficiently active and powerful committee. The political willingness is also needed in order to help pass legislation. On the political level, a strong positive argument is the reduction, described above for Germany, in the very large amounts of money currently spent on screening, diagnosis, and treatment of iodine deficiency thyroid diseases in comparison with the negligible cost of prophylaxis. More studies on the cost-effectiveness of iodine prophylaxis, especially in the developed countries, are, however, needed. There is thus no valid argument against the rapid introduction and strengthening of iodine prophylaxis in Europe. In view of the significant health consequences of iodine deficiency still present today, there is no excuse not to undertake this as a priority. In the developed countries, iodine prophylaxis has been shown to be always effective and its future success is thus unquestionable. The elimination of iodine deficiency disorders (IDD) in Europe over the next few years may help to persuade public health authorities to increase their willingness to introduce control measures aimed at other nutritional diseases.

References

Barsano, C., Skosey, C., De Groot L.J., and Refetoff, S. (1982). Serum thyroglobulin in the management of patients with thyroid cancer. *Arch. Intern. Med.* **142**, 763–7.

Beckers, C., Cornette, C., Georgoulis, A., Souvatzoglou, A., Sfontouris, J., and Koutras, D.A. (1981). The effects of mild iodine deficiency on neonatal thyroid function. *Clin. Endocrinol.* **14**, 295–9.

Bleichrodt, N., Garcia, I., Rubio, C., Morreale de Escobar, G., and Escobar Del Rey, F. (1986). Mental and motor development of children from an iodine deficient area. In *Iodine deficiency disorders and congenital hypothyroidism* (eds G. Meideiros-Neto, R.M.B. Maciel, and A. Halpern) pp. 65-74. Ache, San Paulo.

Bourdoux, P., Delange, F., Filetti, S., Thilly, C., and Ermans, A.M. (1985). Reliability of the iodine/creatinine ratio:a myth? In *Thyroid disorders associated with iodine deficiency and excess* (eds R. Hall and J.K. Kobberling) pp. 145-52. Raven Press, New York.

Burgi, H. and Rutishauser, R. (1986). Iodization of salt and its surveillance. In *Towards the eradication of endemic goitre, cretinism and iodine deficiency* (eds J. Dunn, E. Pretell, C. Daza, and F. Viteri) pp. 155-69. Pan American Health Organization, Washington DC.

Connolly, R.J., Vidor, G.I., and Stewart, J.C. (1970). Increase in thyrotoxicosis in endemic goitre area after iodation of bread. *Lancet* **1**, 500-2.

Delange, F., Heidemann, P., Bourdoux, P., Larson, A., Vigneri, R., Klett, M., Beckers, C., and Stubbe, P. (1986). Regional variations of iodine nutrition and thyroid function during the neonatal period in Europe. *Biol. Neon.* **49**, 322-30.

Demaeyer, E.M., Lowenstein, F.W., and Thilly, C.H. (1979). *The control of endemic goitre*. World Health Organization, Geneva.

Escobar Del Rey, F., Gomez-Pan, A., Obregon, M.J., Mallol, J., Arnao, M.D.R., Aranda, A., and Morreale de Escobar, G. (1981). A survey of schoolchildren from a severe endemic goiter area in Spain. *Quart. J. Med.* **198**, 233-46.

Filetti, S., Squatrito, S., and Vigneri, R. (1985). Iodine supplementation by methods other than iodized salt. In *Thyroid disorders associated with iodine deficiency and excess* (eds R. Hall and J.K. Kobberling) pp. 95-110. Raven Press, New York.

Heidemann, P. and Stubbe, P. (1978). Serum 3, 5, 3'—triiodothyronine, thyroxine and thyrotropin in hypothyroid infants with congenital goitre and the response to iodine. *J. Clin. Endocrinol. Metab.* **47**, 189-92.

Hetzel, B.S. (1983). Iodine deficiency disorders (IDD) and their eradication. *Lancet* **2**, 1126-9.

Horster, F.A., Klusman, G., and Wildmeister, W.W. (1975) Der Kopf: eine endemische Krankheit in der Bundesrepublik? *Deutsch. Med. Wochenschr.* **100**, 8-9.

Lamberg, B.A. (1985). Effectiveness of iodized salt in various parts of the world. In *Thyroid disorders associated with iodine deficiency and excess* (eds R. Hall and J.K. Kobberling) pp. 81-94. Raven Press, New York.

Muzzo, S., Leiva, L., and Carrasco, D. (1986). Influence of a moderate iodine deficiency upon intellectual coefficient of schoolage children. In *Iodine deficiency disorders and congenital hypothyroidism* (eds G. Medeiros-Neto, R.M.B. Maciel, and A. Halpern) pp. 40-5. Ache, San Paulo.

Pfannenstiel, P. (1985). Direct and indirect costs caused by continuous iodine deficiency. In *Thyroid disorders associated with iodine deficiency and excess* (eds R. Hall and J.K. Kobberling) pp. 447-53. Raven Press, New York.

Sava, L., Delange, F., Belfiore, A., Purrello, F., and Vigneri, R. (1984). Transient impairment of thyroid function in newborn from an area of endemic goiter. *J. Clin. Endocrinol. Metab.* **59**, 90-5.

Scriba, P.C., Beckers, C., Burgi, H., Escobar del Rey, F., Gembicki, M., Koutras,

D.A., Lamberg, B.A., Langer, P., Lazarus, J.H., Querido, A., and Thilly, C. (1985). Goitre and iodine deficiency in Europe. Report of the subcommittee for the study of endemic goitre and iodine deficiency of the European Thyroid Association. *Lancet* **1**, 1289-93.

Squatrito, S., Delange, F., Trimarchi, F.S., Lisi, E., and Vigneri, R. (1981). Endemic cretinism in Sicily. *J. Endocrinol. Invest.* **4**, 295-302.

Thilly, C.H., Ramioul, L., and Ermans, A.M. (1973). A collaborative study on the geographical variations of thyroidal uptake in normal subjects of Europe. *Europ. J. Clin. Invest.* **3**, 272.

——, Bourdoux, P., Vanderpas, J., Mafuta, M., Berquist, H., Due, D., Le, M., Delange, F., and Ermans, A.M. (1985). Epidemiology and prophylaxis of endemic goiter in developing countries. In *Thyroid disorders associated with iodine deficiency and excess* (eds R. Hall and J.K. Kobberling) pp. 45-59. Raven Press, New York.

——, —— Swennen, B., Lagasse, R., Luvivila, K., Deckx, H., and Ermans, A.M. (1986). Overall worldwide strategy of goiter control. In *Towards the eradication of endemic goiter cretinism and iodine deficiency* (eds J. Dunn, E. Pretell, C. Daza, and F. Viteri) pp. 130-54. Pan American Health Organization, Washington DC.

Wespi, H.J. (1982). Die Salzjodierung als Vorlofer der Salzfluoridierung. *Schweiz Mschr. Zahnheilk.* **92**, 273-89.

9
Iron deficiency

Peter C. Elwood

SUMMARY
Definitions of iron deficiency and of anaemia are difficult as they are usually based on arbitrary 'lower limits of normal' for variables which are continuously distributed between very wide limits. The most common variable used in such definitions is the circulating haemoglobin concentration, but haematocrit, serum ferritin, and other variables have been used. More meaningful definitions have attempted to define disease in terms of morbidity or impaired function. Studies which have used these have indicated that the prevalence of iron deficiency and of anaemia, of degrees which affect health or function, are probably low throughout Europe. Furthermore, although the evidence is very limited it seems likely that prevalence rates in the general community are falling. A number of countries have introduced strategies for the reduction of iron deficiency by the fortification of foodstuffs with iron. None of these were adequately evaluated before they started and doubt lingers as to their effectiveness. Moreover the balance between costs and benefits of any national fortification programme is complicated by the possibility of iron overload developing in some individuals.

Defining the problem

Definition of anaemia and iron deficiency

Definitions of *anaemia* are usually dependent on the concentration of circulating haemoglobin in the peripheral circulation. For example, the World Health Organization (1972) has defined anaemia as the occurrence of a haemoglobin concentration below 120 g/l in adult, non-pregnant women, or below 130 g/l in adult males. Other criteria are appropriate for children and pregnant women, and other definitions have been proposed (Cavill 1982; Cavill *et al.* 1986).

The definition of *iron deficiency* is much more difficult. First, the focusing of attention on circulating haemoglobin ignores cause completely, and a microcytic and a macrocytic anaemia have nothing in common other than a low circulating haemoglobin concentration. At the same time the causes of macrocytic anaemia, generally a deficiency in B_{12} or folate, are relatively uncommon and so these are ignored in what follows in this chapter.

A more serious difficulty arises in the definition of iron deficiency because, although haemoglobin contains at least 60 per cent of the total body iron, iron stores in ferritin and haemosiderin constitute a major iron pool and these can be depleted without any effect on circulating haemoglobin concentration. The most useful single index of iron status is probably serum ferritin and the only cause of a low concentration is reduced reticulo-endothelial stores of iron (Cavill 1982). Degrees of iron deficiency which do not show in a reduced concentration of circulating haemoglobin will be detected by serum ferritin. While there is no agreed 'lower limit of normal' for serum ferritin, most authors seem to regard 120 μg/l as a diagnostic level (Cavill 1982; Cook et al. 1986).

However, the main difficulty that arises in the use of haemoglobin or serum ferritin concentrations in the definition of iron deficiency arises because the distribution of these, and all other haematological indices, have a continuous distribution, with only a slight negative skewness and kurtosis. Reference to a single concentration of any variable, implying as it does a dichotomy of subjects into 'normal' and 'anaemic' is therefore a procedure with limited clinical usefulness.

There have been several approaches to this problem. The most simple was perhaps that of Garby (1970) who determined the proportion of subjects in a community who responded to iron therapy by showing a rise in circulating haemoglobin (or haematocrit) on being given iron, whatever their initial concentration. He found that, in these terms, the prevalence of iron deficiency is about twice as high as that suggested by the simple application of the World Health Organization (WHO) criteria of anaemia and, moreover, many subjects with concentrations above the WHO criteria showed a rise, while many below did not. The other approach to this problem is to attempt to determine concentrations of haemoglobin which, on the basis of their association with indices of health and function, are clinically normal (Elwood 1970). This is a fundamental approach and, as the results of studies which have used this approach challenge the usual clinical concepts of iron deficiency as discussed later in the chapter, several other matters will be considered first.

Size of the problem

Prevalence of iron deficiency and differences between countries

The prevalence of anaemia, as defined by the use of the WHO criteria, is probably low throughout Europe. There have been numerous surveys in separate countries and it would be difficult to review all of these adequately.

One study is, however, of special interest in the context of this book as this attempted to look at a number of countries (Elwood et al. 1976). Haematological surveys of adult population samples were conducted simultaneously in twelve countries. Haematological estimations on samples from nine of the countries were made in one central laboratory. Differences in the mean concentrations of haemoglobin between countries were found to be relatively small, and the prevalence of concentrations below the arbitrary WHO criteria for anaemia was, on the whole, low. In males, the data showed a fall in haemoglobin concentration throughout adult life, and the fall increased slightly in advanced age. In females, there was no evidence of any important relationship between age and haemoglobin concentration, though, in the elderly, there may have been a slight fall. Tables 9.1 and 9.2 and Figure 9.1 summarize some of the data from this study and suggest that overall the prevalence of anaemia, using the WHO criteria for circulating haemoglobin concentration, is around 1–4 per cent in men and around 4–7 per cent in women.

Little epidemiological work on serum ferritin seems to have been reported. Table 9.3 contains a summary of some unpublished data from a random sample of subjects in a defined area in Wales. Judged by haemoglobin concentrations (WHO criteria) the prevalence of anaemia in this population was 4.8 per cent in males and 9.6 per cent in females, whereas only 1.6 per cent and 7.4 per cent had serum ferritin concentrations below 120 µg/l. The

Table 9.1 Males: mean haemoglobin concentrations (SD) and prevalence of anaemia (using WHO criteria) in representative population samples.

	Number in survey	Mean Hb (SD) (g/l)	Prevalence of anaemia (%)
Wales			
<65 yr	326	155 (11.5)	4.5
65 yr +	71	145 (16.4)	
Finland			
<65 yr	182	156 (16.0)	1.0
65 yr +	17	155 (10.0)	
Norway			
<65 yr	161	150 (10.7)	3.1
65 yr +	39	144 (10.3)	
Poland			
<65 yr	87	159 (14.7)	1.1

Source: Elwood et al. (1976).

Iron deficiency

Table 9.2 Females: mean haemoglobin concentrations (SD) and prevalence of anaemia (using WHO criteria) in representative population samples.

	Number in survey	Mean Hb (SD) (g/l)	Prevalence of anaemia (%)
Wales			
<65 yr	670	137 (12.9)	6.9
65 yr +	188	135 (15.6)	
Finland			
<65 yr	138	140 (15.9)	7.0
65 yr +	19	143 (1.93)	
Norway			
<65 yr	208	135 (10.2)	5.8
65 yr +	30	137 (7.4)	
Poland			
<65 yr	133	144 (18.5)	3.8

Source: Elwood *et al.* (1976).

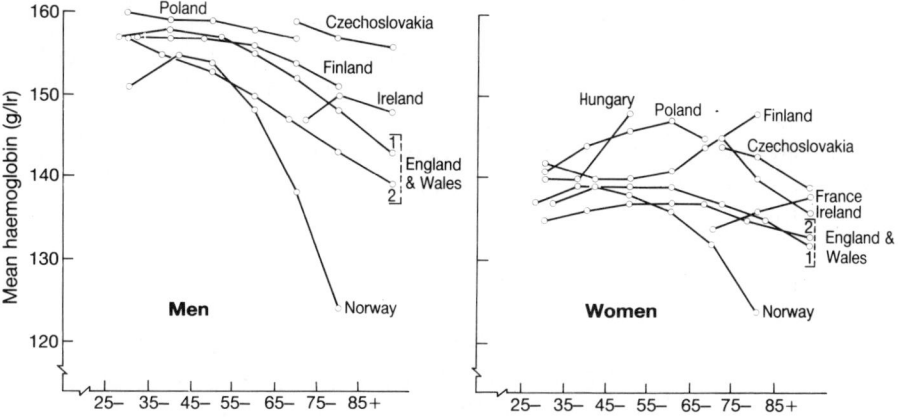

Fig. 9.1 Mean haemoglobin concentrations, by age, in representative samples of subjects in various countries. (Source: Elwood *et al.* 1976.)

correlation ('r') between haemoglobin concentration and serum ferritin was 0.25 ($p < 0.001$). In the subjects judged to be anaemic according to the WHO haemoglobin standards, the mean concentrations of serum ferritin were considerably lower (88 µg/l in males, and 26 µg/l in females) than the overall mean concentrations shown in Table 9.3.

The largest study of serum ferritin to date was based on 2829 of the subjects

Table 9.3 Haematological indices (SD) in a random sample of adult subjects in South Wales (unpublished data).

Variable	Males ($N = 211$): mean (SE)	Females ($N = 124$): mean (SE)
Age (yr)	47 (15.4)	48 (17.4)
Haemoglobin (g/l)	147 (10.2)	133 (11.1)
Haematocrit (%)	43.3 (3.20)	39.7 (3.45)
Serum ferritin (μg/l)[a]	129.8 (116–146)	51.4 (43–62)

[a]The distribution of serum ferritin shows gross positive skew so the geometric means and the 95 per cent probability ranges are shown.

seen in the second National Health and Nutrition Examination Survey (NHANES II) in the United States (Cook et al. 1986). A complex sampling procedure, based on clinical criteria, was used to select subjects for estimation of serum ferritin, and then statistical procedures were used to weight the results and reconstruct distributions appropriate for the general population. While this introduces some uncertainties into the eventual conclusions, these are probably small and the eventual estimates of frequency of deficiencies are likely to be too high rather than too low. The mean serum ferritin concentration in men and women (18–64 years of age) were remarkably close to those shown in Table 9.3, namely 113.0 μg/l and 52.2 μg/l. From these data it was estimated that the prevalence of iron deficiency in the United States was 0.2 per cent in men, 2.6 per cent in pre-menopausal women, and 1.9 per cent in post-menopausal women.

Trends over time

Trends over time are exceedingly difficult to examine because of changes in the selection of subjects in different studies, changes in laboratory methods, and drift within laboratories. The first of these difficulties can be overcome by random sampling of defined communities, and the others can be minimized by the use of standards and quality control techniques within laboratories.

Table 9.4 contains a summary of data from random samples drawn in closely adjacent communities in the South Wales industrial valleys (Elwood et al. 1967; Waters et al. 1969; Caerphilly and Speedwell Collaborative Group 1984). Strict quality control, based on the use of internationally approved haemoglobinometry standards, was exercised in the laboratories in which these estimations were done. Although some uncertainties about estimations made at different times remain, the data give no evidence of any

Table 9.4 Haemoglobin concentration and prevalence of anaemia[a]: a comparison of two surveys in random population samples of adults from similar areas in South Wales.

	Males		Females	
	1968[b]	1980[c]	1967[d]	1984[c]
Numbers of subjects	406	2472	1080	216
Haemoglobin (g/l)	156	154	134	137
(SD)	(13.6)	(11.5)	(16.0)	(12.0)
Prevalence of anaemia (%)	3.0	1.8	11.1	5.6

[a]WHO criteria.
[b]See Waters et al. (1969).
[c]See Caerphilly and Speedwell Collaborative Group (1984).
[d]See Elwood et al. (1967).

important change in mean concentrations. There is, however, some evidence of a reduction over time in the scatter of individual results around the overall mean, and this is confirmed by the fact that the prevalence of concentrations below the WHO criteria fell markedly both in males and in females.

Hallberg and his colleagues (1979) also examined changes in the distribution of haemoglobin concentrations over time in women in Goteborg, Sweden. Their data suggest that the mean haemoglobin concentration around 1963 to 1966 was around 125 g/l whereas in 1974–75 it was around 135 g/l. The prevalence of anaemia, using the WHO criteria, fell from 25–30 per cent in the 1960s to around 7 per cent in 1974–75.

Unfortunately there are very few data like these for other areas so generalizations to other countries cannot be made with any confidence.

Risk factors and vulnerable groups

Apart from the first 10 years of life, the mean haemoglobin concentration is significantly higher in males than in females (Elwood et al. 1976). Following an initial dramatic fall after birth, the haemoglobin concentration rises steadily during childhood. After adolescence, mean haemoglobin concentrations remain remarkably steady throughout adult life. There is, however, a steady fall in males which is probably physiological as most males have considerable iron stores at post-mortem examination (Charlton et al. 1970). In women mean haemoglobin concentrations are about 20 g/l lower than in males, and there is very little change with age, other than perhaps a slight fall at advanced ages (Elwood et al. 1976). It is often stated that anaemia is common in women of childbearing years and in the elderly of both sexes. The epidemiological evidence gives remarkably little support to such statements, and a fall in mean concentrations seems to occur only at very advanced ages. Other groups which are believed to be especially vulnerable to anaemia are immigrants from Third World countries, but one cannot generalize because these do not represent a homogeneous population, and, while some studies have detected a high prevalence of low haemoglobin concentrations in immigrant groups (Elwood et al. 1972), others have not (Britt et al. 1971).

It is in young children that there are the greatest uncertainties about iron deficiency. A recent report from Bradford in England (Erhardt 1986) stated that 12 per cent of white children and 28 per cent of Asian children between 6 and 48 months of age had haemoglobin concentration below 110 g/l on admission to hospital. However data such as these are of little value because children admitted to hospital do not remotely represent the general population.

Clinical interpretation of measures of iron status

Clinical impressions of anaemia differ greatly from those derived from epidemiological investigations based on representative population samples. This is undoubtedly because patients who consult a doctor and who are found to be anaemic are either severely affected, or have either complications or a more severe underlying condition. Ultimately, the importance of a condition must be judged from direct measurements of its effects on health and function. Appropriate studies are difficult, but those which have been done indicate that anaemia of degrees which impair health is rare (Elwood 1970; Elwood et al. 1971; Cook et al. 1986).

Any lowering of haemoglobin concentration will reduce the oxygen-carrying capacity of the blood. It is reasonable, therefore, to expect anaemia to cause symptoms such as fatigue, breathlessness, dizziness, and palpitations. Yet these symptoms are all rather non-specific and occur to some extent in almost all subjects. Anaemia is likely therefore to be frequently used as a scapegoat to explain such symptoms or general malaise, particularly in women or elderly patients. Yet surveys based on representative population samples have failed to detect a significant association between symptoms and circulating haemoglobin concentration (Elwood et al. 1969). Furthermore, randomized controlled trials of the effect of treatment have given evidence suggestive of benefit in terms of an improvement in symptoms only when anaemia is fairly severe, say, around 80 or 90 g/l or lower. Other effects of anaemia, such as cardiac failure, can occur but these too are almost certainly a consequence of a very severe reduction in haemoglobin concentration and are therefore rare.

An association between haemoglobin concentration and work output has been described. Early work in this context was laboratory-based and, although some evidence emerged indicating that circulating haemoglobin concentration could be a limiting factor, it appeared that this only operated at maximal, or near maximal, work outputs (Viteri and Torun 1974). More recent work in real-life situations in developing communities based on sugar workers in Guatemala, latex tappers in Java, weeders in Indonesia, and tea pickers in Sri Lanka (Edgerton et al. 1979) has suggested a beneficial effect from iron therapy. Any relevance of this work to European communities is, however, unlikely because of the very different haematological and general nutritional state throughout Europe.

Another possible effect of iron deficiency, and one which could be of enormous importance, is on behaviour and on mental performance in children. While there is evidence that such effects can occur and that they can be removed by iron therapy (Pollitt et al. 1985; Soemantri et al. 1985; Addy 1986), almost all the relevant studies which have been reported have been based on highly selected groups and have been conducted under laboratory-like conditions. Furthermore, most of the work has been done in developing countries where multiple dietary deficiencies are common. Clearly further epidemiological surveys and randomized controlled trials are urgently needed within Western communities.

In any assessment of the importance of anaemia, associations which suggest beneficial effects must be considered, and possible harmful effects of a high haemoglobin concentration should not be ignored. There are a number of such associations and, while none of these have been adequately worked out, they do merit careful consideration. They include a possible advantage of a low haemoglobin concentration in relation to cardiovascular disease and a raised mortality in subjects with high haemoglobin concentrations (Waters et al. 1969; Elwood et al. 1974; Campbell et al. 1985). Other findings include a greater frequency of electrocardiographic abnormalities in patients with iron overload, a positive correlation between haemoglobin and cholesterol concentrations, and a greater number of coronary anastamoses, or links between major coronary vessels, in anaemic subjects. Other studies have demonstrated beneficial associations of low haemoglobin concentrations with cerebral blood flow (Thomas et al. 1977; Humphrey et al. 1979), wound healing in diabetic patients (Bailey et al. 1979), and the incidence of hypertension and pre-eclamptic toxaemia in pregnancy (Murphy et al. 1986).

An overall assessment of the importance to health of a condition such as anaemia can be obtained from long-term follow-up studies in which haemoglobin concentration is related to subsequent mortality. Several studies have identified raised haemoglobin concentrations as an independent risk factor for ischaemic heart disease (Waters et al. 1969; Cullen et al. 1981; Sorlie et al. 1981). Others have either failed to detect an association, or if one has been found, it has been accounted for by other risk factors such as raised blood pressure, serum cholesterol, or smoking (McDonough et al. 1965; Abu-Zeid and Chapman 1976; Carter et al. 1983; Szatrowski et al. 1984). Although,

Table 9.5 Haemoglobin (g/l) and haematocrit (%) and mortality over the subsequent 11 years in a representative sample of adult women in South Wales[a].

	Number of women	Died (%)
Cause of death: ischaemic heart disease		
Haemoglobin: over 140	190	7.9
under 140	673	3.9
Haematocrit: over 45	150	9.3
under 45	708	3.8
Cause of death: cancer		
Haemoglobin: over 120	899	3.4
under 120	187	8.6
Haematocrit: over 40	832	2.3
under 40	249	11.2

[a]Data for ischaemic heart disease are limited to women who had had no angina at the start of the follow-up period.
Source: Campbell et al. (1985).

therefore, the effect may be indirect, through other risk factors, an association of haemoglobin concentration above 140 g/l with mortality from ischaemic heart disease is certainly marked (Table 9.5). Table 9.5 also shows conversely that there is a relationship between cancer deaths and low haemoglobin concentration (<120 g/l) measured previously. To some extent this must be because women with cancer become anaemic. However, a detailed examination of these data gave evidence that the predictive power of haemoglobin concentration for death by cancer did not diminish significantly with time and an excess risk was still apparent 11 years after the estimation of haemoglobin concentration. This relationship has been observed in other studies (Cullen *et al.* 1983), but its relevance, if any, to community aspects of iron deficiency and to food fortification programmes is unknown.

There is another aspect of iron balance which is relevant to attempts to eliminate iron deficiency by strategies which aim to increase the iron intakes of a total community by the fortification of foodstuffs with iron. This is the chance of promoting iron overload in some subjects. In most subjects unwanted iron will remain unabsorbed and will leave the body in the faeces. In cases of manifest or latent haemochromatosis primary iron overload may occur. The prevalence of haemochromatosis may be low, but in alcoholism, which seems to be occurring with increasing frequency throughout the developed world, iron absorption is enhanced and secondary iron overload can occur (Barry *et al.* 1968; Charlton *et al.* 1970). The balance between the risks of a fortification programme to some individuals and the benefits to others is, therefore, pure conjecture.

More recently, Cook *et al.* (1986) warn that in certain segments of the population the homozygous state for hereditary haemochromatosis is now more common than iron deficiency anaemia. This statement could be challenged on the grounds that the proportion of the population who might derive some advantage from iron added to foods is unknown and estimates range from 2 per cent (Crosby 1977) to 56 per cent (Dallman 1977). Nevertheless, the implications of all this for national programmes to fortify foodstuffs with iron are very serious and far-reaching.

Intervention

Proposals for intervention assume that a need has been demonstrated. In iron deficiency it is doubtful if a case can be made for generalized preventive measures in any European country. However certain aspects of the situation merit more detailed consideration.

Treatment and follow-up

The identification of patients with anaemia and the correction of their deficiency with iron medication is part of modern clinical practice. This is reasonable provided the clinician remembers that iron deficiency in patients who present themselves to a doctor may be a consequence of a serious underlying condition (Cahill *et al.* 1986). At the same time, the number of treatable underlying conditions which are uncovered after population screening for anaemia is probably far too small to justify any screening procedure (Elwood *et al.* 1967).

Infants and young children merit special consideration because iron deficiency may well be of importance in relation to normal growth and development. Case detection of anaemia in normal clinical practice should also be very efficient because of the frequency with which infants and young children are seen by doctors and paramedical workers. If any general measure directed to children is proposed then surveys to determine prevalence, and randomized controlled trials of the effects of the preventive measures proposed, should first be conducted. However, paediatricians themselves have expressed doubts about the advantages of any generalized measure directed towards children (Burman 1972; Addy 1986).

Population strategy: food fortification

As a preventive measure directed at the general community it is the practice in a number of countries to add iron to flour, or to bread and other products of flour (Ministry of Health 1968). In the United Kingdom there has been a policy, since 1952, to 'restore' the amount of iron and several other nutrients in white flour to that which naturally occurs in a high extraction (80 per cent) flour. On the other hand the policy in the USA, Sweden, and certain other countries is one of 'fortification'—that is, amounts of iron are added to flour (or to bread and other products of white flour) which take the eventual concentration of iron above that which occurs naturally. In Sweden this policy of fortification is pursued with remarkable enthusiasm—in the United Kingdom 1.85 mg of iron is added to every kilogram of flour, while 65 mg per kilogram is added in Sweden!

The evidence of an effect of this added iron on iron balance is not convincing. Hallberg (1979) attempted, retrospectively, to attribute the fall in the prevalence of iron deficiency in women in Sweden over a decade to the fortification of flour with iron together with changes in other factors likely to be relevant to iron balance, such as the taking of oral contraceptives. He judged that out of an overall improvement in the iron status of women of 20–25 per cent, about 7–8 per cent could be attributed to iron fortification of flour. However, randomized controlled trials of iron restoration at or around the UK level failed to give any convincing evidence of benefit (Elwood *et al.* 1971; Gershoff *et al.* 1977).

The value of iron fortification of foodstuffs is also questioned in a study of several European countries with differing food fortification practices (Elwood and Barasi 1979). Despite very marked differences in dietary iron intakes, there appears to be a remarkably similar prevalence of anaemia (Table 9.6).

Conclusions

Evidence from population studies indicates that iron deficiency, of a severity which is of clinical importance, is uncommon. The identification and treatment of affected patients is part of normal clinical practice. While doubts arise as to the overall benefit of this, it is probably worthwhile provided the clinician remembers that a low concentration of circulating haemoglobin can be a consequence of serious underlying disease.

Evidence on prevalence and on clinical importance indicates that screening for iron deficiency cannot be justified. Furthermore, there is no convincing evidence of benefit from any procedure aimed at increasing the dietary iron intakes of a Western community.

Table 9.6 Estimates of iron supply and the prevalence of anaemia in some European countries in 1977.

	Sweden	Denmark	England and Wales
Natural food iron mg/person/day	19	19	14
Fortification iron mg/person/day	6.5	5	1.6
Tablet iron mg/person/day	6.6	2.7	2.0
Total iron intake mg/person/day	32	27	18
Percentage of subjects anaemic:			
Women < 120 g/l	7	8	7
Men < 130 g/l	6	6	6

Source: Elwood and Barasi (1979).

References

Abu-Zeid, H.A.H. and Chapman, J. (1976). The relation between haemoglobin level and the risk for ischaemic heart disease. A prospective study. *J. Chron. Dis.* **29**, 395–403.

Addy, D.P. (1986). Happiness is: iron. *Br. Med. J.* **292**, 969–70.

Bailey, M.J., Johnston, C.L.W., Yates, C.J.P., Somerville, P.G., and Dormandy, J.A. (1979). Preoperative haemoglobin as predictor of outcome of diabetic amputations. *Lancet* **2**, 168–70.

Barry, M., Scheuer, P.J., Sherlock, S., Ross, C.F., and Williams, R. (1968). Hereditary spherocytosis with secondary haemochromatosis. *Lancet* **2**, 481–5.

Britt, R.P., Harper, C., and Spray, G.H. (1971). Megaloblastic anaemia among Indians in Britain. *Quart. J. Med.* **40**, 499–520.

Burman, D. (1972). Haemoglobin levels in normal infants aged 3 to 24 months, and the effect of iron. *Arch. Dis. Child.* **47**, 261–71.

Caerphilly and Speedwell Collaborative Group (1984). Caerphilly and Speedwell collaborative heart disease studies. *J. Epidemiol. Comm. Hlth* **38**, 259–62.

Cahill, C.J., Pain, J.A., and Bailey, M.E. (1986). Gastrointestinal investigation of iron deficiency anaemia. *Br. Med. J.* **293**, 269.

Campbell, M.J., Elwood, P.C., MacKean, J., and Waters, W.E. (1985). Mortality, haemoglobin level and haematocrit in women. *J. Chron. Dis.* **38**, 881–9.

Carter, C., McGee, D., Reed, D., Yano, K., and Stemmerman, G. (1983). Haematocrit and the risk of coronary heart disease: the Honolulu Heart Program. *Am. Heart J.* **105**, 674–9.

Cavill, I. (1982). Diagnostic methods. *Clin. Haematol.* **11**, 259–73.

——, Jacobs, A., and Worwood, M. (1986). Diagnostic methods of iron status. *Ann. Clin. Biochem.* **23**, 168–71.

Charlton, R.W., Hawkins, D.M., Mavor, W.O., and Bothwell, T.H. (1970). Hepatic storage iron concentrations in different population groups. *Am. J. Clin. Nutr.* **23**, 358–71.

Cook, J.D., Skikne, B.S., Lynch, S.R., and Reusser, M.E. (1986). Estimates of iron sufficiency in the US population. *Blood* **68**, 726-31.

Crosby, W.H. (1977). Current concepts in nutrition. Who needs iron? *New Engl. J. Med.* **297**, 543-5.

Cullen, K.J., Stenhouse, N.S., and Wearne, K.L. (1981). Raised haemoglobin and risk of cardiovascular disease. *Lancet* **4**, 1288-9.

——, ——, ——, and Welborn, T.A. (1983). Multiple regression analysis of risk factors for cardiovascular disease and cancer mortality in Busselton, Western Australia—13-year study. *J. Chron. Dis.* **36**, 371-7.

Dallman, P.R. (1977). Who needs iron? (letter). *New Engl. J. Med.* **297**, 1238-9.

Edgerton, V.R., Gardener, G.W., Ohira, Y, Gunawardena, K.A., and Senewiratne, B. (1979). Iron deficiency anaemia and its effect on worker productivity and activity patterns. *Br. Med. J.* **2**, 1546-9.

Ehrhardt, P. (1986). Iron deficiency in young Bradford children from different ethnic groups. *Br. Med. J.* **292**, 90-3.

Elwood, P.C. (1970). Some epidemiological aspects of iron deficiency relevant to its evaluation. *Proc. R. Soc. Med.* **63**, 1230-2.

—— and Barasi, M.E. (1979). Iron in flour—do we need it? *Nutr. Bull.* **5**, 98-103.

——, Burr, M.L., Hole, D., Harrison, A., Morris, T.K., Wilson C.I.D., Richardson, R.W., and Shinton, N.K. (1972). Nutritional state of elderly Asian and English subjects in Coventry. *Lancet* **1**, 1224-7.

——, Hughes, J., Abernethy, M., Davies, R., Gough, R., Johnson, A.P., and Dubourg, A.Y. (1976). An international haematological survey. *Bull. World Hlth Org.* **54**, 87-95.

——, Shinton, N.K., Wilson, C.I.D., Sweetnam, P.M., and Frazer, A.C. (1971). Haemoglobin, vitamin B_{12} and folate levels in the elderly. *Br. J. Haematol.* **21**, 557-63.

——, Waters, W.E., Benjamin, I.T., and Sweetnam, P.M. (1974). Mortality and anaemia in women. *Lancet* **1**, 891-4.

——, ——, Greene, W.J.W., and Sweetnam, P. (1969). Symptoms and circulating haemoglobin level. *J. Chron. Dis.* **21**, 615-28.

——, ——, ——, and Wood, M.M. (1967). Evaluation of a screening survey for anaemia in adult non-pregnant women. *Br. Med. J.* **4**, 714-7.

——, ——, and Sweetnam, P. (1971). The haematinic effect of iron in flour. *Clin. Sci.* **40**, 31-7.

Garby, L. (1970). The normal haemoglobin level. *Br. J. Haematol.* **19**, 429-34.

Gershoff, S.N., Brusis, O.A., Niro, H.V., and Huber, A.M. (1977). Studies of the elderly in Boston. 1. The effects of iron fortification on moderately anaemic people. *Am. J. Clin. Nutr.* **30**, 226-34.

Hallberg, L., Bengtsson, C., Garby, L., Lennartsson, J., Rossander, L., and Tibblin, E. (1979). An analysis of factors leading to a reduction in iron deficiency in Swedish women. *Bull. World Hlth Org.* **57**, 947-54.

Humphrey, P.R.D., du Boulay, G.H., Marshall, J., Pearson, T.C., Ross Russell, R.W., Symon, L., Wetherley-Mein, G., and Zilkha, E. (1979). Cerebral blood-flow and viscosity in relative polycythaemia. *Lancet* **2**, 873-6.

McDonough, J.R., Homes, C.G., Garrison, G.E., Stulb, S.C., Lichtman, M.A., and Hefelfinger, D.C. (1965). The relationship of haematocrit to cardiovascular

states of health in the negro and white population of Evans County, Georgia. *J. Chron. Dis.* **18**, 243–57.
Ministry of Health. (1968). *Iron in flour*. Reports on Public Health & Medical Subjects No. 117. HMSO (Her Majesty's Stationery Office) London.
Murphy, J.F., O'Riordan, J., Newcombe, R.G., Coles, E.C., and Pearson, J.F. (1986). Relation of haemoglobin levels in first and second trimesters to outcome of pregnancy. *Lancet* **1**, 992–4.
Pollitt, E., Soemantri, A.G., Yunis, F., and Scrimshaw, N.S. (1985). Cognitive effects of iron-deficiency anaemia. *Lancet* **1**, 158.
Soemantri, A.G., Pollitt, E., and Kim, I. (1985). Iron deficiency and educational achievement. *Am. J. Clin. Nutr.* **42**, 1221–8.
Sorlie, P.D., Garcia-Palmieri, M.R., Costos, R., and Havlik, R. (1981). Haematocrit and risk of coronary heart disease: the Puerto Rico Heart Health Program. *Am. Heart J.* **101**, 456–61.
Szatrowski, T.P., Peterson, A.V., Shimizu, Y., Prentice, R.L., Mason, M.W., Fukunaga, Y., and Kuto, H. (1984). Serum cholesterol, other risk factors, and cardiovascular disease in a Japanese cohort. *J. Chron. Dis.* **37**, 569–84.
Thomas, D.J., du Boulay, G.H., and Marshall, J. (1977). Effect of haematocrit on cerebral blood flow in man. *Lancet* **2**, 941–3.
Viteri, F.E. and Torun, B. (1974). Anaemia and physical work capacity. *Clin. Haematol.* **3**, 609–26.
Waters, W.E., Withey, J.L., Kilpatrick, G.S., Wood, P.H.N., and Abernethy M. (1969). Ten-year haematological follow-up: mortality and haemotological changes. *Br. Med. J.* **4**, 761–4.
World Health Organization (WHO) (1972). *Nutritional anaemias*. Technical Report Series No. 503. WHO, Geneva.

10
Dental caries and periodontal disease

Martin Hobdell and Gerard Gavin

SUMMARY

Dental caries can be virtually eliminated. Dramatic strides in that direction have been made by most European countries in the past 10 to 15 years. However, this general reduction in prevalence has resulted in a wider variation than before between individuals in the intensity of dental caries experience. The residuum of dental caries will only be eliminated if countries adopt a combination of preventive programmes. Indeed those countries which have adopted planned preventive programmes for young children, using a variety of preventive measures, seem to be achieving more rapid decreases in dental caries prevalence than those with little planned activity or those relying on one preventive measure alone. Dental health education and a national nutrition policy which includes reduced sucrose consumption are pre-requisites to achieving further significant increases in the percentage of the population free from dental caries. The prevalence of chronic periodontal disease has declined in recent years in most European countries. It is not now thought to be a major threat to the preservation of a natural dentition throughout life for most individuals whose periodontal health improves with increased levels of oral cleanliness. For a small percentage of the population, however, it will be the major cause of tooth loss. The current level of understanding of this disease does not permit the development of public health programmes which will significantly alter the natural history of the disease for this small percentage of people.

Defining the problem

There have been considerable changes in the prevalence of dental caries in European Countries in the past 10 years. As recently as 1979 Sheiham stated that 'In industrialized countries the two major dental diseases, dental decay (caries) and gum (periodontal) disease, affect every man, woman, and child

... (they) are responsible for a great deal of pain, misery, inconvenience and economic loss'.

While the second part of this statement remains largely true for older population groups, because of the consequences of the earlier high prevalence rates for dental caries, much has changed to modify the first part. The dramatically improved dental health of the young in Europe suggests that there is now a real prospect for a sustained reduction of sizeable proportions within the foreseeable future in many European countries. The total elimination of dental caries, if present trends continue, will be a reality for an increasing percentage of the population. However, for some, more comprehensive preventive programmes than those currently employed will be necessary.

Historically, dental caries grew to be a problem in Europe during the midnineteenth century. Many studies have linked the prevalence of dental caries to the presence of substantial amounts of sucrose in the diet (Gustafsson 1954; Toverud 1957; Takeuchi 1961; Harris 1963; Geddes et al. 1978). Studies of caries prevalence in young European and Japanese populations before, during, and after the Second World War (Toverud 1957; Takeuchi 1961) suggest that limitation of sucrose in the diet is an effective way of controlling caries prevalence. Thus today in many developing countries, where there is a low level of sucrose consumption, the prevalence of dental caries is also low (Frencken et al. 1986; Manji et al. 1986).

The current situation, as far as it is known at a national level, is presented in Table 10.1 for the countries of the European Economic Community and in Table 10.2 for other European countries selected.

The two parameters presented in these Tables are the percentage of the 5–6-year-old population found to be free from dental caries and the mean total number of decayed, missing, and filled teeth (DMFT) at four ages. This latter index has been extensively used in the comparison of the intensity of dental caries experience in different populations (Klein and Palmer 1937; Klein et al. 1938). It is a progressive index and cannot be reversed. It therefore attempts to record past and present dental caries experience. There are, however, a number of shortcomings with the use of both parameters. The fundamental problem is the accurate definition of dental caries and a correspondingly accurate method of diagnosis. Although much has been done in recent years to standardize examiners and reduce inter-examiner variability, and also to simplify and increase the accuracy of the methods used, there is still a need for improvement (Robens Appeal 1986).

With respect to the consequences of dental caries included in the index—that is, the missing and filled teeth—there are also problems. Missing teeth may be missing for reasons other than advanced dental caries. Surprisingly, the reasons for filling teeth are not always explicit to the operator before work is started and the vagaries of treatment decisions made by

Table 10.1 Dental caries in countries of the EEC at different ages as measured by the mean decayed, missing, and filled tooth index.

Country	Caries-free rate (%) age 5–6 yr	Mean DMFT Age (yr)			
		12	18	35–44	65 +
Belgium	N/A	N/A	N/A	N/A	N/A
Denmark	54	3.4	10.7	22	27
France	N/A	3.4[a]	N/A	N/A	N/A
FRG	N/A	6.2	14.0	18.6[b]	N/A
Greece	N/A	N/A	N/A	N/A	N/A
Ireland	45[c]	2.9	N/A	18.8[b]	N/A
Italy	20	4.0	N/A	N/A	N/A
Luxembourg	N/A	N/A	N/A	N/A	N/A
Netherlands	55	2.4	N/A	19.6	22.8
Portugal	N/A	3.8	N/A	10.9	N/A
Spain	N/A	4.2	N/A	N/A	N/A
United Kingdom	52[d]	3.1[d]	N/A	N/A	N/A

Data from World Health Organization, Oral Health Unit, Copenhagen, based upon reports from Chief Dental Officers, and, where indicated, local and national epidemiological surveys.
[a]Cahen et al. 1982.
[b]Arnljot et al. 1985.
[c]Minister of Health, Ireland 1985.
[d]Todd and Dodd 1985.

practitioners are only now coming to light (Elderton and Nuttall 1983; HMSO 1986). At present these measures are the best available and the most widely used, but caution must be exercised in interpreting such data.

The age groupings selected in this chapter and presented in Tables 10.1 and 10.2 are chosen as they represent the age groups specifically mentioned in the six goals for oral health developed by the International Dental Federation and The World Health Organization to be achieved at the global level by the year 2000. Hence it is possible to measure the progress being made towards these goals by member states of the EEC and elsewhere in Europe. For convenience the FDI/WHO Global Goals are reproduced in Table 10.3 (Federation Dentaire Internationale 1982). As the data are more complete for 12-year-olds than any other group much of the rest of this chapter is built around this particular age group.

Table 10.2 Dental caries in non-EEC European countries at different ages as measured by the mean decayed, missing, and filled tooth index.

Country	Caries-free rate (%) age 5–6 yr	Mean DMFT age (yr)			
		12	18	35–44	65+
Austria	N/A	4.0	N/A	N/A	N/A
Bulgaria	19.8	4.5	10.6	N/A	N/A
Czechoslovakia	N/A	5.0	9.8	21.0	28.0
Finland	50	3.0	9.5	22.0	25.0
GDR	25	5.0	10.0	14.0	24.0
Malta	50	2.0	5.6	10.0	20.0
Norway	N/A	4.4	11.5	26.5[a]	N/A
Poland	25	5.1	N/A	21.5[a]	N/A
Sweden	46	3.4	8.0	N/A	N/A
Switzerland	N/A	3.0	N/A	20.0	N/A
USSR	55	3.5	6.0	12.5	N/A

Data from World Health Organization, Oral Health Unit, Copenhagen, based upon local and national epidemiological surveys.
[a]Arnljot et al. 1985.

Current trends

The data presented in Tables 10.1 and 10.2 are the most recently available figures for the countries listed. There are many omissions and not all the data relate to national surveys. There has been much recent interest in the documented improvements in oral health, not least because of the implications of such changes on the need for dentists and other types of oral health workers (Todd 1975; Kalsbeck 1982; von der Fehr 1982; Renson et al. 1985). Figures 10.1 and 10.2 show the size and rapidity of the changes achieved in a number of EEC and other countries. These data raise a number of issues.

First, dental caries, like many aspects of ill health (Davidson and Townsend 1982), is found to be related to social class (Silver 1982; Meyer et al. 1983). While reductions in caries prevalence have been found to a greater or lesser degree in all socio-economic groups, it is frequently the more affluent who have benefited most (Hansen et al. 1982; Bradnock et al. 1984). The net effect of this has, in a number of instances, been to lower the prevalence but increase the distribution of severity found within the population (Poulsen et al. 1982; French et al. 1984). This, however, does not imply that a significant further reduction in mean DMF score for an entire population group of 12-year-old children could be achieved by an individualized preventive programme aimed specifically at the high-risk individuals. The

Table 10.3 FDI/WHO global oral health goals for the year 2000.

Proposed global goals

With the expectation that each country will formulate its own sub-goals or targets, it is proposed that additional indicators of improved oral health be adopted and that they cover the young, the mature and the elderly. The following global goals for the year 2000 are proposed:

Goal 1 50 per cent of 5–6-year-olds will be caries free.

Goal 2 The global average will be no more than 3 DMF teeth at 12 years of age.

Goal 3 85 per cent of the population should retain all their teeth at the age of 18 years.

Goal 4 A 50 per cent reduction in present levels of edentulousness at the age of 35–44 years will be achieved.

Goal 5 A 25 per cent reduction in present levels of edentulousness at the age of 65 years and over will be achieved.

Goal 6 A data-based system for monitoring changes in oral health will be established.

---

reason is that such high-risk individuals form an increasingly small percentage of the total population (Poulsen *et al.* 1982).

Second, in order to appreciate the discussion in relation to the opportunities for a further improvement of dental health and, in particular, a further significant increase in those who remain caries-free, it is necessary to discuss the epidemiology of dental caries in a little more detail. In the past, when most European populations had high prevalences of dental caries, this affected the front teeth and the back teeth and both the biting surfaces (of the back teeth) and the smooth surfaces on the sides of the teeth, particularly where neighbouring teeth touch each other. The decay process is much the same although the bacteria may be different. Decay on the biting surfaces occurs where the bacteria can lurk in the crevices of fissures. On the smooth surfaces the bacteria collect in colonies beneath the point of contact of the adjacent teeth. Where caries prevalence is high—for example, above 4 DMFT—there are likely to be significant proportions of both fissure and smooth surface lesions. Once the score drops below this level fissure caries is the most significant proportion of all the lesions found. To date most preventive measures have concentrated on lowering the caries prevalence for whole populations and hence have been most effective in reducing the amount of smooth surface caries (Backer Dirks *et al.* 1961). As is seen in Figures 10.1 and 10.2 much has been achieved. What remains to be prevented, however, in most populations with relatively low mean DMFT scores is the fissure caries in the back teeth.

Dental caries and periodontal disease

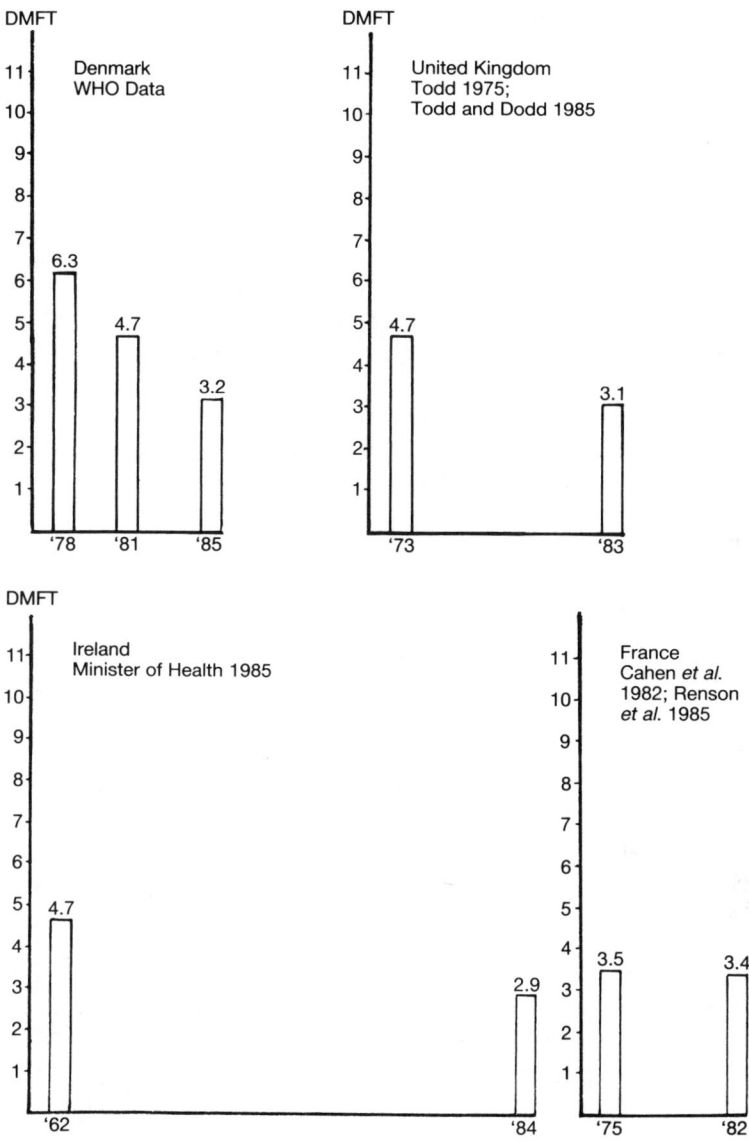

Fig. 10.1 Recent changes in 12-year-old mean DMFT scores.

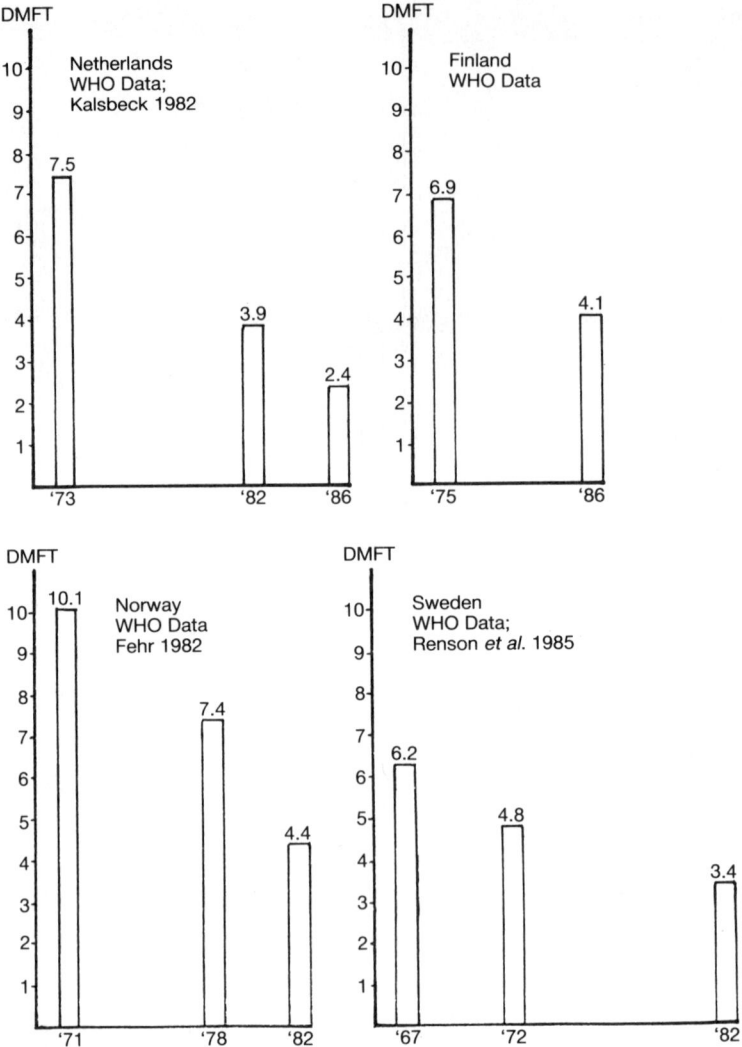

Fig. 10.2 Recent changes in 12-year-old mean DMFT scores.

Interventions

Before discussing the different methods of preventing dental caries it is necessary to describe the pathology of the disease. Like gum or periodontal disease which is discussed later, it develops in relation to the microbial plaque that is found on the teeth and gums.

Dental caries and periodontal disease

Dental caries is the softening and destruction of the tooth caused initially by the dissolution of the calcium salts that form the hard surface enamel of a tooth. The acid, produced by the bacteria that are commonly found in everyone's mouth, is the cause. The initial demineralization is then followed by the bacterial invasion and decomposition of the underlying dentine, which is richer in organic matter, chiefly collagen. This causes the tooth literally to rot away. Current programmes to prevent dental caries focus on two important aspects of the process described above.

Use of fluorides

First, the outer layer and in some programmes the entire substance of the teeth is made less soluble in acid and hence more resistant to attack by the incorporation of minute quantities of fluoride into the tooth substance. There are a number of therapeutic regimes by which the tooth surface can be exposed to fluoride ions. However, the mechanism by which it is incorporated into the tooth and by which it prevents dental caries is disputed. Historically, one of the first methods used in public health programmes was the fluoridation of piped water supplies (Arnold *et al.* 1953). Subsequently fluoridated salt (Toth 1973), fluoride tablets (Marthaler 1969), professionally applied topical fluoride applications (Bibby 1943; Horowitz and Doyle 1972), self-applied fluoride mouth-rinses (Rugg-Gunn *et al.* 1973), and fluoridated toothpaste (Marthaler 1968; Hodge *et al.* 1980; Beiswanger *et al.* 1981; Mainwaring and Naylor 1983) have been the principal methods used. Combinations of different methods have been shown to have additive effects (Heifitz *et al.* 1979). The approximate levels of reduction in dental caries prevalence achieved with these methods have been summarized by Horowitz (1980a) and are presented in Table 10.4. It should be stressed, however, that these data come largely from clinical trials conducted at a time when the prevalence of dental caries in the populations studied was relatively high. Also few of the studies, except perhaps those dealing with water fluoridation, relate to larger population groups.

The efficacy of fluoride supplementation to piped water supplies is greater than that of toothpaste (Table 10.4). However, very few water fluoridation schemes exist. Thus, if the dramatic reduction in dental caries is due to fluoride supplementation, this is more likely to result from toothpaste than from water, given the relatively wider population exposure to the former. An alternative hypothesis is that the improvement has occurred because of a reduction in the virulence of the principal micro-organism (*Streptococcus mutans*) responsible for dental caries. It is interesting to note that in the recent summary of world-wide water fluoridation programmes (Naylor and Murray 1983), of the four community studies that have specifically reported on the effects of fluoridation on 12-year-olds, after a mean of 12.75 years

Table 10.4 Approximate anticipated percentage reductions in dental caries using different fluoride regimes.

Regime	Reduction (%)
Piped water fluoridation	50
Fluoridated salt	50
Daily fluoride tablets (during tooth formation)	40
Mouth rinsing with fluoride solutions	30
Tooth cleaning with brush and fluoridated toothpaste	25

Table 10.5 Four studies reporting on the reduction in dental caries experience in 12-year-old children.

Location	Duration of fluoridation (yr)	Reduction (%)
Grand Junction USA	11	68
Albert Lea USA	14	53
Birmingham UK	13	45
Karl-Marx-Stadt GDR	13	66
Mean	12.75	58

there was a mean reduction in dental caries prevalence of 58 per cent (Table 10.5).

Other preventive methods

The second focus of programmes for the prevention of dental caries has been on the main aetiological factor, namely sucrose. Three approaches have been used—health education for groups and individuals (Health Education Council 1984), and at a national level the development of national nutrition policies (Health Education Council 1983), and fissure sealing (Rock and Evans 1982). This is the painting over of the fissures of the back teeth with rapidly setting resin.

Health education

Health education on dental caries has suffered some of the earlier deficiencies of health education in general. Many programmes concentrated solely on the provision of information that was often inaccurate or contradictory. This problem has been exacerbated because dental health education has often been given in isolation from general health education and other health-promoting activities. More recently attempts have been made to integrate dental health education with other programmes and to focus on educational techniques that will promote behavioural change (Beal 1983).

Nutrition policies

National data on sugar (sucrose) available for consumption have been studied and their relationship to dental caries experience has been explored (Screenby 1982). However questions remain as to the actual distribution of sugar within populations and its pattern of consumption (Hobdell 1980). The inclusion of sugar consumption within national policies on nutrition is increasing and this has the advantage of being associated with the control and prevention of diseases other than dental caries (Department of Health 1984). Apart from the forced food policies engendered by the rationing imposed on large population groups during the Second World War (Toverud 1957; Takeuchi 1961), there have been no studies which have tested the effects of such policies on the incidence of dental caries in peace time and in isolation from other preventive measures such as fluoridated toothpaste.

Fissure sealants

Fissure sealants are now being used more and more in an attempt to eliminate the type of carious lesion found in the fissures of the back teeth. They act by blocking the nutrient supply to the bacteria harboured in the fissures by the painting of a resin over the acid-etched surfaces of the teeth. An attack on this type of carious lesion is essential if significantly more people are to remain caries-free. However doubts have been expressed about the cost-effectiveness of this measure when compared to filling a tooth (Horowitz 1980b). More recent studies showing the relatively short life-expectancy of such fillings would suggest that such cost-effectiveness comparisons are of limited use. Clinical trials of these materials have shown that the *bis*-GMA resins are superior both to the cyano-acrylates and polyurethanes. The results of studies so far have concentrated mainly on the retention of the material on the tooth surface after specified periods of time and a wide range of results have been reported (Gordon 1983). The reasons for the variations reported are attributed to differences in the techniques of application as well as the materials. Despite these difficulties the elimination of dental caries and, particularly, the increasingly important fissure caries would appear to be dependent upon the control of frequent sugar intakes combined with the cutting off of the nutrient supply to the bacteria in the fissures by the widespread use of fissure sealants.

Immunization

Research continues in a number of laboratories around the world to develop a vaccine against dental caries but to date no clinically proven vaccine for human populations for which there is proof of efficacy is commercially available. Recent developments in immunology have provided considerable impetus to this field of endeavour.

Problems in maximizing effectiveness

These different preventive measures or interventions have all been shown to have some effect in preventing dental caries. When used in combination at an individual level, dental caries can be virtually eliminated. However, the level of success within populations has been somewhat varied. While most authorities agree that piped water fluoridation is the most cost-effective method of dental caries prevention in populations (Davies 1974), there remain some obstacles to the maximization of its effectiveness and the total elimination of dental caries from the population. To date relatively few countries have implemented fluoridated water schemes on a wide basis. In some circumstances the other methods of dental caries prevention would appear to have an advantage over water fluoridation.

This can be illustrated by taking Ireland and Denmark as examples. Ireland has had mandatory water fluoridation legislation since 1964. In practice this has meant that an effort has been made to fluoridate the water supplies for all population groups of over 800 people, and at present, some 60–65 per cent of the population have access to fluoridated water supplies. Because the population is very scattered in the rural areas and many households have wells or other private water supplies, the achievement of 100 per cent coverage of the population must await the development of further group water schemes. Although the technology for the dosing of water supplies has developed considerably since 1964 there remain difficulties in the treatment of relatively small quantities of water. The results of the statutory tests of the water supplies carried out in the past few years have been disappointingly at variance with the legal requirements of between 0.8 and 1 part per million of the water (Bell and Lemasney 1986).

In Denmark the dental caries preventive programme is not based upon water fluoridation. Instead dental health education, flouride mouth-rinsing, and fluoride tablets for school-age children have been used.

What is interesting is that the rate of decrease in dental caries prevalence in the two countries has been very different. In Ireland, since 1962, it has dropped from a mean DMFT of 4.7 at 12 years of age to 2.9 DMFT in 1984, whereas in Denmark it had dropped from a mean of 6.3 DMFT at 12 years of age in 1978 to 3.2 in 1985. This means that Ireland has achieved a decrease of 38 per cent in the DMFT at age 12 in 22 years whereas Denmark has achieved a reduction of 49 per cent in eight years. Part of this difference may be as a result of the higher initial DMFT in Denmark, and hence the greater proportion of the lesions being on smooth surfaces which have proved to be the most easily prevented.

What is certain is that both countries are left with a residuum of dental caries in the population which is predominantly in the occlusal surfaces of the back teeth. Apart from dramatic reductions in sucrose consumption in the two countries, fissure sealants are the only known way of eliminating this residuum of dental caries. Denmark, with a well-developed school dental health programme using both dentists and dental auxiliary personnel to run the preventive and treatment programme, is better placed than Ireland to incorporate the widest possible use of fissure sealants into the programme. Ireland, in relying upon water fluoridation alone, has a limited school dental service, which is oriented mainly towards treatment and employs no dental auxiliary personnel who could be trained to provide fissure sealants on a wide scale. Indeed the employment of such personnel would be illegal at present.

The major obstacle to the maximization of the effectiveness of water fluoridation programmes is the reluctance of public authorities to adopt such a policy. Adoption of such schemes requires that they be legal and acceptable within the country and that finance is available to meet the initial capital costs and subsequent recurrent costs. On the cost point, for big water systems the initial capital costs may be quite large. However the actual cost discounted over a number of years together with the running costs still make this the cheapest method for preventing dental decay in populations, and it is considerably cheaper than the costs of treatment.

It is in the achievement of legality for water fluoridation programmes that public opposition is found. There are two general grounds for this opposition—mass medication, or loss of freedom of choice, and hazard to health. The mass medication/loss of freedom of choice issue was the basis for an action in Ireland against the introduction of water fluoridation. The court ruled the fluoridation was constitutional and did not accept that it could be classed as mass medication. This was upheld by the Irish Supreme Court (Ryan *versus* Attorney General for Ireland 1964). The legality and safety of fluoridation were the basis for a more recent case in Scotland (*British Dental Journal* 1983). In this instance, the judge found that fluoridation was then illegal (although the law has now been changed) but could find no evidence to suggest that it was unsafe, caused cancer, mental handicap, or any other disease. This finding gave a legal seal of approval to the scientific report of The Royal College of Physicians investigation which had also concluded that there was no link between cancer and water fluoridation (Royal College of Physicians 1976).

Periodontal disease

Differences in the pattern of chronic periodontal disease exist within European countries, but comparisons between them are difficult because of the problems of developing an internationally acceptable method of measuring its prevalence and severity. Although much has been done recently in this direction not all the difficulties have been resolved (Cushing *et al.* 1986). Because of this only a note on periodontal disease will be given here.

Periodontal or gum disease occurs in both chronic and acute forms. Acute periodontal disease is usually associated with specific infections, microorganisms, or trauma. The chronic inflammation of the soft gum tissue surrounding the teeth is the condition of concern here and this is associated with the mixed bacterial plaque which covers the teeth and gums. A very high proportion of all people living in Europe have some inflammation of the gingival tissue at the necks of the teeth. This gingivitis was once seen as the first stage in a chronic degenerative process which resulted in the loss of both the gums and bone tissue surrounding the teeth.

No specific public health measure has been developed to prevent gingivitis other than the instruction of groups and individuals on how to remove the bacterial plaque from around the teeth and gums with a toothbrush. The net effect of the instructional programmes given by health professionals and through commercial advertising and a general increase in the standard of living seems to have resulted in mouths being generally cleaner and showing less signs of inflammation (Suomi *et al.* 1971). The significance of this change in terms of the retention of natural teeth in populations is currently being questioned because it is no longer certain that all those who have gingivitis will lose the hard and soft supporting tissues of the teeth and ultimately the teeth themselves (Socransky *et al.* 1984). The current belief is that only 5 to 10 per cent of the population will lose significant numbers of teeth because of this advanced destructive and chronic periodontal disease. For the majority periodontal health will be maintained by adequate personal hygiene. For those who have or will have significant tooth loss because of chronic periodontal destruction, current knowledge of aetiology and natural history of the disease does not permit scientifically sound preventive programmes to be developed. It is probable that developments in immunology will, as mentioned briefly earlier in the chapter, have profound importance for this group.

Recommendations

National and local community health goals should be set along the lines of those given in Table 10.3. Preventive programmes which focus on the specific preventive needs of the local community and have local popular support should be adopted. Where possible, water fluoridation should be the backbone of a range of measures at national and local level through the development of nutritional policy and consistent, integrated, and relevant health education programmes. Such programmes should continue to encourage the widest possible use of fluoridated toothpaste for personal oral hygiene.

References

Arnljot, H.A., Barmes, D.E., Cohen, L.K., Hunter, P.B.V., and Ship, L.L. (1985). *Oral health care systems, an international collaborative study*. Quintessence Publishing, London.

Arnold, F.A., Jr, Dean, H.T., and Knutson, J.W. (1953). Effect of fluoridated public water supplies on dental caries prevalence Results of the seventh year of study at Grand Rapids and Muskegon. *Mich. Public Hlth Rep.* **68**, 141-8.

Backer Dirks, O., Horowitz, B., and Kwant, G.W. (1961). The results of 6½ years of artificial fluoridation of drinking water in The Netherlands. The Tiel—Culemborg Experiment. *Arch. Oral. Biol.* **5**, 284-300.

Beal, J.F. (1983). Social factors and preventive dentistry. In *The prevention of dental disease* (ed. J.J. Murray) pp. 313-42. Oxford Medical Publications, Oxford.

Beiswanger, B.B., Gish, C.W., and Mallatt, M.E. (1981). Effect of a sodium fluoride-silica abrasive dentifrice upon caries. *J. Dent. Res.* **60**, 1072.

Bell, J.F. and Lesmasney, J.F. (1986). Fluoridation levels in Ireland. 1974-1984. *J.Dent.Res.* **65**, 569.

Bibby, B.G. (1943). The effect of sodium fluoride applications on dental caries. *J. Dent. Res.* **22**, 207.

Bradnock, G., Marchment, M.D., and Anderson, R.J. (1984). Social background, fluoridation and caries experience in a 5-year-old population in the West Midlands. *Br. Dent. J.* **156**, 127-31.

British Dental Journal (1983). Strathclyde Verdict. Fluoridation Society on the Strathclyde Verdict. *Br. Dent. J.* **155**, 67-8.

Cahen, P.M., Frank, R.M., and Turlot, J.C. (1982). Comparative unsupervised clinical trial on caries inhibition effect of monofluorophosphate and amino fluoride dentifrices after 3 years in Strasbourg, France. *Comm. Dent. Oral Epidemiol.* **10**, 238-41.

Cushing, A.M., Sheiham, A., and Maizels, J. (1986). Developing socio-dental indicators: the impact of Dental Disease. *Comm. Dent. Hlth* **3**, 3-17.

Davidson, N. and Townsend, P. (1982). *Inequalities in health* (The Black Report) pp. 51-75. Penguin Books, Harmondsworth.

Davies, G.N. (1974). *Cost and benefit of fluoride in the prevention of dental caries.* World Health Organization, Offset publication No. 9 WHO, Geneva.
Department of Health. (1984). *Guidelines for preparing information and advice to the general public on healthy eating.* Food Advisory Committee, Department of Health, Dublin.
Elderton, R.J., and Nuttall, N.M. (1983). Variation among dentists in planning treatment. *Br. Dent. J.* **154**, 201-6.
Fédération Dentaire Internationale. (1982). Global goals for oral health in the year 2000. *Int. Dent. J.* **32**, 74-7.
Fehr, F.R. von der. (1982). Evidence of decreasing caries prevalence in Norway. *J. Dent. Res.* **61**, 1331-5.
French, A.D., Carmichael, C.L., Furness, J.A., and Rugg-Gunn, A.J. (1984). The relationship between social class and dental health in 5-year-old children in the North and South of England. *Br. Dent.J.* **156**, 83-6.
Frencken, J., Manji, F., and Mosha, H. (1986). Dental caries prevalence amongst 12 year old urban children in East Africa. *Comm. Dent. Oral Epidemiol.* **14**, 94-8.
Geddes, D.A.M., Cooke, J.A., Edgar, W.M., and Jenkins, G.N. (1978). The effect of frequent sucrose mouth-rinsing on the induction in vivo of caries like changes in human dental enamel. *Arch. Oral Biol.* **23**, 663-5.
Gordon, P.H. (1983). Fissure sealants. In *The prevention of dental disease* (ed. J.J. Murray) pp. 175-91. Oxford Medical Publications, Oxford.
Gustafsson, B.E., Lanke, L.S., Lundqvist, C., Grahnen, H., Bonow, B.E., and Krasse, B. (1954). The Vipeholm dental caries study: the effect of different levels of carbohydrate intake on caries activity in 436 individuals observed for five years. *Acta Odont. Scand.* **11**, 232-364.
Hansen, H., Milen, A., Heinonen, O.P., and Paunio, I. (1982). Carries in primary dentition and social class in high and low fluoride areas. *Comm. Dent. Oral Epidemiol.* **10**, 33-6.
Harris, R. (1963). The biology of the children of Hopewood House, Bowral, V. Observations on dental caries experience proximal lesions. *Austr. Dent. J.* **8**, 521-8.
Health Education Council. (1983). *A discussion paper on proposals for nutritional guidelines for health education in Britain.* National Advisory Committee on Nutrition Education, London.
—— (1984). *Notes on dental health education.* Health Education Council, London.
Heifitz, S.B., Franchi, G.J., MacDougall, O., and Brunelle, J. (1979). Combined anticariogenic effect of fluoride gel trays and fluoride mouthrinsing in an optimally fluoridated community. *J.Clin. Prev. Dent.* **6**, 21-8.
Her Majesty's Stationery Office (HMSO) (1986). *The report of the committee of enquiry into unncecessary dental treatment.* Her Majesty's Stationery Office, London.
Hobdell, M.H. (1980). Dental caries prevalence and estimated sugar consumption: a comparison between the Peoples Republic of Mozambique and the United Kingdom. *Trop. Dent. J.* **4**, 145-50.
Hodge, H.C., Holloway, P.J., Davies, T.G.H., and Worthington, H.V. (1980). Caries prevention by dentifrices containing a combination of sodium monofluorophosphate and sodium fluoride. *Br. Dent. J.* **149**, 193-204.

Horowitz, H.S. (1980a). Established methods of prevention. *Br. Dent. J.* **149**, 311-8.
—— (1980b). Pit and fissure sealants in private practice and public health programmes: analysis of cost-effectiveness. *Int. Dent. J.* **30**, 117-26.
—— and Doyle, J. (1972). The effect on dental caries of topically applied acidulated phosphate-fluoride: results after 3 years. *J.Am. Dent. Assoc.* **82**, 359-65.
Kalsbeck, H. (1982). Evidence of decrease in prevalence of dental caries in the Netherlands: an evaluation of epidemiological caries surveys on 4-6 and 11-15 year old children between 1965 and 1980. *J. Dent. Res.* **61**, 1321-6.
Klein, H. and Palmer, C.E. (1937). Dental caries in American Indian children. *Public Health Bulletin*, No. 239. Government Printing Office, Washington, DC.
——, ——, and Knutson, J.W. (1938). Studies on dental caries, dental status and dental needs of elementary school children. *Publ. Hlth Rep.(Wash)* **53**, 751-65.
Mainwaring, P.J., and Naylor, M.N. (1983). A four year clinical study to determine the caries inhibiting effect of calcium glycerophosphate and sodium fluoride in calcium carbonate base dentifrices containing sodium monofluorophate. *Caries Res.* **17**, 267-76.
Manji, F., Mosha, H., and Frencken, J. (1986). Tooth and surface patterns of dental caries in 12 year old urban children in East Africa. *Comm. Dent. Oral Epidemiol.* **14**, 99-103.
Marthaler, T.M. (1968). Caries inhibiting after seven years of an amine fluoride dentifrice. *Br. Dent. J.* **124**, 510-5.
—— (1969). Caries-inhibiting effect of fluoride tablets *Helv. Odontol. Acta* **13**, 1-12.
Meyer, K., Freitas, E., David, R.K., Freitas, J., and Kristoffersen, T. (1983). Dental health among young Portuguese in relation to socio-economic differences. *Rev. Prot. Estomatol. Gr. Maxillofac.* **24**, 461-78.
Minister of Health, Ireland. (1985). *Children's dental health in Ireland, 1984.* Stationery Office, Dublin.
Naylor, M.N. and Murray, J.J. (1983). Fluorides and dental caries. In *The prevention of dental disease* (ed. J.J. Murray) pp. 83-158 Oxford Medical Publications, Oxford.
Poulsen, S., Amaratunge, A., and Risager, J. (1982). Changes in the epidemiologic pattern of dental caries in a Danish rural community over a 10-year period. *Comm. Dent. Oral Epidemiol.* **10**, 345-51.
Renson, C.E., Crielaers, P.J.A., Ibikunle, S.A.J., Pinto, V.G., Ross, C.B., Sardo-Infirri, J., Takazoe, I., and Tala, H. (1985). Changing patterns of oral health and implications for oral health for oral health manpower: Part 1. *Int. Dent. J.* **35**, 235-51.
Robens Appeal. (1986). Report of the work of the independent Committee on Dental Research set up by Guy's and St. Thomas' Hospitals, London.
Rock, W.P. and Evans, R.I.W. (1982). A comparative study between a chemically polymerised sealant resin and a light cured resin. *Br. Dent. J.* **152**, 232-4.
Royal College of Physicians. (1976). *Fluoride, teeth and health—summary of a report on fluoride and its effects on teeth and health.* The Royal College of Physicians of London, Pitman Medical, London.
Rugg-Gunn, A.J., Holloway, P.J., and Davies, T.G.H. (1973). Caries prevention by daily fluoride mouth rinsing. *Br. Dent. J.* **135**, 353-60.
Ryan, G. *versus* Attorney General for Ireland. Judgement of the Supreme Court,

Ireland, delivered by Chief Justice O'Dalaigh on appeal from Mr. Justice Kenny, July 3 1964.

Screenby, L.M. (1982). Sugar availability, sugar consumption and dental caries. *Comm. Dent. Oral Epidemiol.* **10**, 1–7.

Sheiham, A. (1979). The epidemiology of dental caries and periodontal disease. *J. Clin. Periodontol.* **6**, 7–15.

Silver, D.H. (1982). Improvements in the dental health of 3-year-old Hertfordshire children after 8 years—the relationship to social class. *Br. Dent. J.* **153**, 179–83.

Socransky, S.S., Haffajee, A.D., and Goodson, J.M., and Lindhe, J. (1984). New concepts of destructive periodontal disease. *J. Clin Periodontal.* **11**, 21–32.

Suomi, J.D., Greene, J.C., and Vermillion, J.R., Doyle, J., Chang, J.J., and Leatherwood, E.C. (1971). The effect of controlled oral hygiene procedures on the progression of periodontal disease in adults: results after third and final year. *J. Periodontal.* **42**, 152–60.

Takeuchi, M. (1961). Epidemiological study on dental caries in Japanese children, before, during and after World War II. *Int. Dent. J.* **11**, 443–57.

Todd, J.E. (1975). *Childrens' dental health in the United Kingdom, 1973.* Her Majesty's Stationery Office, London.

—— and Dodd, T. (1985). *Childrens' dental health in the United Kingdom, 1983.* Her Majesty's Stationery Office, London.

Toth, K. (1973). Caries prevention in deciduous dentition using table salt fluoridation. *J. Dent. Res.* **52**, 533–4.

Toverud, G. (1957). The influence of war and post-war conditions on the teeth of Norwegian school children. *Milbank Mem. Fund Quart.* **35**, 373–459.

11
Occupational cancers

Franco Merletti and Nereo Segnan

SUMMARY

Occupational hazards are among the known causes of cancer which are susceptible to regulatory control and thus especially suitable for prevention. Despite these opportunities for intervention, we seem to have identified only those agents that produce a large increase in the risk of a particular cancer or a small increase in the risk of rare cancers. It seems reasonable to assume that many occupational exposures that have induced cancer are as yet undetected and that we have only uncovered the tip of the iceberg. Identification of situations suitable for intervention is, therefore, part of eradication programmes for occupational cancer. Use of experimental data, implementation of monitoring systems, registers of exposed workers, studies of pooled cohorts, and application of job exposure matrices to epidemiological studies seem to be steps to identify specific hazards in occupational carcinogenesis. The most effective measure to prevent occupational cancer is undoubtedly to prohibit the presence of carcinogenic substances in industrial processes. A second major option is to eliminate the contacts between workers and carcinogenic substances when present in the workplace. Any programme designed to reduce or to eradicate occupational cancer needs to concentrate both on the identification of specific excesses and on specific interventions.

Defining the problem

It is difficult to define realistically what can now be achieved in terms of primary prevention of cancer, unless we view environmentally-induced cancer as a series of more or less independent problems. Within this approach, interest in occupationally-induced cancer has increased greatly during the last 10 to 15 years. There seem to be three major reasons for this. First, despite decades of intensive studies and recent major break-throughs, basic research on the mechanism of cancer causation has produced only limited knowledge applicable to preventive measures. Yet it was established long ago that some chemicals are human carcinogens. In fact complex occupational exposures were among the first causes of cancer to be identified, and this led, in many instances, to the identification of specific causal agents.

Second, the perception exists that when specific carcinogenic agents are identified in the occupational environment they can be readily controlled. This is in contrast to aspects of life-style, such as smoking or dietary habits, where control requires modification of cultural and personal behaviour patterns. The final reason for the interest in occupational carcinogenesis is more subtle: it relates to the fact that free personal choice may play a role in contributing to the cancer attributable to some environmental causes. The great majority of lung cancer cases, for instance, are attributable to tobacco smoking and can be prevented by avoiding the habit. Obviously, personal choice plays little or no role in occupational exposures, and thus workers warrant special attention to be given to their protection. Furthermore, occupational cancer tends to be concentrated among relatively small groups of people whose risk of developing the disease may be quite large.

Size of the problem

Population

Caution must be used in attempting to interpret estimates of the size of the occupational cancer problem. Recent estimates for the United States have ranged from 1 per cent to as much as 20–40 per cent of all cancers (Wynder and Gori 1977; Bridbord *et al.* 1978; Higginson and Muir 1979; Doll and Peto 1981).

In early estimates the methods used were not described so that interpretation and evaluation of such figures is not possible. However, in 1978, 10 scientists of the National Cancer Institute, the National Institute of Environmental Health Sciences, and the National Institute for Occupational Safety and Health of the United States released a paper containing an estimate that up to 20–40 per cent of all cancers were the result of occupation (Bridbord *et al.* 1978). This paper described the methods used and thus opened a debate in the scientific community on the validity of such figures. However, the paper contained such methodological weaknesses that the suggested estimate is very difficult to defend, and Doll and Peto (1981) made a detailed criticism of it and gave other 'informed estimates' of 2–8 per cent.

The wide range of these estimates makes it clear that this is an area of uncertainty. However, if a reasonably valid estimate of the proportion of cancer attributable to occupation could be developed, it might serve at least two purposes. First, it could be useful in health education. Second, the estimate might contribute to the establishment of cancer research priorities by permitting major categories of carcinogenic exposures such as smoking, drugs, occupation, and so on to be ranked according to public health impact.

All such proportional estimates are very difficult to develop because they depend both on the proportion of the population experiencing the exposure of interest and the magnitude of the excess risk among such persons. Since each of these figures is itself difficult to estimate, we believe that any single overall summary estimate of the proportion of cancer attributable to occupational exposures will be difficult to defend and interpret. In fact such summary estimates (either 'guessed' or 'informed') may lead to a nonproductive discussion on numbers rather than on problems.

A more satisfactory alternative to any overall estimate is to view occupational cancer as a series of more or less independent problems. This focuses attention on specific occupational experiences that require evaluation and on others where control is indicated. This view should prove useful both for understanding occupational carcinogenesis and for preventing it. For example, it was suggested that in Boston in 1967 and 1968 about 18 per cent of all bladder cancer in men was the result of occupational exposure. Such an estimate is specific for place, time, sex, and cancer site, and its validity and precision can be assessed by evaluating the study that developed it (Cole *et al.* 1972).

More recently, a review of the proportion of bladder cancer attributable to occupation in the general male population has estimated the contribution of occupational exposures to be from 8–10 per cent to 20 per cent (Vineis and Simonato 1986). Here again only studies which were specific for place, time, sex, and cancer site estimates were considered.

The various estimates of occupational cancer have been used by legislators, policy-makers, and others to exaggerate (or, alternatively, to minimize) the importance of the problem. But, occupational cancer should have a high priority in aetiological research and in programmes of cancer prevention, regardless of its proportional importance. There are three pragmatic reasons for this.

First occupational cancer is concentrated among specific groups of people. For these people the risk of developing a particular form of cancer may be very large. For example, an estimate of 3 per cent of total deaths from cancer as a result of occupation in the general population, would immediately become 12 per cent in the still very broad category of male blue collar workers (Nicholson 1984).

Second, among the known causes of cancer, occupational hazards are among the few that are susceptible to regulatory control (this has been done in some countries), and are thus especially suitable for prevention.

Finally, even if only 1 or 2 per cent of the cancer burden is the result of occupational exposure, this represents 8000 to 16 000 preventable cases and 4000 to 8000 preventable deaths each year in the United States alone.

Carcinogens

Another way of looking at the magnitude of the problem of occupational cancer is to consider the 'absolute numbers' of compounds and of industrial processes which are known or suspected to be carcinogenic, and the number of people known to be exposed.

In 1971, the International Agency for Research on Cancer started a programme to try to identify chemical carcinogens through searches and evaluation of published work. Compounds are selected for carcinogenicity evaluation mainly on two grounds: (1) human exposure to the compound is known to occur; and (2) there is some suspicion (derived from human data, animal data, or other laboratory data) that the chemical may be carcinogenic (Saracci 1981). Over the last 14 years this programme has been responsible for the evaluation of 695 chemicals, groups of chemicals, industrial processes, occupational exposures, and cultural habits (Vainio *et al.* 1985). Table 11.1 contains a summary of some of the results of the evaluation programme. Even if one cannot compare the group of compounds hitherto evaluated with a random sample of all chemicals, it is nevertheless striking to note the large proportion of compounds for which an evidence of carcinogenicity is found either in man or in animals.

Table 11.1 Chemicals, groups of chemicals, industrial processes, occupational exposures, and cultural habits considered for evidence of carcinogenicity by the International Agency for Research on Cancer.

Category	N	(%)
Chemicals and exposures causally associated with cancer in humans	39	(5.9)
Chemicals and exposures probably carcinogenic to humans (higher level of probability)	17	(2.6)
Chemicals and exposures probably carcinogenic to humans (lower level of probability)	51	(7.7)
Chemicals and exposure not classifiable as to carcinogenicity to humans	67	(10.2)
Chemicals for which no data in humans were available, but for which the evidence of carcinogenicity in experimental animals was considered to be sufficient	115	(17.5)
Other chemicals for which no data in humans were available	406	(58.4)
Total evaluations	695	(100)

Source: International Agency for Research on Cancer (1972–1985).

Table 11.2 Chemicals and groups of chemicals, entailing occupational exposures and industrial processes carcinogenic for humans.

4-Aminobiphenyl
Arsenic and certain arsenic compounds
Asbestos
Benzene
Benzidine
Bis(chloromethyl)ether and technical-grade chloromethyl methyl ether
Chromium and certain chromium compounds
Mustard gas
2-Naphthylamine
Soots, tars, and mineral oils
Vinyl chloride
Auramine manufacture
Boot and shoe manufacture and repair (certain occupations)
Coal gasification
Coke production
Furniture manufacture
Isopropyl alcohol manufacture (strong-acid process)
Nickel refining
Rubber industry (certain occupations)
Underground haematite mining (with exposure to radon)

Source: International Agency for Research on Cancer (1972–1985).

Even more striking is that, for 115 chemicals for which there was sufficient evidence of carcinogenicity in experimental animals, no data on humans were available. A large number of these agents entail occupational exposures. Tables 11.2 and 11.3 list agents established as causes of occupational cancer and occupations with sufficient evidence of increased cancer risk.

The task of estimating the population at risk to specific exposure is difficult for various reasons. The precise number of persons occupationally exposed to given compounds is often not known. The level of exposure to specific compounds necessary to increase cancer risk is only imperfectly known. Furthermore, estimates are complicated by the varying interactions between length and intensity of exposure. The extent to which workers have changed occupations or activities or both from time-to-time is often not known. Placing or excluding them as at risk to occupation-related cancers at any time in the past or at present is, therefore, difficult.

A few exercises have been conducted to try to estimate populations at risk to specific exposures (Bridbord *et al.* 1978; ASA 1980; Nicholson *et al.* 1982). For asbestos (Nicholson *et al.* 1982), it was estimated that from 1940 to 1979, in the United States, 27 500 000 individuals had potential exposure at work.

Table 11.3 Occupations with sufficient evidence of increased cancer risk[a].

Industry	Occupation	Site	Substance known or suspected as cause
Agriculture, forestry, and fishing	Vineyard workers using arsenical insecticides	Lung, skin	Arsenic
Pesticide, herbicide production	Arsenical insecticides production, and packaging	Lung	Arsenic
Petroleum	Wax pressmen	Scrotum	Polycyclic hydrocarbons
Gas	Coke plant workers	Lung	Benzo(a)pyrene
	Gas workers	Lung, bladder, scrotum	Coal carbonization products, α-naphthylamine
	Gas retort house workers	Bladder	α/β-Naphthylamine
Metal	Copper smelting	Lung	Arsenic
	Chromate producing	Lung	Chromium
	Chromium plating	Lung	Chromium
	Ferrochromium producing	Lung	Chromium
	Steel production	Lung	Benzo(a)pyrene
	Nickel refining	Nasal sinuses, lung	Nickel[b]
Extractive	Arsenic mining	Lung, skin	Arsenic
	Iron ore mining	Lung	Not identified
	Asbestos mining	Lung, pleural and peritoneal mesothelioma	Asbestos
	Uranium mining	Lung	Radon
Rubber	Rubber manufacture	Lymphoid and haematopoietic tissues (leukaemia)	Benzene
		Bladder	Aromatic amines
	Calendering, tire curing, tire building	Lymphoid and haematopoetic tissues (leukaemia)	Benzene
	Millers, mixers	Bladder	Aromatic amines
	Synthetic latex producers, tyre curing, calender operatives, reclaim cable makers	Bladder	Aromatic amines

Industry	Occupation	Site	Substance known or suspected as cause
Leather	Boot and shoe manufacturers, repairers	Nose, haematopoietic tissues (leukaemia), urinary bladder	Leather dust, benzene
Furniture	Furniture and cabinet making	Nose (adenocarcinoma)	Wood dust
Asbestos production	Insulation material production (pipes, sheeting, textile, cloths, masks), asbestos cement manufacturers	Lung, pleural and peritoneal mesothelioma	Asbestos
Construction	Insulators and pipe coverers	Lung, pleural and peritoneal mesothelioma	Asbestos
Shipbuilding, motor vehicles and transport	Shipyard and dockyard workers	Lung, pleural and peritoneal mesothelioma	Asbestos
Chemical	BCME and CMME products and users	Lung (oat cell carcinoma)	*Bis*-chloromethyl ether (BCME) Chloromethyl methyl ether (CMME)
	Vinyl chloride producers	Liver (angiosarcoma)	Vinyl chloride monomer
	Isopropyl alcohol manufacturing (strong acid process) workers	Paranasal sinuses	Causative agent not identified
	Pigment chromate producing	Lung	Chromium
	Dye manufacturers and users	Bladder	Benzidine, 2-naphthylamine, 4-aminodiphenyl
	Auramine manufacture	Bladder	Auramine[c]
Other	Roofers, asphalt workers	Lung	Benzo(a)pyrene

[a]Source: Simonato and Saracci (1983). Reprinted by permission of the authors and the International Labour Organization.
[b]The specific compound(s) responsible for a carcinogenic effect cannot be specified precisely.
[c]Together with the other aromatic amines used in the process.

Of these 18 800 000 had exposure in excess of that equivalent to 2 months employment in primary manufacturing or as an insulator.

The same authors have estimated from these data that approximately 8200 asbestos-related cancer deaths are now occurring annually, and that even if asbestos was removed from the environment today a number of deaths of the same order of magnitude would still occur in the next decades from past exposures.

Recent patterns in discovering occupational carcinogens

By the mid-1960s the discovery of new occupational agents with persuasive human evidence of carcinogenicity was at an ebb. This changed in the early 1970s with the discovery of the carcinogenicity of vinyl chloride and *bis*-chloromethylether. But, since 1973, although many compounds have fallen under suspicion, only in a few (for example, ethylene oxide) is there a convincing association and only for a few industrial processes (for example, coal gasification, coke production, and certain occupations in rubber industry) was there considered to be sufficient evidence of carcinogenicity.

In looking closely at the workplace, we no longer see only those things which are clearly carcinogens but also those the danger or safety of which is difficult to establish. Yet, it is essential to assess whether each of these suspicious carcinogens either is, or is not, a true carcinogen. Their borderline status may result either because they are weak carcinogens, because exposure to them is low, or because, though non-carcinogenic, they have fallen under suspicion for some other reason.

A number of considerations are relevant here. A review of the chemicals and industrial processes carcinogenic for humans (listed in Table 11.2), showed that 9 of these 20 agents and processes had relative risks of from about 50 to 500 for cancer of a specific site among some groups of individuals. Ten had risks between 5 and 50 and only 1 (certain occupations in the rubber industry) had a risk of the order of 2 for cancer at some sites (Nicholson 1984). Any plausible frequency distribution of the relative risks of site-specific occupational cancers would certainly have a large number of points with relative risks less than 5, were they to be known.

The most common element leading to the discovery of carcinogenic effects has been the suspicion that arises in the mind of a clinician or pathologist. Typically, a cluster of cases is noted by the observer and related to a place of employment. Subsequently, the causative factor may be identified through epidemiological or experimental studies. An excellent example of this was the first realization that an occupational exposure was carcinogenic. In 1775, a surgeon linked cancer of the scrotum in chimney sweeps to their exposure to soot (Pott 1775). It was not until much later that a carcinogen, benzo(a)pyrene, was identified in soot (Cook *et al.* 1932).

The same pattern can be seen in two other classical examples. In 1879, Harting and Hesse identified pulmonary cancer as an occupational disease among metal miners in Central Europe, but radioactivity was not identified as the causal agent until almost a century later (Hueper 1966). In 1895, Rehn pointed out that tumours of the urinary bladder had an origin in the German dyestuffs industry (Rehn 1895), but formal epidemiological studies providing strong evidence on the identity of the specific causative agents, primarily benzidine and beta-naphthylamine, were not carried out until 60 years later (Case and Pearson 1954).

Other occupational carcinogens were first identified as a result of experimental studies of animals or epidemiological studies of human beings. Table 11.4 gives examples of carcinogens identified by these methods.

Table 11.4 Occupational carcinogens by site, occupation, and method by which they were first disclosed.

Site	Carcinogen	Occupational group
First noted by clinicians or pathologists		
Scrotum	Polycyclic hydrocarbons	Sweeps
Pleura	Asbestos	Miners
Skin	Ionizing radiation	Radiologists
	Ultra-violet light	Outdoor workers
	Arsenic	Sheep-dip makers
Nose	Wood dust	Furniture makers
	Isopropyl oil	Chemical workers
Nose and bronchus	Nickel oxide	Smelters
Leukaemia	Benzene	Leather workers
Bone	Radium	Luminizers
Bladder	2-Naphthylamine	Dye workers
Bronchus	Chrome pigments	Refiners
	Bichromethyl ether	Ion resins exchange makers
Liver	Vinyl chloride	PVC manufacturers
First noted in work in animals		
Bronchus, nose, larynx	Mustard gas	Chemical workers
Bladder	4-Aminodiphenyl	Chemical workers
First noted by epidemiologists		
Bladder	2-Naphthylamine	Coal gas producers
	2-Naphthylamine	Rubber workers
Nose	Leather dust	Boot and shoe operatives

Source: Acheson (1979) after Doll (1975).

Special circumstances favourable to the discovery of a carcinogen operated in many of the instances listed in Table 11.4. In some instances—for example, hepatic angiosarcoma, nasal cancer, bone sarcoma, and mesothelioma—the baseline frequency of the cancer was so low that the occurrence of even a small number of cases in the experience of one observer was sufficient to bring a cause–effect relationship to attention. In others—for example, nasal sinus cancer—the geographical concentration of the hazardous industry, furniture-making, in a small town caused the association to come to light.

The demonstration of a cause–effect relationship in laboratory animals has rarely been the initial factor leading to the discovery of an effect in man. Doll described only four examples of this: carcinoma of the bronchus in gas retort house workers caused by polycyclic hydrocarbons; respiratory cancer in mustard gas manufacturers; angiosarcoma of the liver in manufacturers of polyvinyl chloride; and bladder cancer in chemical workers using 4-aminodiphenyl (Doll 1975). Similarly, although usually necessary for refining risk estimates, epidemiological studies have only occasionally brought about the initial identification of the existence of a human carcinogen (Acheson 1979).

As Acheson (1979) pointed out, there is no logical reason why carcinogenic effects should manifest themselves predominantly in unusual situations or in terms of tumours that are otherwise rare. It seems reasonable to assume that many occupational exposures that have induced cancer are as yet undetected. Up to now we seem to have detected only those agents that produce a large increase in the risk of a particular cancer or a small increase in the risk of a rare cancer. There have been relatively few systematic approaches to the discovery of occupational carcinogens. Thus, it is possible that any systematic approach (that is, prospective follow-up studies done in the context of large industrial cohorts) will lead to the identification of a number of occupational carcinogens.

Thus it seems that, in terms of accepted human carcinogens, we have identified only the tip of the iceberg.

Prospects for intervention

Four categories of substances or occupations associated with human carcinogenesis can be identified:

1. Well-defined chemicals or occupations for which evidence of carcinogenicity in humans is sufficient, such as asbestos or gas retort house workers.
2. Well-defined occupations or activities for which a causal association with cancer has been demonstrated—at least in some plants and in some

periods—but for which the specific causative agents have not been identified. Extrapolation under these circumstances is more problematic than in (1), as industrial processes have changed over time and may differ between plants. An example is work in the wood industry, which is associated with adenocarcinoma of the nasal sinuses. Nevertheless, the causal agent is unknown and it can only be stated that, at least in England, it was present from 1920 to 1940 (Acheson 1976).

3. Chemicals suspected to be carcinogenic in human beings on the basis of either limited or inadequate information, such as epichlorohydrin.
4. Chemicals considered carcinogenic in animals but for which there are no epidemiological studies (see Table 11.1).

With regard to these four categories it is obvious that before any intervention to reduce or to eradicate occupation-induced cancer it is essential to identify and describe specific problems—first of all who is exposed and where and how does the exposure take place?

Detecting the problem

New compounds are constantly introduced into the occupational environment. Such compounds should be tested for mutagenicity in short-term assay systems. The same should apply to compounds in use which have not been assessed with regard to their carcinogenicity. Testing for carcinogenicity in animals is a much more burdensome task both from the economic and the feasibility points of view and should be implemented according to priority criteria. There has been much debate among scientists and legislators on the use of such laboratory data.

From a regulatory point of view, it has been stressed that '. . . so many thousands of chemicals are active to some extent in one laboratory test or another that it is difficult to know what, if any, practical regulations to enact on the basis of laboratory tests . . . In fact in the absence of direct evidence of the exact quantitative relevance to humans of the findings in long-term animal tests or in any of the short-term tests, blanket restrictions on very large numbers of minor chemical pollutants may be unacceptably expensive . . . A socially acceptable approach would then be to use results of laboratory tests for 'priority setting' to identify, study and if possible reduce the few apparently most extreme human hazards with respect to each particular test, without necessarily requiring human evidence of harm' (Doll and Peto 1981). On the other hand from a scientific point of view there is no doubt that results that can be obtained *in vitro* or *in vivo* correlate well with human experience. All recognized human carcinogens tested in long-term tests—with the single exception of ethanol—are also animal carcinogens (including arsenic and benzene for which new evidence has appeared (Vainio *et al.* 1985)). Furthermore, for certain compounds experimental evidence preceded human evidence of carcinogenicity. For these reasons we believe the extrapolation of the results from long-term carcinogenicity tests in animals to be a valid means of predicting carcinogenic risk to humans even in the absence of other means of demonstrating human risk. Substances suspected to be carcinogenic with either limited animal evidence or positive in short-term tests, should be studied further, and, in the meanwhile, action should be taken to limit exposure. Short-term tests can also be useful to establish priority between chemical products to be subjected subsequently to long and costly tests on animals. From a public health point of view this approach introduces 'priority setting' in intervention and regulation, according to different levels of scientific evidence of carcinogenicity, but it does also stress the importance of experimental carcinogenicity studies in the primary prevention of cancer.

A shortcoming of experimental studies is that work environments involving exposures to complex mixtures cannot be reproduced in the laboratory. This is particularly relevant since hazards may derive from a combination of exposures each of which on its own may be innocuous. This is where the idea of monitoring—defined as an ongoing system of recording of health data as well as exposure data—comes in. Monitoring implies that excesses of cancer would be detected as soon as they develop on the basis of the ongoing surveillance programmes. Furthermore, keeping records of exposure data would permit retrospective epidemiological investigations on groups of workers.

The problem of quantifying the who, where, and how of exposure to occupational carcinogens requires different strategies. One is the implementation of the ILO (International Labour Organization) Convention No. 139 of 1974, concerning the prevention of occupational hazards caused by carcinogenic substances and agents (International Labour Organization 1974). This Convention recommends the establishment of registries of workers exposed to occupational carcinogens. To our knowledge the only country which has established such a registry at national level is Finland (ASA 1980), although countries such as Canada, Italy, and the Federal Republic of Germany (Costa *et al.* 1982) have developed limited experience towards doing so. Only, however, by applying such systematic approaches, will it be possible to recognize excesses of cancer risks from occupation of around two-fold—that is, much smaller than those so far detected.

Another approach important in the identification of occupational cancer is to pool cohorts exposed to the same substance to increase the possibility of detecting an existing risk. Such an approach can lead logically to the registration of exposed workers.

In recent decades the number of chemical substances used in industry has increased rapidly, and the nature of industry and technology has become more complex. As a consequence the number of exposures associated with particular job titles has increased, and the number of jobs in which the nature of the exposure is obvious from the title has declined. Many epidemiological studies, therefore, have to rely on information on job titles as a substitute for information on chemical agents used in that job.

To overcome this problem recent efforts have been made to develop job exposure matrices (Siemiatycki 1981; Medical Research Council 1983), which may be defined as a cross-classification of a list of job titles with a list of agents to which persons carrying out the job are exposed. Recently, lists of job titles associated with known hazards, such as asbestos and certain aromatic amines, have been made available for epidemiological research workers, and a number of industries have compiled job exposure matrices, some of which have linked data about exposure to data about sickness and death. Two of the principal potential uses of such matrices are the identification of previously undisclosed hazards and the location of jobs in which workers are exposed to known hazards. An example of such application can be found in the compilation of a matrix of job titles associated with aromatic amines (Hoar *et al.* 1980). Such a matrix was used to reanalyse the data of a classical study (Cole *et al.* 1972) where certain occupational categories had been found associated with bladder cancer. Data were reanalysed using exposure rather than job title as the basis for classification. As indicated in Table 11.5, a higher relative risk was found for persons aged 20–59 years exposed to aromatic amines than to any of the industrial categories in the original paper. This was because the analysis by exposure had the effect of excluding some subjects in 'suspicious' industrial categories who had not in fact been exposed to aromatic amines. In other words the use of the matrix reduced the number of persons misclassified by the indicator of exposure previously used and increased discriminating power. It seems likely that a number of associations between factors in the workplace and a disease remains undisclosed because of inadequacies of job titles as indicators of exposure (Acheson 1983).

Table 11.5 Relative risks for bladder cancer in occupational settings identified by a conventional epidemiological study[a] and by the application of a job exposure matrix[b].

	Relative risk	95% confidence limits
Occupational category		
Dyestuffs	2.2	0.7–7.6
Rubber etc.	1.6	1.0–2.4
Leather etc.	2.0	1.4–2.9
Exposure category		
Aromatic amines	8.6	6.2–12.0

[a]Cole *et al.* (1972).
[b]Hoar *et al.* (1980); Acheson (1983).

Interventions

We have seen that in the case of specific occupational cancer much has still to be done to inquire below the tip of the iceberg to identify problems in the form of specific causative agents. Once this has been done, as for most of the agents listed in Tables 11.2, 11.3, and 11.4, then intervention can be implemented.

As already mentioned, occupational hazards are among the few known causes of cancer that are susceptible to regulatory control and thus especially suitable for prevention. The most effective measure to prevent occupational cancer is undoubtedly to prohibit the use of carcinogenic substances in industrial processes. Together with the removal of carcinogens from industrial processes, research on substances to be used as substitutes should be developed. Most industrialized countries have general laws dealing with toxic substances, and in a few of these the legislation includes special provision for carcinogens. The first country to prohibit the manufacture of certain chemicals because of their carcinogenicity was the United Kingdom with regard to aromatic amines. After unsuccessful attempts in the 1930s to have it included in the Workmen's Compensation Act, bladder cancer caused by exposure to aromatic amines was included in the 1962 Prescribed Industrial Diseases Regulation. Finally, in 1967 specific legislation prohibiting the manufacture of 2-naphthylamine, benzidine, 4-aminodiphenyl, 4-nitrobiphenyl, and their salts was enacted. It is worth noting that in 1921 the ILO (International Labour Organization) had already recognized that 2-naphthylamine and benzidine were causes of bladder cancer. A few industrialized countries followed the example of the United Kingdom, namely Ireland, Japan, the USSR, and the United States, but not all give consideration to banning the importation of carcinogens whose manufacture is prohibited (Tomatis 1982).

With regard to the European Economic Community (EEC) only a few member states currently have legislation specifically for carcinogenic substances, and those that do often have it incorporated in the more comprehensive regulations for toxic substances. However there is an increasing tendency to regulate the sector of carcinogens at work by means of specific provisions. Examples are the code of practice regarding vinyl chloride in the United Kingdom or the EEC directives on vinyl chloride and asbestos. Only in a few cases and only in a minority of member states of the European Community, was production of these two substances actually prohibited. Of about 100 substances or production activities known to have carcinogenic effects on man, only a few have been totally prohibited. It is more common to find provisions prohibiting their use in particular sectors (foodstuffs, medicine, cosmetics, pesticides, and so on). Greater use has been made of prohibitions and permits in the Nordic countries and, in particular, in Sweden and

Finland. In national and international legislation a clause is often inserted to the effect that the substance must be replaced, but with the rider 'where possible' (Benvenuti 1986).

A second major option is to eliminate the contacts between workers and carcinogenic substances when present in the workplace. This includes three aspects: (a) production and transportation of carcinogens in a closed system; (b) control of the working environment by monitoring levels of exposure and installation of air-conditioning systems effective even in cases of emergency; (c) personal protective equipment for those workers at highest risk of coming into contact with carcinogenic substances (Simonato and Saracci 1983).

In the scientific community it is widely accepted that, given the present state of knowledge on carcinogenic mechanisms, the definition of a threshold 'safe' level of exposure to a carcinogen is not possible (Crump et al. 1976). Nevertheless, in the absence of other preventive measures one should take into account the simple fact that any appreciable reduction in the levels of exposure to a carcinogen helps to diminish the risk for the exposed population.

There are examples of successful intervention in industrial occupational cancer. In the nickel industry, for instance, the excess risk of nasal sinus cancers seems to have disappeared after changes were made in the manufacturing process (Doll 1977).

In reviewing published reports on occupational cancer, it is surprising to see that only a very small number of studies have dealt with the assessment of effectiveness of intervention. This reflects both intrinsic difficulties regarding effectiveness of intervention for diseases with very long induction periods and lack of use of the epidemiological approach to evaluate results in the occupational setting. Among the few exceptions is an American study on the assessment of the effect of improved working conditions on bladder tumour incidence in a benzidine manufacturing facility (Ferber et al. 1976) which is described below.

In a large dye manufacturing facility, all cases of bladder tumours occurring among workers exposed to benzidine, but not to other known carcinogens, were traceable to operations of the original process installed in 1915. In 1950 studies were set up to devise processes and procedures which could drastically reduce the possibilities of exposure to benzidine in any form.

The studies culminated in the development, installation, and successful demonstration, in 1955, of a new fully enclosed wet process for benzidine sulphate. A number of industrial hygiene controls were also put into effect. After 20 years of operation of the new process, objective evidence of effectiveness of the improved design of the plant process and controls was sought. Since the average induction period of occupationally induced bladder tumours is around 18 years (Case and Pearson 1954), any earlier comparison would have been unconvincing. In the study population exposed to benzidine, beta-naphthylamine, and other aromatic amines before 1955, 115 cases of bladder cancer (36 among workers exposed only to benzidine) had developed. In the group first exposed since 1955 no case developed. Even if no estimate of person-years at risk was given, the data are convincing with regard to the effectiveness of the intervention.

Similar results were found for the workers employed in the British rubber and cablemaking industries where in 1950 the use of known carcinogenic aromatic amines was stopped. An analysis of the mortality for bladder cancer over the period 1967–76 showed no overall evidence of a continued excess risk of neoplasms of the bladder in people who entered the industry after 1949 (Fox *et al.* 1974; Fox and Collier 1976; International Agency of Research on Cancer 1982).

In Table 11.6 some intervention possibilities for elimination of certain occupational cancers are presented. Aspects essential to the implementation of prevention strategies are classified with (+) if information or positive evidence are available. We considered target organs, chemical carcinogens, exposed population, preventive measures, evidence for effectiveness of intervention and need for epidemiological research, as fundamental. In the case of asbestos, target organs, modes of exposure, preventive methods, and their effectiveness are all well known. The eradication of asbestos-induced cancer is related purely to economic, social, and political constraints, not to scientific and technical problems as such.

On the contrary, the excess of buccal cavity cancer in boot and shoe manufacture (International Agency for Research on Cancer 1981) has not been explained in terms of either chemical agent or job title and work area. From a public health point of view, it is extremely difficult to adopt preventive measures in such a situation.

Other examples fall between the two just described. In the printing industry, the excess of multiple myeloma has been observed in a specific occupational title group—compositors. In the rubber industry a work area—tyre assembly—may be related to brain cancer. In both instances, preventive measures by means of industrial hygiene controls in the specific groups and areas are possible.

Knowledge of target organs is not strictly necessary to adopt preventive measures. The effects of exposures to carcinogens with different levels of evidence in experimental animals can be prevented if we know where exposures occur. For instance, no convincing evidence exists that carbon tetrachloride (CCl_4) causes cancer in humans (Merletti *et al.* 1984). Nevertheless, exposure in laundry dry cleaners can be avoided. Finally in the last line of the table, the need for epidemiological research to evaluate the effectiveness of intervention and to identify in more detail patterns of causation of cancer is presented and should be stressed. Mortality surveys in the case of asbestos and pleural mesothelioma would be an adequate approach for evaluating the

Table 11.6 Intervention possibilities for elimination of occupational cancer at different sites.

	Target organs				
	Lung pleura	Buccal cavity	Brain		Multiple myeloma
Carcinogen	Asbestos	Unknown	Unknown	Carbon tetrachloride	Unknown
Exposed population					
Job title	+	–	–	Laundry dry cleaners	Compositors
Work area	+	–	Tyre assembly	–	–
Type of industry	+	Boot and shoe manufacture	+	–	Printing
Preventive measures					
Evidence for effectiveness	+	Unknown	+	+	+
Epidemiological methods	Ongoing mortality survey	Aetiological and evaluation research	Aetiological and evaluation research	Ongoing mortality survey by job titles	Aetiological and evaluation research

+ : information or positive evidence available.
– : information or positive evidence not available.

effectiveness of preventive measures whereas aetiological studies are necessary to identify the carcinogenic agent(s) responsible for buccal cavity cancer in boot and shoe manufacture.

Constraints and problems in eliminating occupational cancers

We have not discussed screening programmes, but it is important to warn again that screening is not to be relied upon as an occupational cancer control activity. Screening is obviously not a primary preventive measure and, more importantly, there is no real evidence that screening for occupationally-induced cancer brings about any benefit. If screening is conducted, it should be done only under circumstances where its effects can be evaluated. This recommendation is made because screening in this context has the potential to do more harm than good (Cole and Morrison 1978).

Another important issue is that, even in absence of immediate intervention to remove a carcinogenic hazard, workers are always entitled to know the likely long-term health effects of their exposures in so far as such information exists. This has not only an 'ethical' relevance, but it also has implications for intervention. The pressure that society and workers use to change the working environment may be very different according to the knowledge available to them regarding risk.

Finally we have not covered the issues of cost–benefit analysis. When a cost–benefit analysis is made at the individual level with regard to life-style exposures, such as tobacco or alcohol, part of the benefit and of the cost refers to the same individual. He can then decide—based partly on individual choice and partly on societal and cultural influences—what risk to run for what benefit. But in the case of occupational cancer, the workers exposed to carcinogenic substances run a risk which is not counterbalanced by an individual benefit. In fact, if a benefit exists, it is to the advantage, at the best, of society at large. This also implies that the issue of occupational cancer, regardless of its relative importance and of the difficulties of implementing programmes of elimination, is somehow unique and deserves particular attention and priority.

Conclusions and recommendations

The implementation of preventive measures to eradicate occupational cancers contains contradictory aspects. On the one hand such cancers are susceptible to regulatory control and are thus especially suitable for prevention. On the other hand, social, political, and economic constraints have prevented the removal of many carcinogenic substances from industrial processes. Furthermore, although only the tip of the iceberg of occupational cancer is known, there are methodological and practical problems in identifying the specific excesses of cancer in the exposed groups. Any programme designed to reduce or to eradicate occupational cancer needs, therefore, to concentrate both on identification of new problems and on specific interventions. The approaches we have mentioned, aimed at the identification of situations suitable for intervention as part of eradication programmes for occupational cancer, include:

1. Testing for mutagenicity in short-term assay systems of compounds used or introduced in the working environment; testing for carcinogenicity in animals on a subset of these compounds according to priority criteria.
2. Development of ongoing systems for recording of health data as well as exposure data: maintaining records of employees for many decades (even after retirement); establishing registers of workers exposed to occupational carcinogens, following the ILO Convention 139; linking exposed workers to incidence and mortality statistics using some kind of national identification number such as the pension or the national health service number.
3. Development of job exposure matrices to cover some inadequacies of job titles as indicators of exposure.
4. Studies of large or pooled industrial cohorts.

With regard to intervention, the prohibition of substances or production activities known to have carcinogenic effects on man is undoubtedly the only and most effective method of preventing occupational cancer. Nevertheless, any appreciable reduction in the levels of exposure to a carcinogen by elimination of contacts between workers and carcinogenic substances present in the workplace helps to diminish the risk for the exposed population.

References

Acheson, A.D. (1976). Nasal cancer in the furniture and boot and shoe manufacturing industries. *Prev. Med.* **5**, 295–315.
—— (1979). Record linkage and the identification of long-term environmental hazards. *Proc. R. Soc. Med. London* **205**, 165–78.
—— (1983). What are job exposure matrices? In Medical Research Council—Environmental Epidemiology Unit—Scientific Report No. 2. *Job exposure matrices*, pp. 1–4. Proceedings of a conference held in April 1982 at the University of Southampton. Southampton General Hospital, Southampton.
ASA, 1980. (1982). Data from the register of employees occupationally exposed to

substances and working processes possibly causing cancer risk in Finland in 1980. Institute of Occupational Health, Helsinki.

Benvenuti, F., Hunter, W.J., and Rossi, L. (1986). Carcinogens at work; scientific and regulatory aspects. Proceedings of the international conference, Rome, 13-14 June, 1985. *Med. Lav.* 77, 323-479.

Bridbord, K., Decoufle, P., Fraumeni, J.F., Hoel, D.G., Hoover, R.N., Rall, D.P., Saffiotti, U., Schneiderman, M.A., and Upton, A.C. (1978). *Estimates of the fraction of cancer in the United States related to occupational factors.* National Cancer Institute, National Institute of Environmental Health Sciences, and National Institute for Occupational Safety and Health, Bethesda, Maryland.

Case, R.A.M., and Pearson, J.T. (1954). Tumours of the urinary bladder in workmen engaged in the manufacture and use of certain dyestuff intermediates in the British chemical industry. II. Further considerations on the role of aniline and of the manufacture of auramine and magenta (Fuchsine) as possible causative agents. *Br. J. Ind. Med.* 11, 213-6.

Cole, P. and Morrison, A.S. (1978). Basic issues in cancer screening. In *Screening in cancer* (ed. A.B. Miller) pp. 7-39. UICC Technical Report Series 40, Geneva.

——, Hoover, R., and Friedell, G.H. (1972). Occupation and cancer of the lower urinary tract. *Cancer* 29, 1250-60.

Cook, J.W., Hieger, I., Kennaway, E.L., and Maynard, W.V. (1932). The production of cancer by pure hydrocarbons: Part I. *Proc. R. Soc. Ser. B*, 111, 455.

Costa, G., Merletti, F., Segnan, N., and Vineis, P. (1982). Territorial maps of occupational exposures to chemicals with sufficient evidence of carcinogenicity on human and/or experimental animals. In *Prevention of occupational cancer*, pp. 281-90. International Labour Office, Geneva.

Crump, K.S., Hoel, D.G., Langley, C.H., and Peto, R. (1976). Fundamental carcinogenic processes and their implications for low dose risk assessment. *Cancer Res.* 36, 2973-9.

Doll, R. (1975). Pott and the prospects for prevention. *Br. J. Cancer.* 32, 263-72.

—— (1977). Strategy for detection of cancer hazards to man. *Nature* 37, 589-96.

—— and Peto, R. (1981). The causes of cancer: quantitative estimates of avoidable risks of cancer in the United States today. *J. Nat. Cancer Inst.* 66, 1193-308 and Oxford University Press, Oxford.

Ferber, K.H., Hill, W.J., and Cobb, D.A. (1976). An assessment of the effect of improved working conditions on bladder tumour incidence in a benzidine manufacturing facility. *Am. Ind. Hyg. Assoc. J.* 37, 61-8.

Fox, A.J. and Collier, P.F. (1976). A survey of occupational cancer in the rubber and cablemaking industries: analysis of deaths occurring in 1972-74. *Br. J. Ind. Med.* 33, 249-64.

——, Lindars, D.C., and Owen, R. (1974). A survey of occupational cancer in the rubber and cablemaking industries: results of five year analysis, 1967-71. *Br. J. Ind. Med.* 31, 140-51.

Higginson, J. and Muir, C.S. (1979). Environmental carcinogenesis. Misconceptions and limitations to cancer control. *J. Nat. Cancer Inst.* 63, 1291-8.

Hoar, S.K., Morrison, A.S., Cole, P., and Silverman, D.T. (1980). An occupation and exposure linkage system for the study of occupational carcinogenesis. *J. Occup. Med.* 22, 722-6.

Hueper, W.C. (1966). *Occupational and environmental cancers of the respiratory system*. Springer Verlag, New York.
International Agency for Research on Cancer. IARC Monographs on the evaluation of the carcinogenic risk of chemicals to humans. Vol. 1-36. International Agency for Research on Cancer, 1972 to 1985, Lyon.
—— (1981) IARC Monographs on the Evaluation of the Carcinogenic Risk of Chemicals to Humans, Vol. 25, *Wood, leather and some associated industries*. IARC, Lyon.
—— (1982). IARC Monographs on the Evaluation of the Carcinogenic Risk of Chemicals to Humans, Vol. 28. *The rubber industry*. IARC, Lyon.
International Labour Organization. (1974). Convention No. 139. *Concerning the prevention of occupational hazards caused by carcinogenic substances and agents*. International Labour Organization, Geneva.
Medical Research Council—Environmental Epidemiology Unit. (1983). Scientific Report No. 2. *Job exposure matrices*. Proceedings of a conference held in April 1982 at the University of Southampton. Southampton General Hospital, Southampton.
Merletti, F., Heseltine, E., Saracci, R., Simonato, L., Vainio, H., and Wilbourn, J. (1984). Target organs for carcinogenicity of chemicals and industrial exposures in humans: a review of results in the IARC Monographs on the evaluation of the carcinogenic risk of chemicals to humans. *Cancer Res.* **44**, 2244-50.
Nicholson, W.J. (1984). Quantitative estimates of cancer in the workplace. *Am. J. Ind. Med.* **5**, 341-2.
——, Perkel, G., and Selikoff, I.J. (1982). Occupational exposure to asbestos: population at risk and projected mortality. 1980-2030. *Am. J. Ind. Med.* **3**, 259-311.
Pott, P. (1775). *Chirurgical observations*. Hawes, Clarke and Collings, London.
Rehn, L. (1895). Blasengeschwulste bei Fuchs—Arbeitern. *Arch. Klin. Chir.* **50**, 588-600.
Saracci, R. (1981). The IARC Monograph Program on the evaluation of the carcinogenic risk of chemicals to humans as a contribution to the identification of occupational carcinogens. In *Quantification of occupational cancer* (eds. R. Peto and M. Schneiderman), pp. 165-76. Cold Spring Harbor Laboratory.
Siemiatycki, J., Day, N.E., Fabry, J., and Cooper, J.W. (1981). Discovering carcinogens in the occupational environment: a novel epidemiologic approach. *J. Nat. Cancer Inst.* **66**, 217-25.
Simonato, L. and Saracci, R. (1983). Occupational Cancer. In *ILO encyclopedia on occupational health*, pp. 369-75. ILO, Geneva.
Tomatis, L. (1983). Cancer, occupational (legislation). In *ILO encyclopedia on occupational health*. pp. 376-7. ILO, Geneva.
Vainio, H., Hemminki, K., and Wilbourn, J. (1985). Data on the carcinogenicity of chemicals in the IARC Monographs programme. *Carcinogenesis* **6**, 1653-65.
Vineis, P. and Simonato, L. (1986). Estimates of the proportion of bladder cancers attributable to occupation. *Scand. J. Work Environ. Hlth* **12**, 55-60.
Wynder, E.L., and Gori, G.B. (1977). Contribution of the environment to cancer incidence. An epidemiologic exercise. *J. Nat. Cancer Inst.* **58**, 825-32.

Section II

Screening to eliminate childhood morbidity

12
Down syndrome and neural tube defects

Janine Goujard

SUMMARY

Down syndrome and neural tube defects (NTD) are two of the most severe congenital anomalies, affecting approximately 3 in every 1000 births. Prenatal diagnosis, based on the examination of amniotic fluid for abnormality of the karyotype in Down syndrome and raised concentrations of both alpha-fetoprotein (AFP) and acetylcholinesterase in NTD, has made it possible to terminate affected pregnancies and so reduce the incidence of these disorders.. Prenatal screening for Down syndrome has been based on two well-established risk factors: a family history of chromosomal anomaly (present in very few pregnant women) and high maternal age. However, screening based on maternal age has its limitations. First, the sensitivity of the test is low—about 30–35 per cent for a maternal age cut-off level of 35 years and over. Second, success is strongly dependent on the availability of screening facilities and the acceptance rate among eligible women. If its effectiveness is proved, a combination of maternal age and low serum AFP concentration might lead to an improvement in the efficacy of screening in younger women. For NTD, primary prevention by multivitamin therapy appears to be premature. Screening in high-risk areas, such as in the United Kingdom, has been based on maternal serum AFP measurement. However, screening by ultrasound has become a serious alternative: one of the advantages being its role in routine antenatal care. The level of ascertainment would be at least 80–85 per cent for spina bifida, and practically 100 per cent for anencephaly. In both cases, perfect co-ordination between the different disciplines involved and an improvement in health education are absolutely essential.

Defining the problem

In most European countries, congenital anomalies are the second most common cause of infant mortality—for example, in 1980 they were responsible for 31 per cent of infant deaths in the Netherlands, 27 per cent in England and Wales, and 22 per cent in France (Blondel et al. 1984). However, the problem of major congenital anomalies cannot be assessed solely in terms of mortality since morbidity and handicap must also be taken into account. Thus, in Europe the birth prevalence of all congenital anomalies is about 22 per 1000 (Eurocat 1986). The current trend towards limiting family size has increased public pressure to reduce the risk of a future handicapped child. This is reinforced by better access to genetic counselling, education on risk, and by the development of techniques of prenatal diagnosis, allowing for a possible selective abortion. The possibilities now offered by prenatal diagnosis are particularly relevant to the identification of two types of severe and disabling malformations—Down syndrome and neural tube defects (NTD)—which represent 15 per cent of all cases of congenital anomalies. It seems important to evaluate the possibilities and also the limits of prenatal diagnosis for these anomalies with a view to better control in the future.

Down syndrome
Size of the problem

Occurrence

Like all other congenital defects, the prevalence of Down syndrome can be studied only if specific surveys or special registers based on geographically defined populations are used, such as those recently developed in Europe for monitoring birth defects (Flynt et al. 1979; Eurocat 1985a). It is clear that the real (total) prevalence is dependent on the ability of each registry to cover therapeutic abortions performed as a result of prenatal diagnosis. Most European registers, regional as well as national, tend to monitor neonatal birth defects and are only reliable for birth prevalence. Even so, the under-reporting of cases cannot be completely eliminated. This renders geographical comparisons unreliable. The size of the population monitored could also play an important role in the accuracy of the rates, although complete ascertainment is more difficult to obtain in a large population.

There are two forms of Down syndrome. In the most common situation, 95 per cent of cases, there is so-called non-dysjunction. The other 5 per cent of cases consist mainly of those with unbalanced Robertsonian translocation but the normal number of 46 chromosomes.

The prevalence rate of Down syndrome at birth (live or stillborn babies) recorded for the years 1979–82, in 18 regional registers involved in the Eurocat Project (1985b, 1986), (a sample size of 200 000 annual births) is indicated in Figure 12.1a. The data is corrected for centres in which prenatally diagnosed (and aborted) fetuses with Down syndrome are registered.

These data yield a mean birth prevalence rate of 12.0 per 10 000 births. Differences are observed between countries, but the rates within a country are more homogeneous. The impact of prenatal diagnosis on the prevalence of Down syndrome among births appears clearly in the data from Paris and Glasgow. Data from other sources of information, such as those recorded during the same period in the International Clearinghouse for Birth Defects Monitoring System (1982–84), generally on a nationwide level, lead to equivalent rates (Figure 12.1b). The impact of prenatal diagnosis on birth prevalence is perhaps most important in Denmark.

On the whole, the highest birth prevalence rates are currently observed in Spain (hospital-based nationwide data) where there are 15.1 cases per 10 000 births, in Italy, where the rates range from 13.4 per 10 000 (hospital-based nationwide) to 16.6 per 10 000 births (regional level), and in Dublin (regional-based data) where there are 16.8 cases per 10 000 births. The lowest recorded rates are those registered in Denmark (population-based national data): 7.3 per 10 000 births and in England and Wales: 7.7 per 10 000 births (population-based national data). When cases of aborted fetuses are also registered, the highest prevalence rates are observed in Sweden (nationwide level): 16.7 per 10 000 births for the period 1980–82.

Trends

The registration of congenital anomalies in the Eurocat Project began in January 1979, and it is still too early to evaluate trends. Moreover, the small number of births covered each year by the majority of centres cannot always allow a rigorous analysis. Most of the European programmes of the International Clearinghouse for Birth Defects Monitoring Systems use relatively recent base-line periods which also makes it more difficult to detect changes in the rates. However, the study of the 5-year specific ratios of observed to expected numbers of Down syndrome illustrates the current trends for 1980–83 (Figure 12.2).

Owens et al. (1983) in collating data from the Liverpool Congenital Malformations Registry allow trends to be followed over a 19-year period. From 1961 to 1979, the authors have registered a gradual but significant fall in the incidence of Down syndrome in the Liverpool and Bootle areas: 16.2 per 10 000 live births for 1961 to 1963 to 10.9 per 10 000 live births for 1977 to 1979.

According to the rates in the Copenhagen area in 1970 (Mikkelsen et al. 1976) and the trend towards a younger age of pregnancy in Denmark from 1960 to 1980, a decrease in the number of all liveborn children with Down syndrome from 1960–61 to 1979–81 of 23.4 per cent would have been expected (Mikkelsen et al. 1983). Further, the expected decrease in the total number of affected births for mothers aged 35 years and over should have

184 *Elimination or Reduction of Diseases?*

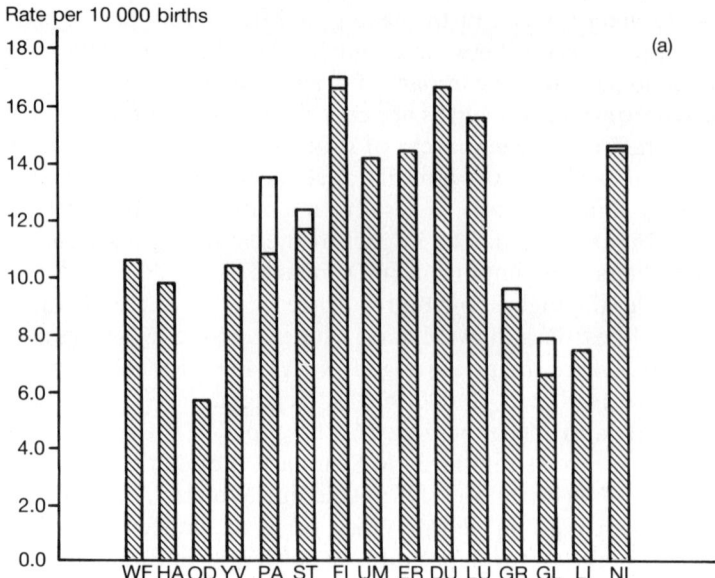

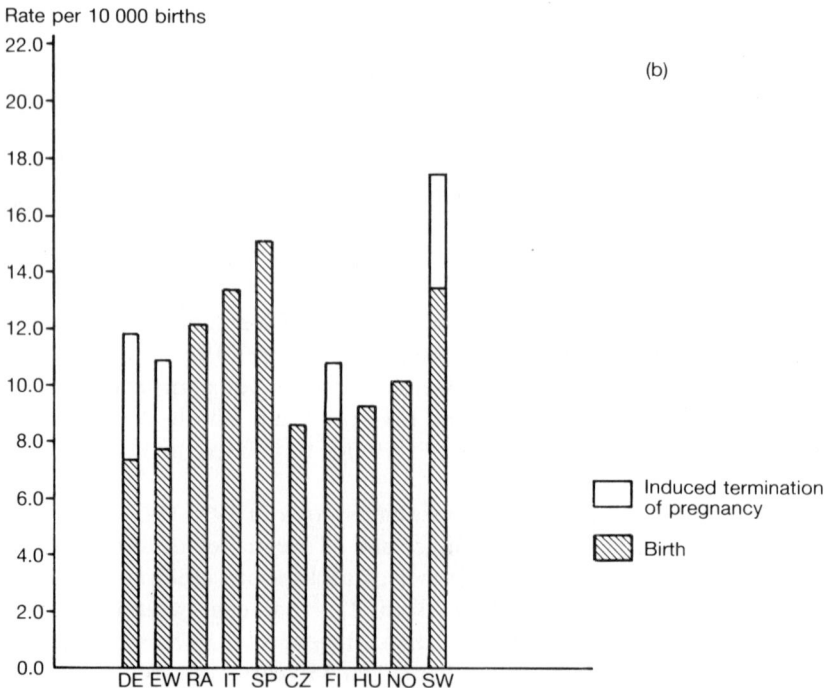

been higher at 68 per cent, but because of an apparent increase in the maternal incidence in some age groups, there was no significant decrease in the overall birth prevalence.

The interpretation of these two apparently contradictory trends will be discussed later.

Fig. 12.1 Prevalence rate (corrected for termination) per 10 000 live and stillbirths of babies with Down syndrome: (a) in Eurocat centres 1979–82; (b) in other European registers of the International Clearinghouse for Birth Defects Monitoring Systems 1980–82.

EEC Countries

—EUROCAT Centres:
West Flanders	W F
Hainaut	H A
Odense	O D
Yvelines	Y V
Paris	P A
Strasbourg	S T
Firenze	F I
Umbria	U M
Emilia Romana	E R
Dublin	D U
Luxembourg	L U
Groningen	G R
Glasgow	G L
Liverpool	L I
Belfast and Northern Ireland	N I

—International Clearinghouse for Birth Defects Monitoring Systems:
Denmark	D E
England & Wales	E W
France: Rhône-Alpes	R A
Paris	see above
Strasbourg	see above
Italy	I T
Spain	S P
Northern Ireland	see above

Other European countries of the International Clearinghouse
Czechoslovakia	C Z
Finland	F I
Hungary	H U
Norway	N O
Sweden	S W

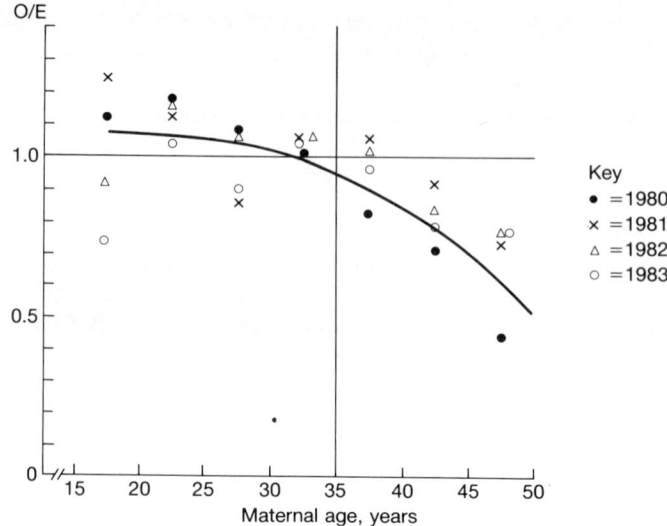

Fig. 12.2 Ratios of observed to expected numbers (O/E) of Down syndrome by maternal age class for all monitoring systems that provided age-specific data. (Source: International Clearinghouse for Birth Defects Monitoring Systems *Annual Report* (1983).)

Risk factors

The most important risk factor for Down syndrome is maternal age, although, more recently, an increased risk from advanced paternal age has been suggested. The increased risk with *maternal age* is well known and has been previously quantified (Hook and Lindsjo 1978; Trimble and Baird 1978; Golbus *et al.* 1979; Milunksy 1979; Galjaard 1980).

Data from nine Eurocat registries, giving the distribution of 5-year age group specific rates in the 1980–83 period (Eurocat 1986), updated this knowledge (Figure 12.3), and emphasized the increased rate of Down syndrome in mothers aged 35 years and over. For the age group 35–39 years, a particularly crucial group, rates range from 17.7 per 10 000 births in West Flanders to 44.0 per 10 000 births in Glasgow. In the same way, rates observed in the other European monitoring programmes of the International Clearinghouse, for women aged 35–39 years, range from 10.0 per 10 000 births in Denmark (period 1980–81) to 45.8 per 10 000 births in Sweden (period 1973–77). Six monitoring programmes out of ten record a rate of over 35.0 per 10 000 births.

When the relationship between maternal age and translocation is studied, a marked age dependency is also observed, but in this case the risk appears

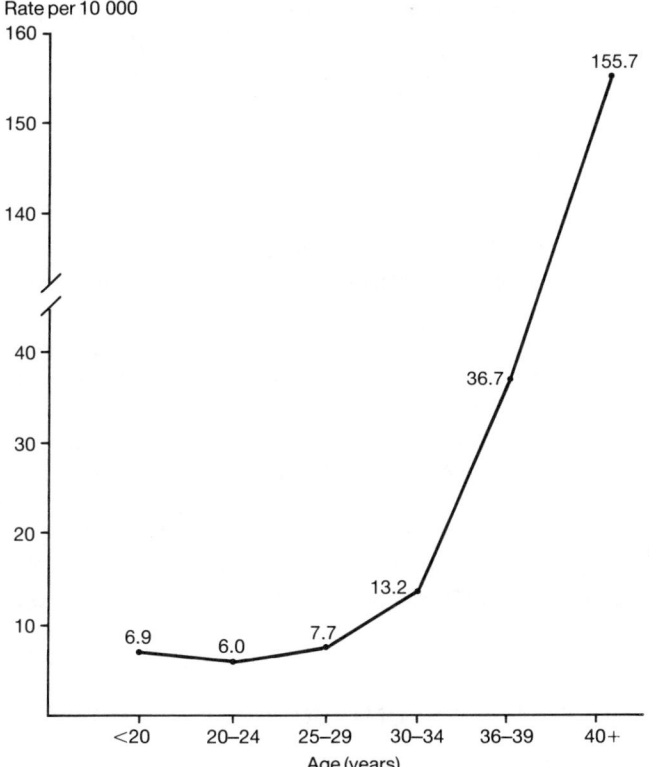

Fig. 12.3 Maternal age-specific incidence of Down syndrome (per 10 000) in 12 Eurocat registries. (Adapted from *EUROCAT* (1986).)

higher for young mothers: from the data recorded in the monitoring programmes of the International Clearinghouse, for the period 1980–84 (in press), the percentages of translocation among reported cases were 5.2 per 100 (25/389) for mothers under 25 years, 5.2 per 100 (51/980) for those aged 25–34 years, and 1.7 per 100 (8/585) for mothers aged 35 years and over.

The *paternal-age* effect has been noted in two studies (Erickson 1979; Stene *et al.* 1979) which demonstrated that men above 55 years of age have a significantly increased risk of having children with Down syndrome. The effect seems to be more evident from the age of 41 years, independent of maternal age, but stronger when the mother is older than when she is younger (Stene *et al.* 1981). Most of the monitoring programmes are not yet able to evaluate the magnitude of this risk as this variable is not systematically collected.

The other major risk factor is the *recurrence risk* after the birth of a child with Down syndrome—one of the parents being a balanced carrier of a structural rearrangement, usually a translocation or an inversion. This risk, affecting a very small part of a population of pregnant women, has been very well documented (Galjaard 1980): in the case of a regular trisomy 21, the prevalence rate is estimated at 1 or 2 per cent of all births.

Nature of the intervention

All the countries of the EEC, apart from the Republic of Ireland, have programmes aimed at reducing the incidence of Down syndrome. These programmes are based on prenatal diagnosis, using amniocentesis and the culture of cells from the amniotic fluid to identify affected fetuses. Termination of pregnancy is then offered to women of 35 years and over (38 years and over in France and Italy). This procedure is also available to mothers who have already given birth to children with chromosomal disorders, and to those with a family history of chromosomal anomalies. More recently, less invasive techniques such as serum alpha-fetoprotein (AFP) measurement (Cuckle *et al.* 1984; Merkatz *et al.* 1984; Spencer *et al.* 1985), trophoblast biopsy (Modell 1985), and the detection and analysis of fetal cells in the maternal circulation (Herzenberg *et al.* 1979; Schroder *et al.* 1980) have been developed. However, the feasibility and effectiveness of these new techniques have not yet been established.

Evidence for the effectiveness of intervention

Methods of antenatal screening for Down syndrome are based on the two well-established risk factors: maternal age and family history of chromosomal abnormality.

In Europe, there is variation in the effectiveness of intervention at regional or national level (Figures 12.1a and b). Thus in Denmark 37 per cent of cases of Down syndrome were prenatally diagnosed in 1981, 40 per cent in 1982, 37 per cent in 1983; in England and Wales: 30 per cent in 1981, and 29 per cent in 1982; in Finland: 23 per cent in 1981, 21 per cent in 1982 and 14 per cent in 1983; and in Sweden: 16 per cent in 1980, 19 per cent in 1981, 25 per cent in 1982 and 24 per cent in 1983 (International Clearinghouse data 1985).

There is evidence that this effectiveness is based mainly on the identification of women at risk by age at the beginning of pregnancy, which constitutes, at present, the major method of antenatal screening. The problem is then the choice of a specific cut-off age for access to the diagnostic test, and this is closely related to the public health policy of each country. In Table 12.1 we have calculated the distribution of total births in 12 Eurocat registers for the period 1980–83, according to six maternal age groups, and the corresponding distributions of the observed normal births and affected cases. This Table shows that 41.5 per cent of cases of Down syndrome are registered

Table 12.1 Distributions of births (Total, Down syndrome cases, and non-affected children), by maternal age, in 12 EUROCAT registries, 1980–83.

Maternal age (years)	Total births surveyed	Observed number of Down syndrome cases		Distribution of observed numbers of Down syndrome cases (%)	Distribution of non-Down syndrome births (%)
		B	IA		
<20	4203	28	1	3.4	0.7
20–24	185000	111	0	13.1	30.1
25–29	224675	170	3	20.3	36.5
30–34	140151	180	5	21.7	22.7
35–39	50954	176	11	22.0	8.3
40+	10662	126	40	19.5	1.7
Total	615645	791	60	100.0	100.0

Adapted from Eurocat report (1986).
B = Births.
IA = Induced abortions.

among mothers aged 35 years and over (that is, the screening sensitivity for this cut-off level), but using this age cut-off level includes 10.0 per cent of the population that are unaffected and are falsely regarded as being at risk (that is, a screening specificity of 90 per cent); for mothers aged 40 years or more, the figures are 19.5 and 1.7 per cent, respectively, and that leads to a screening sensitivity of 19.5 per cent and a specificity of 98.3 per cent. Interestingly, only 14 per cent of cases registered among mothers aged 35 years and over were aborted fetuses. This is in contrast to the conclusions of Mikkelsen *et al.* (1983) for Denmark, in 1979–80, which show that the estimated number of Down syndrome cases averted by unrestricted abortion will be twice the number prevented by amniocentesis. The proportion of Down syndrome cases identified at birth is a useful guide to the success of the screening policy.

An estimation of the sensitivity and the specificity of screening for Down syndrome using different maternal age cut-off levels has been calculated based on the maternal age structure of (i) French pregnancies and (ii) Eurocat registrations (Table 12.2). Thus 6.7 per cent of the French mothers in 1981 were 35-years-old or more compared to an estimated European rate of 10 per cent. Thus the sensitivity of screening is dependent on the maternal age distribution in a population.

The governmental policy of each country plays an important role in deciding a specific cut-off age. For example, in Paris (Goujard *et al.* 1983) where criteria of access, and maternal age in particular, have remained the same

Table 12.2 Estimations of the sensitivity and specificity of screening for Down syndrome using different maternal age cut-off levels.

Maternal age cut-off levels (years)	Model I[a]			Model II[b]		
	Proportion of all pregnancies (%)	Sensitivity (%)	Specificity (%)	Proportion of all pregnancies (%)	Sensitivity (%)	Specificity (%)
⩾34	9.2	34.4	90.8	13.0	44.9	87.0
⩾35	6.7	31.0	93.3	10.0	41.5	90.0
⩾36	4.8	27.9	95.2	7.5	38.0	92.5
⩾37	3.4	24.3	96.6	5.6	33.8	94.4
⩾38	2.4	20.8	97.6	4.0	29.1	96.0
⩾39	1.7	17.9	98.3	2.8	24.7	97.2
⩾40	1.1	14.5	98.9	1.7	19.3	98.3
	N = 811 508			N = 811 508		

[a]Based on the distribution of births in France in 1981 (Rumeau-Rouquette et al. 1984) and applying the prevalence of Down syndrome in each maternal age established by Galjaard (1980).
[b]With the same total number of births and same basis for the estimation of the number of Down syndrome by maternal age but with a different distribution of the maternal age (applying the Eurocat distribution observed in Table 12.1).

since 1980 (aged 38 years and over at the date of amniocentesis), the proportion of Down syndrome births registered among the total number of cases recorded did not change at all from 1981 to 1985, approximately 74 per cent each year (unpublished data).

The recent demonstration of an association of low maternal serum AFP with Down syndrome is of potential importance. Cuckle *et al.* (1984) have calculated that about 20 per cent of all affected pregnancies should be identified by maternal serum AFP screening at 14–20 weeks. They have estimated that if amniocentesis were offered to all women aged 38 years or more and, in addition, to younger women with serum AFP concentrations below specified maternal age-dependent cut-off levels, 40 per cent of Down syndrome pregnancies would be identified. This policy would imply that amniocentesis should be performed in about 7 per cent of pregnancies—that is, twice more often than for age only. The extra resource input this would require has to be considered against the impressive potential reduction of Down syndrome cases. But these conclusions may be premature. Spencer and Carpenter (1985) have pointed out the wide population variance of published reports for the median maternal serum AFP concentration—the latter normally expressed as multiple of the median (MoM)—for Down affected pregnancies. From their survey on 27 064 pregnancies, a 4-year retrospective survey, in which 27 affected pregnancies were identified, the median MoM maternal serum AFP concentration was 0.82 (range 0.33–1.59), considerably higher than previous reports; a strategy in which the serum AFP concentration was a 0.5 multiple of the median for all age groups leads to a poor discrimination between affected and unaffected pregnancies: 14.8 per cent and 8.6 per cent, respectively.*

Problems in maximizing effectiveness in populations

There are three reasons why antenatal screening and perinatal diagnosis in developed countries might not affect the incidence of Down syndrome at birth.

First, the incidence of Down syndrome is dependent on the maternal age structure of the population. The experience of the Liverpool Congenital Malformation Registry (Owens *et al.* 1983) illustrates this phenomenon very clearly. Indeed, if there has been an important decline in Down syndrome births from the period 1961–64 to 1975–79, there has been a concurrent fall over the same period in mean maternal age of Down syndrome, from 36.7 years in 1961 to 29.0 years in 1979 (not observed after 1979), and a decrease in mean maternal age in the population. The percentage of women having

* Editors note. Recent work, at present unpublished, suggests that other serum markers such as oestriol and HCG might increase discrimination further (Cuckle, personal communication).

antenatal diagnosis during this period is too low to explain the decrease. Further, as the termination of pregnancy only became legal in the United Kingdom from 1968, the conclusion of Owens *et al.* that the fall in incidence is explained by the fall in maternal age is unlikely. Similar changes in maternal age distribution have also been observed in France between 1972 and 1976 (Rumeau-Rouquette *et al.* 1984) and in Denmark where the number of live births for women over 35 year has fallen by 36 per cent between 1950 and 1970 (Mikkelsen *et al.* 1983).

Secondly, access to prenatal diagnosis is selective. The use of amniocentesis was studied in France during the period 1972–81 and, particularly, in the Ile de France (Paris Region), in 1979, where 46.5 per cent of all prenatal diagnosis in France was performed (Gardent *et al.* 1984a, b). These data showed an important under-representation of women of lower socio-economic class seeking prenatal diagnosis. This was so even among those over 40 years of age who were, at that time, eligible to receive this service as a routine part of their care. On the whole, the uptake rate among mothers over 40 years of age was low, and varied widely according to the place of residence (15 per cent at national level, 26 per cent in Paris area). This situation is in agreement with results from Denmark by Mikkelsen *et al.* (1983). Further, prenatal diagnosis does not always result in a therapeutic abortion in the case of an affected fetus, either because of the legislation (termination of pregnancy is not legal in Belgium, Northern Ireland, or Eire) or for individual reasons. Thus, either for significant inequalities of access—a phenomenon commonly observed at the time of starting a particular medical innovation—or for personal freedom—to choose whether or not to undergo amniocentesis and termination of pregnancy—a not inconsiderable percentage of anomalies elude prevention. Furthermore, because fertility rates are much higher in younger women, even although the incidence of Down syndrome is low, more than half of the cases (between 55 to 65 per cent) occur in mothers under the age of 35 years (Table 12.3). Therefore, since it is unthinkable to perform amniocentesis in all pregnancies, and because the less invasive techniques, mentioned above, have not been thoroughly tested in terms of reliability and feasibility, an important percentage of Down syndrome cases cannot be eliminated. Indeed indications for amniocentesis, other than maternal age or evidence of chromosomal anomaly, are proportionately rare (Figure 12.4).

The last observation is related to the fact that the risk of Down syndrome has also been reported in young women (under 25 years of age) in the Nordic countries (International Clearinghouse for Birth Defects Monitoring Systems 1982–1984, 1985). Such women are considered as low-risk and are excluded from antenatal screening mainly based on maternal age. This might explain the results reported by Mikkelsen *et al.* (1983) which showed that in Denmark, in contrast to the calculated effect of screening based on the age of pregnant women, there was no change in the birth prevalence of Down syndrome between 1960–61 and 1970–80.

Table 12.3 Births and prenatally diagnosed fetuses with Down syndrome. Total cases and cases with maternal age over 35 years in five European countries.

Country	Period	Total cases of Down syndrome registered	Cases with maternal age over 35 years			
			Total		Births	Prenatally diagnosed fetuses
Denmark	1983	78	29 (37%)[a]		6 (21%)[b]	23
England and Wales	1982	739	317 (43%)		125 (39%)	192
Finland	1983	76	28 (37%)		17 (61%)	11
France: Paris	1983	76	34 (45%)		18 (53%)	16
Sweden	1983	174	80 (46%)		44 (55%)	36

[a] Percentage of cases with maternal age over 35 years.
[b] Percentage of births among mothers with age over 35 years.
Adapted from International Clearinghouse for Birth Defects Monitoring Systems (1985). Annual report 1983.

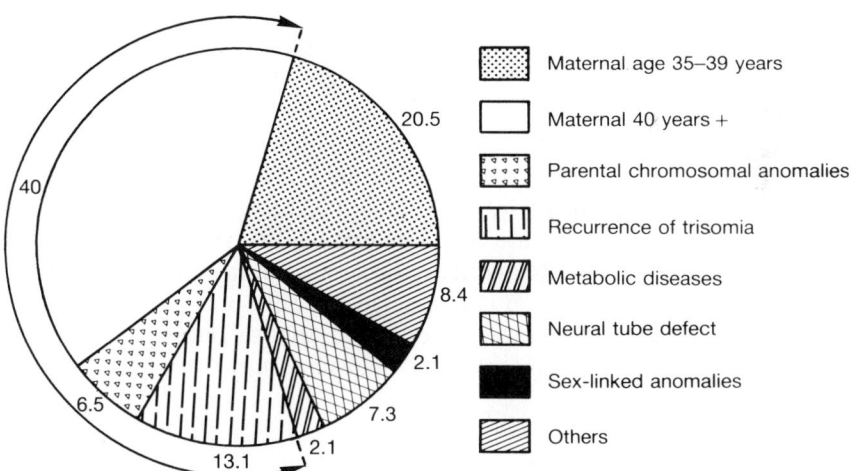

Fig. 12.4 Percentage distribution of medical criteria for prenatal diagnosis in French diagnostic centres (1979). (Source: Gardent *et al.* (1984).)

Costs and benefits of screening

In France, since 1981, much progress has been made in the field of antenatal diagnosis. In 1985 about 40 per cent of eligible pregnant women had access to antenatal diagnosis, and 7880 antenatal diagnosis tests were performed (CEBIOP data). Of course, this strategy has to depend on the financial resources of each country. In their survey on the economics of the spread of prenatal diagnosis by amniocentesis in France, Gardent et al. (1984b) have shown that a policy aiming by the year 2000 to achieve a 50 per cent uptake rate for women aged 38 years and more, instead of the 15 per cent observed at the time of the survey (1981), would prevent 89 cases of Down syndrome each year. In France there are about 800 000 births registered each year, and this would mean an annual increase of 8851 antenatal tests which would double the actual capacity available.

In their analysis of financial costs and benefits, Stene and Mikkelsen (1984), reporting the results of a Danish cost-benefit analysis performed in 1977, have shown that an antenatal screening programme for Down syndrome yielded a net financial saving from 35 years of age. In Europe, the number of live births in women aged 35 years and over is expected to increase in the future. For France, in the survey mentioned above, it has been calculated that lowering the age level for antenatal diagnosis to 35 years might prevent 125 cases of Down syndrome each year, but 21 624 supplementary prenatal diagnostic tests would be necessary. Taken to extreme, lowering the incidence in the target population of women over 35 years of age to the level of the younger population (where the risk is less than 1 per 1000) would imply an unrealistic uptake rate of at least 80 per cent and 51 031 annual supplementary acts.

Table 12.4 is a cost–benefit simulation, applying different policies for the same number of amniocentesis tests performed. It is obvious from this that the detection rate for Down syndrome can be increased more by a policy aiming to increase the uptake rate in the oldest women than by lowering the maternal age cut-off level. The combination of maternal age and serum AFP leads to a similar conclusion. But, to be effective, this policy requires an adequate administrative structure to organize the screening. The French experience (Boué 1981b) is interesting to consider in this context.

Neural tube defects
Size of the problem

Occurrence

There are two problems in interpreting incidence data. First, as for Down

Table 12.4 Cost–benefit estimation of a screening programme for Down syndrome (DS): comparison of the efficacy of different policies.

Basic hypothesis[a] Annual amount of financial resources accredited for this specific national screening programme: 8 000 000 FF.
Cost of one antenatal diagnosis for chromosomal anomaly: 1 010 FF.
Total number of antenatal diagnoses possibly to be performed: 7920.

Maternal age (years)	Distribution of pregnancies[a]	Prevalence rate of DS[b] (‰)	Expected DS cases	H_1 Usage rate of 41.2%[a] among eligible women (≥ 38 years)		H_2 Usage rate of 80% in the highest risk group (≥ 40 years)		H_3 Cut-off level reduced to 36 years; usage rate of 21%		H_4 Usage rate of 21% in the eligible group and 11% of amniocentesis among pregnancies under 38 years with low serum AFP level[c]	
				No. of amniocenteses performed	No. of DS detected	No. of amniocenteses performed	No. of DS detected	No. of amniocenteses performed	No. of DS detected	No. of amniocenteses performed	No. of DS detected
≥ 40	8 724	16.6	145	3 594	60	6 979	116	1 832	30	1 832	30
39	4 874	7.1	35	2 008	14	941 ⎤	3	1 024	7	1 024	7
38	5 644	5.4	31	2 325	13	⎦	3	1 185	6	1 185	6
37	7 700	4.3	33					1 617	7	3 879 ⎤	22
36	10 780	3.3	36					2 264	8	⎦	
≤ 35	732 278	0.9	691								
Total	770 000	1.26	971	7 927	87	7 920	122	7 922	58	7 920	65

[a] Close to the situation in France in 1985 (7880 amniocenteses performed for maternal age ≥ 38 (Cost: 7 958 800 FF, and 769 070 births).
[b] From Galjaard's data (1980).
[c] From Cuckle et al. (1984): among pregnancies ≤ 37 years, 4.7% could be selected for amniocentesis on the basis of AFP level and 20% of pregnancies with Down syndrome could be detected.

syndrome, the increase in screening for NTD and consequent termination of affected pregnancies, in most areas of Europe, has led to an underestimation of the real incidence since birth prevalence rate only is registered. Second, incidence rates derived from regional centres may overestimate the population occurrence if there is selective referral of high-risk cases.

Four main types of NTD can be identified—anencephaly, spina bifida, encephalocele, and iniencephaly—anencephaly and spina bifida accounting for about 90 per cent of all NTD (Eurocat 1986). The prevalence of babies with anencephaly and spina bifida registered in several European areas within recent years are indicated in Figures 12.5a (Eurocat registers) and 12.5b (other sources), the latter being corrected registrations of induced abortions. From Eurocat data, the mean birth prevalence rates were 6.9 per 10 000 births for anencephaly and 10.7 per 10 000 births for spina bifida for 1979-82. Encephalocele is rare (forming approximately 9 per cent of the total number of cases of NTD), and the prevalence rate is about 1.8 per 10 000 births.

As observed in previous studies, reviewed by Elwood and Elwood (1980), the prevalence of NTD remains much higher in the British Isles than in continental Europe, with the pattern of geographical variation being on the whole similar for both anencephaly and spina bifida. High rates are seen in Dublin and in Northern Ireland (40 per 10 000 births). Conversely, in England and Wales (nationwide data) as in Liverpool (regional-based data), there are high prevalence rates of spina bifida (10–12 per 10 000 births), but rates of anencephaly (4–6 per 10 000) are similar to those found on the continent. In the rest of Europe, prevalence rates of NTD vary between 4.6 (Finland, 1980–82) and 13.5 per 10 000 births (Hungary, 1980–82) (International Clearinghouse for Birth Defects Monitoring Systems 1982–84).

Trends

Evidence of recent change can be derived from Eurocat data once the rate of NTD at birth is corrected for terminations (Figure 12.5a). In addition, current trends in birth prevalence can also be assessed from the 1983 data from the International Clearinghouse, as compared to the expected rate based on no screening programme. Data are available for anencephaly, spinal bifida, and encephalocele (Table 12.5). Using this analysis, most of the European programmes demonstrate a relative reduction in the expected birth prevalence ($O/E < 1$).

Particularly interesting are the impressive results observed between 1961 and 1979 from the Liverpool and Bootle register (Owens *et al.* 1981). In Liverpool there was a progressive decline in the incidence of NTD, from 79.1 per 10 000 total births in 1961 to 24.0 in 1979 (and 12.8 in 1983), followed by a greater decline after 1974. Furthermore the incidence of anencephaly

Down syndrome and neural tube defects 197

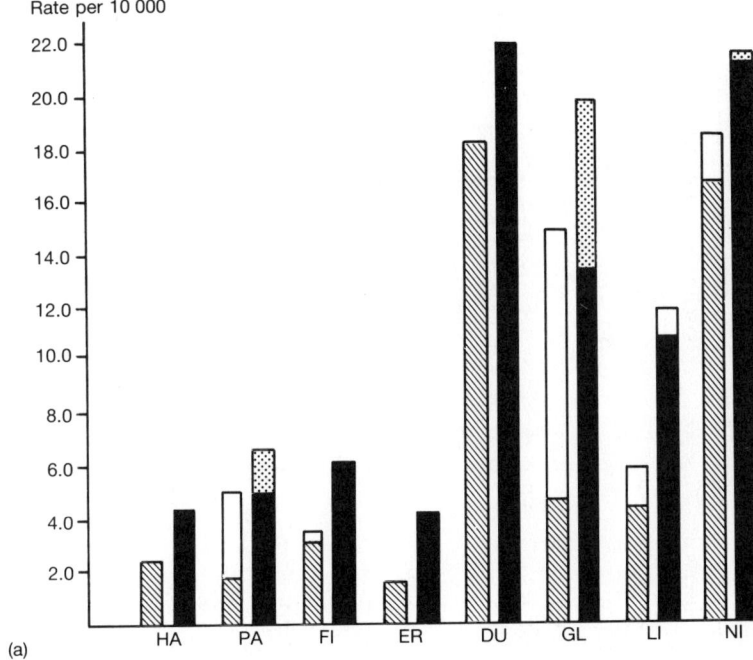

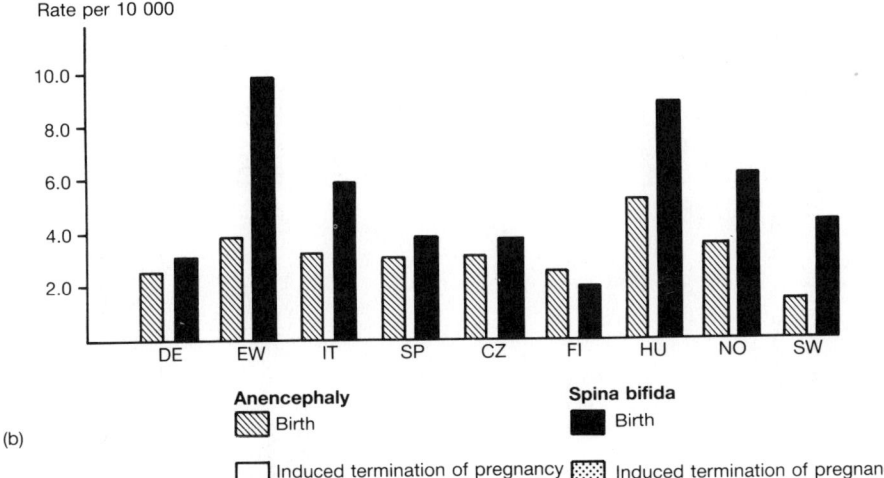

Fig. 12.5 Prevalence rate (corrected for termination) per 10 000 live and stillbirths of babies with NTD: (a) in eight Eurocat centres, 1979–82; (b) other European registries of the International Clearinghouse for Birth Monitoring Systems 1980–82.

Table 12.5 Ratio of observed (O) and expected (E) cases in neural tube defects in European programmes of the International Clearinghouse for Birth Defects Monitoring Systems.

Monitoring programmes	Baseline period	Anencephaly 1983			Spina bifida 1983		
		Baseline rate per 10 000 (E)	Observed rate per 10 000 (O)	O/E	Baseline rate per 10 000 (E)	Observed rate per 10 000 (O)	O/E
Czechoslovakia	1961–1980	3.0	1.9	0.63	3.6	3.6	1.01
Denmark	1978–1981	3.0	1.2	0.39	3.3	4.5	1.36
England and Wales	1978–1980	6.9	1.8	0.26	12.8	6.7	0.52
Finland	1977–1979	2.5	0.6	0.24	2.0	2.8	1.41
France: Rhone-Alps Auvergne	1980–1982	1.4	1.4	0.99	3.7	3.2	0.87
France: Paris	1978–1981	3.6	1.3	0.35	5.2	4.5	0.87
France: Strasbourg	1979–1980	1.0	3.2	3.20	2.6	5.6	2.15
Hungary[a]	1980–1982	5.3	6.2	1.16	9.0	11.2	1.25
Italy: 140 hospitals	1978–1981	4.0	2.9	0.72	4.8	2.9	0.60
Northern Ireland	1977–1979	19.8	9.1	0.46	29.8	15.7	0.53
Norway	1967–1971	4.9	3.6	0.73	5.5	4.8	0.87
Spain: 32 hospitals	1978–1982	3.3	2.3	0.71	3.9	3.9	1.00
Sweden	1973–1977	4.1	1.8	0.45	5.5	7.5	0.86

[a]Includes cases of encephalocele.
Adapted from International Clearinghouse for Birth Defects Monitoring Systems (1985). Annual Report 1983.

declined faster than that of spina bifida. These results are consistent with data from the Office of Populations, Censuses and Surveys (DHSS, 1979, OPCS 1980) showing a decline in NTD rate of 50 per cent in the United Kingdom between 1974 and 1982. Factors that might explain this trend will be analysed later.

Risk factors

The aetiology of NTD is multifactorial. Unlike, for example, cleft lip, genetic factors are less clear, but are nonetheless relevant.

Family data suggest 63-85 per cent inheritability (Leck 1983). This leads to a risk in other siblings of approximately 5 per cent in British populations, which is higher than in other parts of Europe, particularly France (less than 2 per cent) (Boué 1981a). In most communities, anencephaly and spina bifida are more frequent in females than in males. This remains unexplained although a complex genetic model of the sex distribution has been considered (Elwood and Elwood 1980).

The non-genetic risk factors, which explain almost 95 per cent of NTD cases, include both maternal age: U-shaped distribution—and parity: higher risk in primiparae and multiparae. More instructive in terms of prevention are the relationship between NTD and a previous history of spontaneous abortions and stillbirths, the seasonal variation in NTD (high risk in winter), secular trends (increased incidence reported in births around 1940 and 1955), and socio-economic level of the family (highest risks are observed with low parental status and in poor communities). Such risk factors might indeed reflect an association with diet, either poor nutrition in general or vitamin deficiency in particular.

Nature of the intervention

There are two possible approaches to the prevention of NTD. The first is primary prevention, currently based on vitamin supplementation. This is, however, still speculative, and thus the other, surely more feasible, approach is by secondary prevention based on prenatal screening.

Primary prevention

In 1980, Laurence pointed out the possible benefit of dietary counselling to the risk of recurrence of NTD (Laurence *et al.* 1980). Subsequently, Smithells *et al.* (1980) and Laurence *et al.* (1981) published the results of surveys suggesting that multi-vitamin therapy both before and after the beginning of a pregnancy might prevent the formation of NTD. These two surveys were performed among women at high risk (as defined by a previous history of NTD). The first survey (a clinical one) was based on multi-vitamin and iron supplementation; the second, a randomized clinical trial, compared folate administration to placebo. Their results were in agreement and have shown a protective effect: in the first survey, one out of 178 (0.6 per cent) babies of treated women developed NTD, compared with 13 out of 260 (5.0 per cent) in the untreated mothers; in the second survey, the numbers were two out of 60 (0.3 per cent) compared with four out of 63 (0.6 per cent), respectively. Both studies have attracted some criticism. In Smithells' survey, possible sampling biases have been suggested—better education and more health concern in women who did comply. In Laurence's clinical trial, the analysis has been criticized and the number of women participating was small. Any accurate evaluation of the efficacy of vitamin supplementation must be undertaken on a large scale. Three randomized controlled trials are in progress and their results should indicate whether or not vitamins are really successful in reducing the incidence of NTD. However, in many places, the practice of systematic supplementation has become routine and is unlikely to be reversed by negative findings.

Secondary prevention

Intervention based on antenatal screening is at present the most effective way of preventing NTD. It is mainly based on the detection of elevated AFP in maternal serum or amniotic fluid, or both, in early pregnancy. In all cases, the optimal time for screening is between 16 and 18 weeks of pregnancy. More recently, antenatal ultrasound examination has been considered as a possible substitution for serum AFP in some centres.

Evidence for the effectiveness of intervention

The effectiveness of the antenatal screening policy established in Europe during the last 10 years, as judged by the rate of prenatally diagnosed cases, is very promising (Figure 12.5a, Table 12.5).

There are two possible strategies. The first is the high-risk screening of individuals with a previously affected child or positive family history. Only 5 per cent of cases of NTD in the population of the British Isles, and 1 or 2 per cent in other parts of Europe could be detected in this way. The second is total population screening, attempting to cover each pregnancy.

In the first instance, the risk is large enough to justify amniocentesis and AFP amniotic fluid measurement. When the procedure is successfully undertaken, with careful localization of the placenta by ultrasound and the withdrawal of a clear amniotic fluid sample, amniotic fluid AFP determination is a very accurate test for NTD : the false-positive rate is at most 0.1 per cent, the false-negative rate has been estimated at 0.2 per cent (European collaborative study, Lindsten *et al.* 1976); moreover the risk of fetal loss is minimal : 1.0 to 1.5 per cent (Elwood and Elwood 1980; UK Collaborative Study 1979).

In the second instance, mass screening techniques only might be considered: either maternal serum AFP or antenatal ultrasound or both.

Screening for NTD by measuring maternal serum AFP has a detection rate of approximately 80 per cent. All studies agree that the discriminating power appears higher between 16–18 weeks of gestation than before this time, and for anencephaly rather than for spina bifida. From the retrospective data of the UK Collaborative Study Group (mid-1974–June 1977) (UK Collaborative Study 1977), the detection rates for the British Isles among screened pregnancies, at 2.5 times the normal median, were 88 per cent for anencephaly, 79 per cent for open spina bifida, and 38 per cent for closed or unclassified spinal bifida.

From the two large prospective surveys performed in Scotland (Edinburgh—Brock *et al.* 1978—and Glasgow—Ferguson-Smith *et al.* 1978) between 1975 and 1977, the detection rates in the screened group were 93 per cent (53/57 cases) for anencephaly and 54 per cent (21/29) for open spina bifida, but none of the 24 closed spina bifida cases were picked up. Detection rates of 96 per cent (Scriver 1985) for anencephaly and 78 per cent (25/32) for spina bifida were reported in more recent data from Edinburgh (1979–1981) (supplied by Brock in Scriver 1985). The sensitivity of maternal serum screening was always very low for closed spina bifida.

The results are closely related to the selection of the optimum cut-off point. Table 12.6 shows the likelihood of having a fetus with open spina bifida for different maternal serum AFP concentrations. When cut-off levels of 2.0, 3.0, 4.0 multiples of the normal median are considered at 16–18 weeks of gestation, the calculated odds are 1:40, 1:10, and 1:3, respectively. As has been shown by Wald and Cuckle (1984), for an individual woman the odds of having a fetus with open spina bifida with the actual AFP values 2.0, 3.0, and 4.0 MoM are not comparable being, for the same prevalence of 2 per 1000, 1:400, 1:59, and 1:13, respectively (UK Collaborative Study 1982). Lowering the cut-off level to include nearly all affected pregnancies would include a large proportion of unaffected pregnancies. On the other hand, raising the cut-off level would not only reduce the false-positive rate but also the detection rate of anomalies. In the UK Collaborative Study, when the cut-off level point used was 2.5 times the normal median maternal serum AFP concentration, the rate of unaffected pregnancies was 3.3 per cent. Using an extreme cut-off level equal to four times the normal median leads not only to a very low false-positive rate (0.3 per cent) but also to a very low detection rate (76 per cent of anencephaly and 38 per cent of all spina bifida).

The potential for improving screening by repeat AFP testing has been analysed in the fourth UK Collaborative AFP Study Report (1982). However, it appears that there is little value in testing a second maternal sample.

Antenatal ultrasound is an alternative screening tool which has recently become more refined and more widely used. In France, for example, the percentage of pregnant women who had a scan rose from 11 per cent in 1976 to 82 per cent in 1981 (Rumeau-Rouquette et al. 1984). Ultrasound is used routinely during pregnancy in most European countries. Further, as a screening test for NTD, ultrasound scanning offers the only non-invasive option. With this method, results, such as those observed in Oxford (Gough 1984), are extremely encouraging. These indicate that ultrasound is more sensitive than amniotic fluid AFP alone, but less specific. All 23 cases of anencephaly that occurred were detected by ultrasound whereas only 22 were discovered using AFP; out of 17 cases of open spina bifida, 17 were detected by ultrasound, and 16 by AFP. However, among 201 unaffected fetuses with elevated maternal serum AFP (false-positives), there were 6 cases falsely detected by ultrasound and only 4 cases by AFP. In our registration of congenital anomalies in Paris (Goujard et al. 1983) where screening by maternal serum AFP is not undertaken but ultrasound examinations are widely used, the downward trend observed for the period 1979-82 (Figure 12.5a) is confirmed, and in 1985, only 15 per cent of the total number of NTD cases were registered as live or stillbirths.

Until recently, ultrasound scanning has been used as an adjunct to AFP screening for measurement of biparietal diameter to correct gestational age errors, or as a complementary screening or diagnostic test. The advantage of this combination, in terms of the sensitivity of screening, has been shown (Persson et al. 1983), particularly for the detection of small NTD. However it has recently been suggested that ultrasound alone should be used. There are, however, no reliable data on the sensitivity or specificity of routine screening by ultrasound for congenital anomalies although a prospective multi-centre survey involving EEC countries is under way. There are also no clinical trial data to suggest that ultrasound is effective in screening. Again trials are planned. It is also extremely important to realize that the extension of ultrasound scanning as routine screening for fetal anomalies implies an increase in the number of trained staff using good equipment. In such an ideal situation (Campbell et al. 1985), the level of ascertainment would be 80 to 85 per cent of all fetal structural abnormalities. But, even if optimal technical conditions prevail there are limitations, the major problem being closed spina bifida and small area spina bifida. In the Danish screening project (Norgaard-Pedersen et al. 1985), for example, 14 out of 16 cases of spina bifida could not be verified by ultrasound scan even after abnormal AFP results.

Finally, screening may not fully explain recent trends. The decline in the birth prevalence of NTD registered in England and Wales over the period 1965–1981 was studied by Owens et al. (1981) for the Liverpool and Bootle areas. However, the small number of selective abortions for NTD registered over this period could not explain the fall in incidence. Second, no single demographic or social factor, such as falling birth rate, change in social class, maternal age distribution, or limitation of births because of previously affected children, could be identified. The recurrence rate was also apparently unchanged (3.4 per cent in 1961–65; 5.0 per cent in 1980–83) (Owens et al. 1985) suggesting an environmental hypothesis for the fall. Among the possible environmental factors is periconceptional vitamin supplementation although the effect is impossible to analyse because of the uncontrolled way it is distributed.

Problems in maximizing effectiveness in populations

Despite improvements in the management of open spina bifida, it remains a severely handicapping birth defect and the main method of prevention is still fetal diagnosis and selective abortion.

The effectiveness of prenatal screening for NTD depends on three well-known parameters, common to all fetal disorders: the detection rate of the screening methods, the establishment of the programme, and its acceptability. A fourth parameter, the incidence of the defect in the population, is particularly important to consider in the case of NTD because of the wide regional variation in Europe. Indeed the positive predictive value of a test depends on the prevalence of the defect—the lower the prevalence, the lower the positive predictive value. From the UK Collaborative Study data (Table 12.6), it has been calculated that the chances of having a fetus with NTD for women with serum AFP concentrations of 2.5 times the normal median, were 1:42 when the prevalence rate was 1 per 1000 births, 1:21 when the prevalence rates was 2 per 1000 births, and 1:10 for a prevalence rate of 8 per 1000 births. Thus, in countries where the incidence of NTD is low, the expected proportion of fetuses with NTD among pregnant mothers with raised concentrations of AFP is also low. This increases the risk of false interpretation, which could easily reverse the value of such screening in a low-risk population. Screening must, therefore, be highly accurate to obtain a reasonable cost–benefit advantage.

According to several studies, it appears that the acceptance of screening for all NTD is of the order of 80 per cent. Data supplied by Brock (in Scriver 1985) have indicated that, multiplication of the parameters of eligibility for screening (estimated at 80 per cent for open spina bifida), sensitivity of the test (about 80 per cent if AFP maternal serum is considered), and acceptance plus delivery of the programme (80 per cent) leads to an index of preventive

Table 12.6 Chances of women with serum AFP levels equal to or greater than specified cut-off levels at 16–18 weeks of gestation having a fetus with an NTD or open spina bifida[a].

Cut-off level (MoM)[b]	All neural tube defects					Open spina bifida				
	Birth prevalence[c] per 1000 births					Birth prevalence[c] per 1000 births				
	2	4	6	8	10	1	2	3	4	5
2.0	1:41	1:21	1:14	1:10	1:8	1:79	1:40	1:26	1:20	1:16
2.5	1:21	1:10	1:7	1:5	1:4	1:42	1:21	1:14	1:10	1:8
3.0	1:10	1:5	1:3	1:2	1:2	1:20	1:10	1:7	1:5	1:4
3.5	1:4	1:2	2:3	1:1	1:1	1:9	1:5	1:3	1:2	1:2
4.0	1:3	1:1	1:1	3:2	2:1	1:7	1:3	1:2	2:3	1:1

[a]Multiple pregnancy was excluded by ultrasound.
[b]MoM = multiple of the median.
[c]In the absence of antenatal diagnosis and selective abortion.
Source: Wald et al. (1984).

effectiveness of 64 per cent for open spina bifida. This overall efficacy is far less than expected (the equivalent calculation for Down syndrome leads to an index of effectiveness of 25 per cent). This failure was previously noted by Roberts. et al. in 1983. This index would be higher using ultrasound as a screening test. These results provide a strong argument in favour of screening for NTD, probably even in areas where the incidence is lower than that observed in the British Isles.

Recommendations

Recent developments in the field of antenatal diagnosis have been considerable, perhaps to the detriment of other programmes or other areas of public health. The consequences of screening are serious since a positive result implies the elimination of the affected fetus. Therefore, cost–benefit analyses (Henderson 1982) and discussions on ethics (Elwood and Elwood 1980; Engel and Tran-Ngoc 1981) have been numerous—is the prevention of the birth of an abnormal child of 'benefit' to society? Is it even a serious medical problem since the number of children involved is at the most 30–40 in 10 000? These aspects have been discused by Wald (1984).

Down syndrome

In high-risk groups, such as those where one parent carries a translocation or where there is a previously affected child, the question of benefit of an amniocentesis is not raised. Moreover, the number of women who have to be examined is small.

In other cases, where the risk of anomaly is low, the discussion might be approached in cost–benefit terms. Screening begins based on the simple identification of the age of the pregnant women.

1. The first step should be an increase in access to prenatal diagnosis among eligible women—age 35 or 38 years, according to country. This should be possible with the better training of health professionals (to detect the risk factors and to inform parents on antenatal diagnosis) and if women themselves are better informed about the disorder and its risk through more effective health education. This programme should be the responsibility of public health authorities, departments of preventive medicine, and medical and paramedical staff.

2. The second step should be for each country to review the maternal age cut-off level to achieve higher test sensitivity. In most European countries the actual level, at present, is 35 years of age.

3. A third step could be an extension of access to antenatal screening and diagnosis to include women with risk factors other than those accepted at present. Among such factors are a previous history of spontaneous abortion, vaginal bleeding in the first trimester of pregnancy, severe and unexplained intra-uterine growth retardation, and diagnosis of structural anomalies by ultrasound (Table 12.7). A multi-centre study is now in progress in France to evaluate the efficacy of screening based on these extra risk factors.

Table 12.7 Potential risk factors for congenital anomaly.

	Chromosomal disorders	Other congenital anomalies
	Relative risks	Relative risks
Vaginal bleeding in the first trimester[a]		
maternal age <35 yr	1.1	1.8
>35 yr	2.4	1.8
Early growth delay observed by ultrasound[b] (95% confidence intervals)	20.0 (4.6–87.4)	25.0 (8.2–73.7)
Previous histories of spontaneous abortions >2[c]	2.5	2.3

[a]Prospective survey: 9525 pregnancies (Rumeau-Rouquette et al. 1971).
[b]Case-control survey: (Tchobroutsky et al. 1985).
[c]Prospective survey: 12 764 pregnancies (Rumeau-Rouquette et al. 1978).

4. Finally, Cuckle *et al.*'s (1984) proposal that a combination of maternal age and serum AFP might be a better screening tool than age only, must also be reconsidered in countries or centres already using maternal serum AFP to screen for NTD. This will require pilot surveys on the effectiveness in practice and new analytical techniques to measure low and high AFP concentrations with similar precision and accuracy.

Neural tube defects

The initial difficulty is that there is no simple maternal variable to identify an at-risk group in the general population of pregnant women. The solution is therefore to use more sophisticated investigations—blood samples for maternal serum AFP estimation and ultrasound are the alternatives, with amniocentesis as the diagnostic procedure.

Some countries, such as the United Kingdom, give greater prominence to maternal serum AFP screening; others, such as France, concentrate on ultrasound. Maternal serum AFP screening has not been used in Europe as widely as it might have been. On the contrary, routine ultrasound examination is becoming more and more an accredited part of prenatal care. Anencephaly and severe open spina bifida might be detected by routine ultrasound examination and with sufficient confidence to avoid amniocentesis. But, this technique is still insufficiently sensitive to detect small NTD. The detection of those less severe anomalies requires the use of focused ultrasound examination and this in turn requires experienced ultrasonographers who have the appropriate equipment and time.

1. In the British Isles, where the prevalence of NTD is high, the cost of AFP screening appears cheap (Scriver 1985; Wald and Cuckle 1984) and its practice is well developed. AFP maternal serum screening should therefore be done as primary screening, followed systematically by ultrasonography in cases of elevated serum AFP. The addition of the ultrasound examination leads to an acceptable increase of the initial cost (3–5-fold according to prevalence). The selection of a cut-off level (Wald 1984) must be a compromise based on the resources available to carry out ultrasound examination and amniocentesis. The use of AFP testing requires high quality medical and laboratory work and good coordination for follow-up testing (focused ultrasound examination, amniocentesis, and abortion services).

2. In low-risk populations screening by AFP maternal serum alone has a lower priority in cost-effective terms than screening by routine ultrasound, (Persson *et al.* 1983). It is now a priority to stimulate evaluative population-based studies, at regional or national level, on the per-

Down syndrome and neural tube defects

There are three recommendations applicable to both Down syndrome and NTD. First, genetic counselling must be developed, and the acceptability of screening must be discussed. There is also a need for continuing research into adequate primary prevention measures in order that the financial balance of research between primary and secondary preventions may be maintained.

Second, in each case of an abnormal fetus, it is absolutely essential to arrange a multidisciplinary consultation between the echographist, the obstetrician, the paediatrician, the geneticist, and the surgeon in order that the final decision, taken with the parents, is fully evaluated.

Finally, any extension of antenatal diagnosis has to be strictly controlled since extension without planning or control would increase the risk of errors.

References

Blondel, B., Darchy, P., and Kaminski, M. (1984). Mortalité foeto-infantile et maternelle. In *Naître en France* (eds C. Rumeau-Rouquette, C. Du Mazaubrun, and Y. Rabarison) pp. 19–31. Doin, Paris.

Boué, A. (1981a). In *Médecine périnatale. 10èmes Journées Nationales* (eds G. Barrier and J.M. Thoulon) pp. 162. Arnette, Paris.

—— (1981b). Le diagnostic prenatal des anomalies du foetus. Son organisation. In *Médecine périnatale. 10èmes Journées Nationales* (eds G. Barrier and J.M. Thoulon) pp. 131–4. Arnette, Paris.

Brock, D.J.H., Scrimgeour, J.B., Stenen, J. Barron, L., and Watt, M. (1978). Maternal plasma alpha-fetoprotein screening for neural-tube defects. *Br. J. Obstet. Gynaecol.* **85**, 575–81.

Campbell, S., Allan, L., Griffin, D., Little, D., Pearce, J.M., and Chudleigh, P. (1985). Early diagnosis of fetal structural anomalies. In *Prevention of physical and mental congenital defects. Part B: Epidemiology, early detection and therapy, and environmental factors* (ed. M. Marois). New York, Alan R. Liss.

Cuckle, H.S., Wald, N.J., and Lindenbaum, R.H. (1984). Maternal serum alpha-fetoprotein measurement: a screening test for Down's syndrome. *Lancet* **1**, 926–9.

Department of Health and Social Security. (1979). Working Group on the Screening for Neural Tube Defects. Report. Her Majesty's Stationery Office, London.

Elwood, J.M., and Elwood, J.H. (1980). *Epidemiology of anencephalus and spina bifida.* Oxford University Press, Oxford.

Engel, E. and Tran-Ngoc, T. (1981). Résultats et perspectives de l'amniocentèse et du foeto-diagnostic préventifs. In *Génétique médicale. Acquisitions et perspectives.* (ed. J. Feingold). Flammarion, Paris.

Erickson, J.D. (1979). Paternal age and Down's syndrome. *Am. J. Hum. Genet.* **31**, 489-97.
Eurocat (1985a). *The beginnings of Eurocat* (ed. J.A.C. Weatherall). Cabay, Louvain La Neuve.
—— (1985b). *Registration of congenital anomalies in Eurocat Centers 1979-1983.* Cabay, Louvain La Neuve.
—— (1986). *Surveillance of congenital anomalies. Years 1980-1983. An EEC concerted action project.* Bruxelles.
Ferguson-Smith, M.A., Rawlinson, H.A., May, H.M., Kate, H.A., Vince, J.D., Gibson, A.A.M., Robinson, H.P., and Ratcliffe, J.G. (1978). Avoidance of anencephalic and spina bifida births by maternal serum alpha-fetoprotein screening. *Lancet* **1**, 1330-3.
Flynt, J.W. and Hay, S. (1979). International Clearinghouse for Birth Defects Monitoring Systems. *Contributions to epidemiology and biostatistics* (eds M.A. Klingberg and J.A.C. Weatherall) pp. 44-52. Karger, Basel.
Galjaard, H. (1980) *Genetic metabolic diseases.* Elsevier, Amsterdam.
Gardent, H., Goujard, J., Fardeau, M., and Crost, M. (1984a). Analyse économique de la diffusion d'une innovation médicale: l'exemple du diagnostic prénatal par amniocentèse préoce. 1ère partie: les fondements épidémiologiques, médicaux et socio-économiques. *Rev. Epidemiol. Santé Publ.* **32**, 88-96.
—— Fardeau, M., Lanoe, J.L., and Kerleau, M. (1984b). Analyse économique de la diffusion d'une innovation médicale: l'exemple du diagnostic prénatal par amniocentèse précoce. 2ème partie: L'aide à la décision en Santé Publique pour la diffusion optimale d'une innovation. *Rev. Epidemiol. Santé Publ.* **32**, 97-106.
Golbus, M.S., Loughman, W.D., Epstein, C.J., Halsbach, G., Stephens, J.D., and Hall, B.D. (1979). Prenatal genetic diagnosis in 3000 amniocenteses. *New Engl. J. Med.* **300**, 157-63.
Gough, J.D. (1984). Ultrasound. In *Antenatal and neonatal screening* (ed. N.J. Wald). Oxford University Press, Oxford.
Goujard, J., Maillard, F., Ancelin, C., Du Mazaubrun, Ch., and André, F. (1983). Enregistrement des malformations congénitales à Paris. Bilan et perspectives de l'étude placée sous l'égide de la CEE. *J. Gynecol. Obstet. Biol. Reprod.* **12**, 805-17.
——, ——, Passavy, A.M., and Du Mazaubrun, C. (1986). The impact of prenatal diagnosis on the prevalence rate of birth defects. *Eur. J. Epidemiol.* **2**, 321.
Henderson, J.B. (1982). Measuring the benefits of screening for open neural-tube defects. *J. Epidemiol. Comm. Hlth.* **36**, 214-9.
Herzenberg, L.A., Bianchi, D.W., and Schroder, J. (1979). Fetal cells in the blood of pregnant women: detection and enrichment by fluorescence-activated cell sorting. *Proc. Nat. Acad. Sci. (Washington)* **76**, 1453-5.
Hook, E.B. and Lindsjo, A. (1978). Down's Syndrome in live birth by single year maternal age interval in a Swedish study: comparison with results from a New-York State study. *Am. J. Hum. Genet.* **30**, 19-27.
International Clearinghouse for Birth Defects Monitoring Systems (1982, 83, 84). Annual Reports 1980-1981-1982. Garnisonstryckeriet, Stockholm.
—— (1985). Annual Report 1983. V.R. Ward, Wellington.
Laurence, K.M., James, N., Miller, M., and Campbell, H. (1980). Increased risk of

recurrence of pregnancies complicated by fetal neural-tube defects in mothers receiving poor diets, and possible benefit of dietary counselling. *Br. Med. J.* **281**, 1592–4.

—, —, —, Tennant, G.B., and Campbell, H. (1981). Double-blind randomised controlled trial of folate treatment before conception to prevent recurrence of neural-tube defects. *Br. Med. J.* **282**, 1509–11.

Leck, I. (1983). Fetal malformations. In *Obstetrical epidemiology* (eds S.L. Barron and A.M. Thomson) pp. 298–318. Academic Press, London.

Lindsten, J., Zetterstrom, R., and Ferguson-Smith, M. (1976). Prenatal diagnosis of genetic disorders of the fetus. *Acta Paediat. Scand.* **259**, 1–99.

Merkatz, I.R., Nitowsky, H.M., Makri, J.N., and Johnson, W.E. (1984). An association between low maternal serum alpha-fetoprotein and fetal chromosomal abnormalities. *Am. J. Obstet. Gynecol.* **148**, 886–94.

Mikkelsen, M., Fischer, G., Stene, J., Stene, E., and Petersen, E. (1976). Incidence study of Down Syndrome in Copenhagen, 1960–71: with chromosome investigation. *Ann. Hum. Genet.* **40**, 177–82.

Mikkelsen, M., Fischer, G., Hansen, J., Pilgaard, B., and Nielsen, J. (1983). The impact of legal termination of pregnancy and of prenatal diagnosis on the birth prevalence of Down syndrome in Denmark. *Ann. Hum. Genet.* **47**, 123–31.

Milunsky, A. (ed.) (1979). *Genetic disorders and the fetus. Diagnosis, prevention and treatment*. Plenum Press, New York.

Modell, B. (1985). Tropoblast biopsy for fetal diagnosis. In *Prevention of physical and mental congenital defects. Part B: Epidemiology, early detection and therapy, and environmental factors* (ed. M. Marois) pp. 138–40. Alan R. Liss, New York.

Norgaard-Pedersen, P., Bagger, P., Bang, J. Fischer-Rasmussen, W., Gad, C., Hasch, E., Helkjaer, P.-E., Jacobsen, J.C., Kjeldsen, J., Kjaersgaard, E., Petersen, P.L., Philip, J., Thisted, J., and Toftager-Larsen, K. (1985). Maternal serum alpha-fetoprotein screening for fetal malformations in 28062 pregnancies. *Acta Obstet. Gynaecol. Scand.* **65**, 511–4.

Office of Population Censuses and Surveys. (1980). *Congenital malformations*. Her Majesty's Stationery Office, London.

Owens, J.R., Harris, F., McAllister, E., and West, L. (1981). Nineteen year incidence of neural tube defects in area under constant surveillance. *Lancet* **2**, 1032–5.

—, —, Walker, S., McAllister, E., and West, L. (1983). The incidence of Down's syndrome over a 19-year period with special reference to maternal age. *J. Med. Genet.* **20**, 90–3.

—, Simpkin, J.M., and Harris, F. (1985). Recurrence rates of neural tube defects. *Lancet* **1**, 1282.

Persson, P.H., Kullander, S., Gennser, G., Grennert, L., and Laurell, C.B. (1983). Screening for fetal malformations using ultrasound and measurements of alpha-fetoprotein in maternal serum. *Br. Med. J.* **286**, 747–9.

Roberts, C.J., Hibbard, B.M., Elder, G.H., Evans, K.T., Laurence, K.M., Roberts, A., Woodhead, J.S., Robertson, I.B., and Hoole, M. (1983). The efficacy of a serum screening service for neural-tube defects: the South Wales experience. *Lancet* **1**, 1315–8.

Rumeau-Rouquette, C., Goujard, J., and Etienne, C. (1971). Relation entre les metrorragies du début de la grossesse et les malformations congénitales. Résultat d'une enquête prospective sur 9 525 grossesses. *Gynecol. Obstet.* **70**, 557–62.

——, ——, Huel, G., and Kaminski, M. (1978). *Malformations congénitales. Risques périnatals.* INSERM, Paris.

——, Du Mazaubrun, Ch., and Rabarison, Y. (eds) (1984). *Naître en France.* Doin, Paris.

Schroder, J. and Herzenberg, L.A. (1980). Fetal cells in maternal circulation. In *Genetic disorders and the fetus. Diagnosis, prevention, and treatment.* (ed. A. Milunsky) pp. 541–55, Plenum Press, New York.

Scriver, Ch. R. (1985). Population screening: report of a workshop. In *Prevention of physical and mental congenital defects. Part B: Epidemiology, early detection and therapy, and environment factors* (ed. M. Marois). Alan R. Liss, New York.

Smithells, R.W., Sheppard, S., Schorah, C.J., Seller, M.J., Nevin, N.C., Harris, R., Read, A.P., and Fielding, D.W. (1980). Possible prevention of neural tube defects by periconceptional vitamin supplementation. *Lancet* **1**, 339–40.

Spencer, K. and Carpentier, P. (1985). Screening for Down's syndrome using serum alpha fetoprotein: a retrospective study indicating caution. *Br. Med. J.* **290**, 1940–3.

Stene, J. and Mikkelsen, M. (1984). Down's syndrome and other chromosome disorders. In *Antenatal and neonatal screening* (ed. N.J. Wald). Oxford University Press, Oxford.

——, Fischer, G., and Stene, E. (1977). The paternal age effect in Down's syndrome. *Ann. Hum. Genet.* **40**, 299–306.

——, Stene, E., Stengel-Rutkowski, S., and Murken, J.D. (1981). Paternal age and Down's syndrome. Data from prenatal diagnoses (DFG). *Hum. Genet.* **59**, 119–24.

Tchobroutsky, C., Bréart, G., Rambaud, D.C., and Henrion, C. (1985). Correlation between fetal defects and early growth delay observed by ultrasound. *Lancet* **1**, 706.

Trimble, B.K. and Baird, P.A. (1978). Maternal age and Down's syndrome: age-specific incidence rates by single-year intervals. *Am. J. Genet.* **2**, 1–5.

First Report of the UK Collaborative Study on alpha-fetoprotein in relation to neural tube defects. (1977). Maternal serum alpha-fetoprotein measurement in antenatal screening for anencephaly and spina bifida in early pregnancy. *Lancet* **1**, 1323–32.

Second Report of the UK Collaborative Study on alpha-fetoprotein in relation to neural tube defects. (1979). Amniotic fluid alpha-fetoprotein measurement in antenatal diagnosis of anencephaly and open spina bifida in early pregnancy. *Lancet* **2**, 652–62.

Fourth Report of the UK Collaborative Study on alpha-fetoprotein in relation to neural-tube defects. (1982). Estimating and individual's risk of having a fetus with open spina bifida and the value of repeat alpha-fetoprotein testing. *J.Epidemiol. Comm. Hlth* **36**, 87–95.

Wald, N.J., and Cuckle, H.S. (1984). Open neural-tube defects. In *Antenatal and neonatal screening* (ed. N.J. Wald). Oxford University Press, Oxford.

Wald, N.J. (ed.) 1984. *Antenatal and neonatal screening.* Oxford University Press, Oxford.

13
Thalassaemia

Eleni Petridou and Dimitris Loukopoulos

SUMMARY
The prevention of thalassaemia and other inherited haemoglobin disorders remains the only realistic way to effectively eliminate their impact, in spite of the considerable recent advances in transfusion therapy, iron chelation, bone marrow transplantation, and gene replacement. Preventive programmes for thalassaemia have been running over the last two decades in high-prevalence countries (Greece, Italy, Cyprus) as well as in countries with large numbers of immigrants of Mediterranean origin (France, the United Kingdom, Belgium, etc.). These programmes include increasing awareness, education of health professionals, and organization of laboratories providing carrier identification and prenatal diagnosis. The effectiveness of these programmes is manifested by a dramatic decrease in the expected number of newborn homozygotes, which has already reached minimal numbers in some areas. However, the fact that these programmes have not been uniformly successful, highlights the need for the wider application of this approach, mainly at a public policy level.

Defining the problem

The name thalassaemia comes from the Greek word 'thalassa' (sea) and means literally 'anaemia of the sea'. This derives from its common occurrence among people in the countries around the Mediterranean. The term Cooley's anaemia is normally reserved for the severe form of the disorder, after the first medical description of the disease by Dr Thomas Cooley in 1925. The thalassaemias are a group of genetically related autosomal recessive disorders that share one common feature: the absence or decreased synthesis of one of the globin chains of normal haemoglobin.

Four types of globin chain are most pertinent to the study of the thalassaemias, these being the α, β, γ, and δ chains (Wintrobe 1974; Orkin and Nathan 1976) which combine in different forms of haemoglobin. Normal adult erythrocytes contain mainly haemoglobin A (approximately 98 per cent) and haemoglobin A_2 (approximately 2 per cent). Traces of the fetal haemoglobin (haemoglobin F), which is the major haemoglobin in the fetus can also be found. Haemoglobin A consists of two α and two β polypeptide chains ($\alpha_2\beta_2$); the structures of haemoglobin A_2 and haemoglobin F being $\alpha_2\delta_2$ and $\alpha_2\gamma_2$ respectively. The relative amounts of the different globin chains change from fetal to adult life.

Any abnormality of the delicate mechanism which results in a decreased production of one or more globin chains corresponds to a distinct type of thalassaemia. There are two globin genes one from each chromosome for each globin chain and hence defective production can result in one of two outcomes. Thalassaemia *traits* exist when a gene for thalassaemic haemoglobin is inherited from one parent and a gene for normal haemoglobin from the other. This is the so-called carrier state or heterozygous state. Thalassaemia *disease* (homozygous state) exists when a gene for thalassaemic haemoglobin is inherited from both parents.

Severity of the problem

Genetic classification of thalassaemia syndromes

On the basis of the affected chain, thalassaemias have been broadly classified as α, β, δ, and $\beta\delta$ thalassaemia, respectively (Bank 1978). In practice, only the α and β thalassaemias are of clinical importance. Because α chains are present at all stages of development, any disease affecting their synthesis would affect the embryo and fetus, as well as the adult. Thus complete absence of the α-gene function in both chromosomes (homozygous state) results in the lethal hydrops fetalis. Conversely, β chains are produced in significant quantity only after birth; therefore, diseases affecting their synthesis begin during the first year of life (Weatherall and Clegg 1981). Beta-thalassaemia displays both genetic and biochemical heterogeneity. There are different sub-types varying from complete deletion of genes to defective transcription, processing, or translation of the β m-RNA.

In addition, other haemoglobinopathies, such as the sickle cell syndromes, may coexist with the heterozygote form of β-thalassaemia.

Clinical classification of thalassaemia syndromes

The thalassaemias are divided into three groups based on their clinical severity. These are, in order of decreasing severity, thalassaemia major, intermedia, and minor. The most severe form of β-thalassaemia, thalassaemia major, is characterized by marked anaemia from infancy, often in the range of 4 to 6 g/dl. Thalassaemia intermedia implies more moderate anaemia and jaundice, and those affected may survive into adult life even without blood transfusions. Approximately 7 to 10 per cent of these patients can spontaneously maintain concentrations of haemoglobin in the range of 6 to 8 g/dl without regular transfusion. Thalassaemia minor is an asymptomatic illness, with mild or no anaemia, but with prominent morphological abnormalities of the erythrocytes.

Clinical status cannot be used to define precisely the genotype of a patient although individuals with thalassaemia major are homozygous for the β-thalassaemias (some, however, may have more than one genetic abnormality of haemoglobin synthesis), whereas those with thalassaemia minor are usually heterozygous for the trait. Thalassaemia intermedia can result from a variety of genetic disorders of β-chain synthesis.

Clinical versus laboratory definition

Homozygotes

The appearance of patients with full-blown clinical Cooley's anaemia is so characteristic that a presumptive diagnosis may be made on examination. The syndrome is characterized by a severe progressive anaemia, varying degrees of jaundice, hepatosplenomegaly, marked bone abnormalities, and progressive heart failure leading to a shortened life-span. However, clinical manifestation of the disease varies considerably, and definitive diagnosis of homozygous β-thalassaemia requires laboratory confirmation.

Haemoglobin studies, indicating a decreased or total absence of haemoglobin A and elevated haemoglobin F, support the diagnosis. Haemoglobin A_2 may be decreased, normal, or increased in homozygotes, but is characteristically elevated in heterozygotes. Family studies documenting the heterozygous state in parents and siblings provide the final clues to the diagnosis (Nathan and Oski 1974; Wintrobe 1974; Weatherall and Clegg 1981).

The diagnosis of Cooley's anaemia in a child generally means a shortened life that is dependent on repeated blood transfusions and chelation therapy, procedures that are associated with considerable expense, inconvenience, and unpleasantness. A shortened life-span, often of only 15 to 20 years, has been the rule; life-expectancy, under current and more aggressive management regimes (Logothetis *et al.* 1972) has not yet been established, but presumably extends beyond the third decade. New approaches to treatment have been reported, such as bone marrow transplantation from HLA identical donors (Milunsky 1975) and activation of the γ-globin genes by various agents, but as yet they remain at the experimental level. Physicians and other health workers who undertake the care of these patients should provide not only the medical care for the child, but also emotional support and counselling for the family that must face years and even decades of physical, psychological, and financial stress.

The scale of the health problem posed by thalassaemia arises both from its high prevalence in some ethnic groups and the need for long-term therapy. Current treatment of β-thalassaemia major is intense, requiring comprehensive health care services. A child with thalassaemia major requires 20–30 units of blood annually and hence a conservative estimate in Greece is that the annual direct expenses per case are in the range of US$ 4000–5000. These figures include the cost of processing and administering the blood, hospitalization, special tests, and treatment. The cost becomes significantly higher when lost working days and transportation expenses are taken into account. In the United States, where the standard of living is higher, families without insurance report annual expenses in the range of $10 500. Treatment expenses will increase as survival improves.

Carriers

The clinical presentation of β-thalassaemia heterozygotes varies from a totally symptom-free state to one of moderately severe disease. The most common form is not, however, associated with symptoms or abnormal physical findings, but presents an abnormal haematological picture (WHO 1983). Expression of the heterozygous state also differs somewhat in different racial groups. Clinical varieties of β-thalassaemia carriers appear to segregate within families (US. DHHS 1981).

Although typical heterozygous β-thalassaemia is generally a benign condition, its identification is important for at least two reasons. First, it permits genetic counselling of persons at risk of having children with major thalassaemia; second, the hypochromic microcytic anaemia found in heterozygotes may be misdiagnosed as iron deficiency anaemia. Identification of the heterozygous state is based on a series of parameters among which MCH, MCV, and haemoglobin A_2 have the major discriminatory power. Simplified flow sheets have been proposed (WHO 1983; Loukopoulos and Kaltsoya-Tassiopoulou 1983); yet relevant diagnostic procedures seem to depend partially on the types of thalassaemia prevailing in each area. For mass screening the aim is to proceed by exclusion or confirmation from simple and inexpensive tests to those which are more sophisticated.

Size of the problem

Occurrence and risk factors

It has been estimated that there are about 60 million heterozygotes for the β-haemoglobinopathies worldwide and that about 300 000 homozygotes or compound heterozygotes are born annually. European heterozygotes number more than 6 million and the number of homozygotes or compound heterozygotes (mainly thalassaemia major and sickle cell disease) born per year is more than 1500 (WHO 1984, 1985). The estimates are much less reliable for the α-thalassaemia traits.

The major risk factor is ethnic group. α-thalassaemia is most commonly found in South-east Asians and to a lesser degree in those of Mediterranean and African origin. β-thalassaemia is frequently found in people of the Mediterranean basin (Greece, Cyprus, and Italy), the Middle East (Iran, Israel, and Turkey), and the Far East (China, India, Thailand, and the Philippines). It is also found to a lesser degree in people of African ancestry. As other haemoglobin disorders (for example, sickle cell trait) are also found in these populations, people may have more than one abnormality. There is increasing evidence that major problem areas exist in other EEC countries, including Portugal and Spain, as well as in other European countries like Albania and Western Yugoslavia. Thalassaemia is rare in native English, French, and German people; however, since the thalassaemia gene is prevalent in the Mediterranean basin extending through Africa and the Middle East to South-east Asia, migration and subsequent intermarriage results annually in a number of homozygous β-thalassaemic children in the United Kingdom, France, and West Germany.

Despite several population surveys in high prevalence areas, few true prevalence figures are available because relatively sophisticated laboratory tests are required to characterize fully the different forms of β-thalassaemia. Most surveys have been conducted with only one or two parameters, such as the erythrocyte osmotic fragility test or electrophoretic haemoglobin A_2 determination. In Greece, Italy, and Cyprus, where detailed mapping has been carried out the distribution of the β-thalassaemia gene is uneven. For example, in Greece the prevalence of heterozygotes is reported to be 7.4 per cent but with a range of 3–15 per cent between regions of the country. In addition, there are a few clusters of haemoglobin S carriers. Based on the assumption that for a rare recessive gene with a gene frequency of q, the frequency of heterozygotes (carriers) is $2q$ and the frequency of homozygotes q^2, it can be calculated that a total of 150 homozygous births would be expected in Greece annually. The prevalence of homozygotes may be derived by multiplying the birth prevalence by mean life-expectancy. This results in 3200 homozygous individuals who need chronic treatment.

In Cyprus 1 in 7 of the population carry the β-thalassaemia trait, 1 in 49 marriages is at risk, and thus 1 in 196 newborns is expected to be a homozygote. The current prevalence of homozygotes in the population is 1 in 1000 since there are 600 affected individuals in a population of 600 000. Given an annual increase of 68–70 cases and the increased survival rates, it was estimated that the prevalence would rise to 1:200 in about 50 years, causing a

300–400 per cent increase in blood requirements and a 600–700 per cent rise in the cost of treatment. The implementation of a national prevention programme therefore seemed essential.

Trends

Recent trends in the birth prevalence of homozygotes following the implementation of preventive programmes are encouraging. The incidence of homozygotes has been reduced by more than 50 per cent in Greece, 62 per cent in Italy, and 97 per cent in Cyprus. Programmes in other countries have been less successful either because the disease is less common and the problem of lower priority (United Kingdom) or the necessary facilities and health services infrastructure are lacking (Kuliev 1986). The population prevalence of homozygotes has not shown a similar reduction because of the gradual increase in life-expectancy. Finally, on theoretical grounds, even in the absence of preventive programmes, one may expect a minimal increase in the frequency of the defective genes, because of a possible reduction in the intermarriage of heterozygotes. In addition the availability of prenatal testing will reduce pregnancy abstinence in married heterozygotes.

Nature of intervention

The control of hereditary anaemia, such as thalassaemia, requires both community education and involvement. The specific interventions consist of prospective screening for carriers in defined population groups by blood testing and subsequent genetic counselling; prenatal diagnosis and possible termination of homozygous fetuses. None of the above procedures is adequately effective when carried out alone and they need to be incorporated as an integral part of a comprehensive programme requiring on-going evaluation and quality control.

In some regions such as Cyprus, Greece, Sardinia, and several regions of continental Italy, preventive programmes have been implemented since 1970. The programmes are based on a central reference unit and several peripheral ones. The central one is responsible for the organization of carrier identification and also undertakes prenatal diagnosis and the investigation of atypical cases; the peripheral units, situated in the smaller cities, are responsible for local heterozygote diagnosis. A similar programme aimed towards Cypriot, Asian, Indian, and Pakistani couples was also introduced to Britain in 1977 (Modell *et al.* 1980).

Public education and community involvement

The most successful preventive programmes require community involvement from the outset, even in the planning phase. Intensive media coverage before the start of the screening procedure helps both the population at risk, and the public at large, to understand the disease and its prevention through such programmes. Before any large-scale health education campaign starts it is essential that adequate facilities be provided in order to meet the potentially increasing demand for carrier screening and prenatal diagnosis.

Some educational procedures which have been successfully implemented include the following:

1. Consultation with, or formation of, parents' associations and other voluntary organizations which are extremely useful in community education and informal genetic counselling. Such associations can play a crucial role in promotion of community education through the organization of public campaigns and the distribution of literature.
2. Consultation with community leaders to inform them of the nature of the programme, enlist their co-operation, and receive their advice; formation of village or community clubs.
3. Meetings with physicians, particularly paediatricians and obstetricians, and other health workers to discuss the best possible approaches. In most genetic conditions a major source of suffering is the misinformation given to individuals by uneducated health workers.
4. Formal education on the inherited anaemias was introduced into the school curriculum in Greece as well as in Cyprus.
5. Presentation of the programme to the general public by means of television, radio, newspapers, information booklets, and posters, followed by intensive publicity campaigns in high-incidence areas. A lower profile can clearly be adopted by communities where the disease is less prevalent.
6. Information leaflets on where and how to report for examination should be made available to prospective couples—for example, at marriage registry offices, general practitioners' premises, and family planning clinics.

It is clear that all these components are more effective when adjusted to the cultural values and religious beliefs of the population. For example, the Orthodox Church in Cyprus contributed substantially to the overall success of the programme thereby encouraging premarital testing and genetic counselling in heterozygote couples. In Sardinia, on the other hand, the Catholic Church apparently ignored the preventive campaign, whose main message was in apparent contrast to its recommendation on pregnancy interruption.

As current medical management prevents the development of profound deformities of the affected homozygotes, the continuous sensitization obtained by confrontation with the sick children is being lost, so there is a need for new approaches to maintain community awareness.

Screening for carriers

Screening by blood tests for the presence of the thalassaemia carrier state permits the identification of prospective parents who may be at risk of having children with thalassaemia major.

The ideal time to offer screening to people who are at risk is determined by a number of factors. Ideally, screening should be incorporated as part of an individual's routine health care with genetic counselling provided for positive subjects (Editorial 1980). Other times for screening include the neonatal period (as part of prenatal care), during sponsored ethnic community programmes, and for immigrants and refugees at the time of first arrival into the host country.

Neonatal screening

Screening of newborn infants, using a blood sample from the umbilical cord, is an effective way to identify sickle cell disease and trait, α-thalassaemia trait, and other abnormal findings such as haemoglobin E trait. The disadvantages of neonatal screening are that it is unsuitable for detecting β-thalassaemia trait and further it is likely that the information will be 'lost' by adulthood, particularly as testing in this age group cannot be accompanied by appropriate health education.

It should be stressed, however, that the main advantage of neonatal screening is the detection of the heterozygous state in the parents. This may lead to prenatal diagnosis in subsequent pregnancies.

Screening during pregnancy

Screening during pregnancy would theoretically provide an opportunity for prenatal diagnosis, although the spouse may not be available and time may be a limiting factor. Many women come for their first prenatal visit well into their pregnancy, and it may be too late both to screen their partner and to provide prenatal diagnosis if indicated. Accurate carrier indentification during pregnancy may be complicated because of the associated folic acid and iron deficiency anaemia and the potential increase of fetal haemoglobin in the blood of the pregnant mother. Lastly, screening at this time may generate unnecessary anxiety and precipitate a crisis regarding the question of pregnancy interruption.

Despite all these ethical, medical, and financial difficulties, screening during pregnancy is still used as an approach to carrier identification, because the target group is easily accessible. However, as the population-based programmes gradually expand and become more successful, there is a shift to the screening of other target groups, notably single people.

'Prospective' screening

When first launched, most preventive programmes involved the so-called 'retrospective screening', namely, screening of couples who had already had affected children before prenatal diagnosis was available. Such carrier couples tended to refrain from having further children and often decided on an abortion because of the fear of producing a homozygote. That method of prevention proved successful in the sense that families with more than one affected child are now extremely rare. However, although retrospective diagnosis is useful on an individual basis, it has only limited population effectiveness. Therefore 'prospective carrier diagnosis' in the sense of assessing the carrier state of couples at or before the first pregnancy was implemented in a second stage.

There is no optimal way of encouraging prospective parents to seek testing, since conditions differ so much between communities. So far, the community approach has been studied only in high-incidence areas of Europe. Such an approach relies on the individuals or couples to request testing when they are best prepared to absorb information.

Screening of recruits during military service

An alternative approach is to test single persons as they enter the reproductive age, for example school leavers. As the production of a homozygous fetus requires both parents to be carriers, the first round of screening can be restricted to males. For example, in countries with obligatory military service, screening can be offered to army recruits during the initial training period. The results will be stored under strict confidentiality and will be released only to the individuals concerned. There are some substantial advantages in this approach including the following:

1. The population is concentrated, available, and in a sense 'captive', thus considerably simplifying the logistical problems. It appears that the *per capita* cost of screening in the army is about one-tenth of the corresponding cost of examining a similar number of individuals in the general population. Moreover, army laboratory facilities can be used and quality control can be easily assured. Effective thalassaemia control may thus be achieved by examining only one member of a prospective couple, plus the prospective spouse of any identified heterozygotes. A substantial reduction of the laboratory burden may thus be achieved by concentrating screening among male recruits.

2. Many people among the less educated segments of the population cannot understand the difference between the heterozygous state and the

particular disease. It is therefore, common for heterozygotes to feel stigmatized by the fact that they have been found to be carriers of the defective gene. Genetic discrimination is part of the larger problem of how society responds to an individual who suffers or simply is at increased risk for bearing sick children. We may therefore need to explore statutory solutions to prevent genetic discrimination or alleviate its consequences. In traditionally male-dominated societies, like those in the Mediterranean basin where thalassaemia is common, stigmatization can be more important for a girl than a boy and the suggested approach could reduce the problem by concentrating screening among males. It is perhaps indicative of the psychological dynamics of these societies that the Greek word 'stigma' is still being used to describe the carrier state.

3. Thalassaemia screening in the army may also facilitate blood donation, screening for other conditions, and some research activities.
4. Screening in the army provides an ideal opportunity for integrating abstract notions of health education with personal concerns and identifiable problems.

Genetic counselling

Genetic counselling should be provided to all persons screened (or in the case of children to their parents or guardians). Once the screening procedure has been completed and the individual has been properly informed, any mandatory measure restricting his or her freedom should be carefully avoided. Experience in Greece and Cyprus has shown that such action has produced negative responses (Angastiniotis et al. 1986). Counselling aims to provide the individual with the various options in deciding his or her reproductive behaviour—namely, mate selection, birth control, avoidance of childbearing, adoption, fetal testing, or artificial insemination by donor. Counselling for those couples who carry the common genotype of thalassaemia is relatively simple and can be addressed by well-trained social workers or health visitors, while in the case of pregnant women or of rare genotypes of thalassaemia a senior member of the staff should be personally involved. Genetic counselling may be effective on its own or in conjunction with prenatal diagnosis; the latter has been widely accepted by Greek and Greek Cypriots, but Sardinian couples and Pakistani Muslims in the United Kingdom have shown a higher refusal rate. Many of the objections were linked to actual or perceived medical hazards or were religious in nature.

Prenatal diagnosis

Prenatal diagnosis of thalassaemia and the subsequent termination of pregnancy has now been accepted as an effective measure to reduce the impact of the disease in high-prevalence populations. The diagnostic procedure is carried out either at the protein level (that is, with determination of the β/α globin chain production ratio which is considered normal for the corresponding stage of pregnancy) or at the gene level (that is, with determination of whether globin genes or the adjacent DNA sequences appear normal or display characteristics of the disease). For the protein studies a sample of fetal red cells is necessary, and this can be aspirated from the placenta, usually, by the 18–20th week of pregnancy. For gene studies any fetal cells which provide an adequate amount of DNA can be used; these can be obtained by amniocentesis or chorionic villus biopsy. Chorionic villus sampling is a relatively new procedure and has an advantage over fetoscopy in that it can be performed earlier in the pregnancy, usually by the 10th week (Weatherall et al. 1985).

Evidence for the efficacy of intervention

As previously indicated, there are three approaches to reduce the incidence of thalassaemia—avoidance of carrier marriage, avoidance of conception, or deliberate termination of high-risk pregnancies. At the clinical level, the first approach is 100 per cent effective, provided that the diagnosis of the carrier state is valid or at least highly sensitive. The sensitivity of modern screening techniques in the laboratory may exceed 98 per cent; however, these techniques require more sophisticated procedures such as family and biosynthesis studies and gene mapping and are thus not readily applicable to most screening programmes. By contrast, routinely applicable screening procedures have a sensitivity of approximately 95 per cent, depending on the experience of the laboratory, other external conditions, and the relative frequency of the underlying genetic patterns.

Avoidance of conception, given the correct ascertainment of the carrier state, is limited only by the effectiveness of the available contraceptive procedures which is known to be very high under strictly controlled conditions. Prenatal misdiagnosis of affected fetuses with the currently available fetal blood testing is now extremely rare ($<$ 1 per cent). Similar or even lower figures are expected with the method of gene mapping on chorionic villus DNA.

Evidence for population effectiveness

Evaluation of a thalassaemia control programme is based on monitoring of homozygote births. Controlling thalassaemia by genetic counselling of heterozygotes has not proved effective. It has been repeatedly shown for other genetic disorders (Berman *et al.* 1986) as well as for thalassaemia itself, that a very small proportion of prospective couples modify their marriage plans on the basis of the results of the screening programmes. More often carrier couples tend to refrain from having children and often decide on abortion because of the fear of giving birth to a homozygote.

While adequate genetic counselling, provided to couples at risk, aimed to modify their reproductive patterns, the advent of fetal diagnosis signalled a new way for disease elimination, by allowing conventional marriage and reproductive behaviour (Modell *et al.* 1980). The latter seems to have been quite successful as the proportion of children born with thalassaemia major has fallen in those countries where such preventive programmes have been implemented—97 per cent of the expected homozygous births were prevented in Cyprus, 60 per cent in Italy, and more than 50 per cent in Greece. Moreover, the number of families with more than one diseased child is now extremely rare. The greater success of the preventive programme in Cyprus is probably the result of the smaller target population and its geographical concentration, two factors permitting easier organization and delivery of services on the one hand, and more effective penetration of the preventive philosophy on the other. Other factors that appear to have contributed to the increased population effectiveness of the screening programme in Cyprus are the high standards of health care already provided as well as the positive attitude and active involvement of the Orthodox Church. A factor which was found to increase population effectiveness of the preventive programme at their initial stages is the so-called 'inductive screening', based on heterozygote testing among relatives of other identified carriers. The magnifying effect of their approach may be particularly useful in countries where the disease prevails in some minority ethnic groups.

In Britain thalassaemia major births have fallen by 60 per cent in Cypriots and by 20 per cent in South-east Asians but not at all in Pakistanis. This discrepancy is probably the result of different religious attitudes in these populations concerning mid-trimester diagnosis and termination of pregnancy.

Problems in maximizing effectiveness in populations

The control of thalassaemia represents a situation where a tool exists with a very high clinical efficacy but a questionable population effectiveness. Therefore thalassaemia control is a public health problem with complex methodological, social, and financial aspects, whereas at the molecular, clinical, and laboratory level substantial progress has already been made and the early targets have been achieved.

According to several health belief models, people take preventive measures under only certain specific circumstances. They must believe that the disease in question is a serious one, that their family is susceptible to the disease, and that the benefits of undertaking the preventive measure outweigh the burdens of doing so. Therefore compliance is expected only in high-risk populations or ethnic groups and only when thalassaemia is perceived as a major problem.

Currently the successful treatment of thalassaemia minimizes deformities whereas the partial success of preventive programmes progressively reduces the numbers of affected individuals; both results lead to a reduction in the frequency and intensity of signals that would reinforce the health education message. The perceived seriousness of thalassaemia may be lower among ethnic immigrants because of cultural beliefs, implying that the disease is a natural part of life or because the language barriers may interfere with understanding the seriousness of the disease. Perceived burdens of prevention may also be higher among poor immigrant minorities because they value large families and are unfamiliar with or distrustful of the health care system. Other factors that may counteract the successful implementation of screening programmes are the stigmatization of carriers, the difficult conceptualization of the disease and its transmission, and the frequent dissociation of the relevant campaign from other health education activities.

Identification of carriers is necessary but is not sufficient for thalassaemia control. It must be accompanied by genetic counselling which in turn requires psychosocial support and the availability of family planning facilities. All factors that affect the psychosocial dynamics and family planning education and delivery are therefore important for the successful implementation of genetic counselling in thalassaemia control. Furthermore, genetic counselling requires a level of sophistication which is not always available or welcomed and may clash with traditional family attitudes or religious beliefs. Fetal diagnosis is the most recent and perhaps most effective of the preventive strategies for thalassaemia control. Refusals were based either on religious beliefs or on perceived risks associated with the second trimester intervention. The recent introduction of chorionic villus sampling and the shift of diagnosis to an earlier stage in pregnancy has reduced the risk and therefore increased the acceptability of the procedure and eventually the population effectiveness of the whole programme.

Costs of programme

The annual cost of running a successful prevention programme in Cyprus (1984 figure) has been estimated to be equivalent to the cost of treatment of all heterozygotes during any 8-week period of the same year. In Greece the cost of prevention has been estimated to be equivalent to the cost of treating newly born patients for 1 year (WHO 1983). A similar approach used in Cagliari in Sardinia disclosed that in 1980 the actual costs of treatment were US$978 000 and those of prevention $284 000 suggesting that the prevention of thalassaemia is the cost-effective solution to the medical and financial burden associated with the disease in high-prevalence countries.

The high population effectiveness of thalassaemia control programmes combining the above strategies has been empirically demonstrated and allows reasonable optimism for practical elimination of disease in the near future. It is true that we are approaching the point of limiting returns in the cost-effectiveness curve of the disease control, in the sense that the prevention of an additional case now requires a larger investment per head than in the earlier stages of the campaign. Nevertheless, given the favourable cost–benefit ratio of prevention programmes in thalassaemia, there seems to be a financial as well as a moral imperative for intensification of the related programmes in the EEC countries.

Recommendations

At the European level, prevention of thalassaemia and HbS syndromes is important not only in countries with high prevalence but also in countries with large numbers of immigrant workers from the Mediterranean basin. These population groups need extensive counselling through health workers, preferably of the same origin and language as themselves, and through community or church leaders.

Acknowledgement

We would like to thank Dr C. Papanicolaou for her helpful comments and constructive criticism.

References

Angastiniotis, M., Kyriakidou, S., and Hadjiminas, M. (1986). How thalassaemia was controlled in Cyprus. *World Hlth Forum* **7**, 291–7.

Bank, A. (1978). The thalassaemia syndromes. *Blood* **51**, 369–84.

Berman, L., Crocker, A., Fosburg, M., and Sallan, D. (1986). Carrier screening for thalassemia. *The genetic resource*. Massachussetts Department of Public Health, **3**, 16–19.

Editorial. (1980). Population screening for carriers of recessively inherited disorders. *Lancet* **2**, 679–80.

Kuliev, A.M. (1986). Thalassaemia can be prevented. *World Hlth Forum* **7**, 286–90.

Logothetis, J., Loewenson, R.B., Augoustaki, O., Economidou, J., and Constantoulakis, M., (1972). Body growth in Cooley's anemia (homozygous beta thalassaemia) with a correlation study as to other aspects or the illness in 138 cases. *Paediatrics* **50**, 92–9.

Loukopoulos, D. and Kaltsoya-Tassiopoulou, Fessas Ph. (1983). Prevention of thalassaemia. *Schweiz. Med. Wochenschr.* **113**, 1419-27.
Milunsky, A. (ed). (1975). *The prevention of genetic disease and mental retardation.* W.B. Saunders Co, Philadelphia.
Modell, B., Petrou, M., Ward, R.H.T., Fairweather, D.V.I., Rodeck, C., Varnavides, L.A., and White, J.M. (1980). Effect of fetal diagnostic testing on birth-rate of thalassaemia major in Britain. *Lancet* **2**, 1383-6.
Nathan, D.G. and Oski, F.A. (eds) (1974). *Hematology in infancy and childhood.* W.B. Saunders Co. Philadelphia. First Edition.
Orkin, S.H. and Nathan, D.G. (1976). Current concepts in genetics: the thalassemias. *New Engl. J. Med.* **295**, 710-14.
US Department of Health and Human Services. (1981). *Cooley's anemia: a medical review.* US DHHS Publication No. (HSA), 81-5125.
Weatherall, D.J. and Clegg, J.B. (1981). *The thalassaemia syndromes.* Blackwell Scientific Publications, Oxford.
——, Old, J.M., Thein, S.L., Wainscoat, J.S., and Clegg, J.B. (1985). Prenatal diagnosis of the common haemoglobin disorders. *J. Med. Genet.* **22**, 422-30.
Wintrobe, M.M. (1974). *Clinical Haematology* (7th edn). Lea and Febiger, Philadelphia.
World Health Organization (WHO) (1983). Community control of hereditary anaemias: memorandum from a WHO meeting. *Bull. WHO* **61**, 63-80.
—— (1985). *Update of the progress of haemoglobinopathies control.* Report of the third and fourth annual meetings of the WHO working groups on the community control of hereditary anaemias. Milan, 1984; Bangkok 1985.

14
Congenital hypothyroidism

Takis Panayotopoulos

SUMMARY

Congenital hypothyroidism is a disorder which, untreated, has devastating effects on a child's growth and development. Prompt diagnosis is essential and cannot be based on clinical grounds since signs and symptoms usually develop after the neonatal period. Biochemical changes, notably changes in concentrations of thyroxine (T4) and thyroid stimulating hormone (TSH) in the blood, occur early, and measurement of these are the two main approaches to the national screening programmes now run by most European countries. Both approaches have their limitations. However, the most effective present method of reducing mental retardation caused by congenital hypothyroidism in Europe is to achieve maximum coverage of the newborn by screening, and a major step towards this would include studies in regions with established programmes where the coverage rate has stabilized below the lower limit of acceptability. Other recommendations are increased quality control and monitoring of the screening procedure with publication of guidelines, and the promotion of automated data processing to minimize human error and increase the statistical usefulness of the large amounts of data available.

Defining the problem

Congenital hypothyroidism (CH) is a disorder which may cause mental retardation and can, therefore, create an enormous burden for individuals and societies. The effects of untreated CH on a child's growth and development are devastating. Imbecility, short stature, coarse features with protruding tongue, broad flat nose, widely set eyes, sparse hair, dry skin, and protuberant abdomen are the main classical characteristics of the untreated cretin.

When a deficiency in thyroid hormone was identified as 'the cause' of cretinism in the later part of the nineteenth century, and replacement therapy was proposed and appeared effective, there was great hope for the elimination of the disease (Osler 1897). Nevertheless, it gradually became clear that the effectiveness of replacement therapy depends not only on the availablity of thyroid hormone, but also on early diagnosis and beginning of treatment. Association of normal intelligence quotient with early onset of treatment is a consistent finding in relevant studies, although there is evidence that relatively subtle motor or neurological abnormalities may remain (Hulse et al. 1982; Glorieux et al. 1983; NECHC 1984).

This essential prompt diagnosis of CH cannot be based on clinical grounds, because the signs and symptoms of the disease usually develop after the neonatal period. In Sweden, with one of the best networks of services for the care of infants, it was shown that before the start of screening for CH, in 1977–78, more than half of the newborns with CH were diagnosed after 3 months of age (Alm et al. 1984). On the other hand, biochemical changes and notably changes in thyroxine (T4) and thyroid stimulating hormone (TSH) concentrations in blood occur very early. In the early 1970s, radioimmunassays for the measurement of T4 and TSH, which could be performed on blood collected on a filter paper, became available. Large-scale screening programmes in the neonatal period became possible and these were rapidly developed in many countries in the hope that universal neonatal screening could achieve virtual elimination of this cause of mental retardation. Indeed, screening for CH has proved to be an extremely successful example of preventive endocrinology, despite the rarity of the condition. Its success is probably related, at least in part, to the potent emotional consequences and the enormous cost posed by any child with CH that is not diagnosed and treated in time.

Neonatal deficiency of thyroid hormones, however, has many causes (Table 14.1). Transient hypothyroidism caused by iodine deficiency is discussed in Chapter 8. In 90 per cent of cases, primary hypothyroidism is the result of thyroid dysgenesis in the first trimester of fetal life. This primary hypothyroidism is characterized by low serum T4 and high serum TSH concentrations and is a realistic target for neonatal screening. Other rarer subtypes of the condition include secondary and tertiary hypothyroidism, are caused by pituitary gland and hypothalamic abnormalities, respectively, and both are associated with a low TSH concentration (Fisher and Klein 1981).

Size of the problem

Before screening programmes, the incidence of CH was estimated, from retrospective studies in a few European countries, to be around 1 in 6–7000 live births (De Jonge 1976; Alm et al. 1978). Since the establishment of

Table 14.1 Main thyroid disorders in the neonate and their birth prevalence.

Disorder	Birth prevalence
Permanent disorders	
Primary hypothyroidism	1:3800 to 4000
Thyroid dysgenesis	90% of primary hypothyroidism
ectopia	2/3 of thyroid dysgenesis
aplasia or hypoplasia	1/3 of thyroid dysgenesis
Dyshormonogenesis	10% of primary hypothyroidism
Secondary and tertiary hypothyroidism	1:100 000
Pituitary aplasia or hypoplasia	
TSH deficiency	
Hypothalamic dysplasia	
TRH deficiency	
Transient disorders	
Hypothyroxinaemia	Variable
Hyperthyrotropinaemia	(more common in areas with iodine
Hypothyroidism from:	deficiency and in premature infants)
iodine deficiency	
iodine excess	
anti-thyroid compounds	

Source: Fisher and Klein (1981); Fisher (1983).

screening, much information on the epidemiology of CH has been gathered. The world-wide incidence of primary CH has been estimated to be 1 in 3800–4000 infants, following the screening of about 25 million infants all over the world (Fisher 1983). The incidence of CH in Europe (Table 14.2) has remained fairly constant—1 in 3500 after the screening of 11.8 million infants (Illig 1983). Primary CH is more frequent in females than in males. The female-to-male ratio is approximately 2:1 and this is a consistent finding in many studies (Pantelakis et al. 1983). The combined incidence of secondary and tertiary hypothyroidism is approximately 1 in 100 000.

The difference between the birth prevalence of CH identified by retrospective studies and that identified by screening, is probably the result of the greater number of mild cases of CH (mainly infants with ectopic thyroid gland) and of transient hypothyroidism detected by screening. There might therefore be some unnecessary treatment in children with transient hypothyroidism, and the practice of allowing a period off treatment and re-evaluating the children detected as hypothyroid is justified (Dunger and Grant 1986).

Seasonal variation of the incidence of CH has been reported at least in two

Table 14.2 Incidence of congenital hypothyrodism in various European countries, 1977–81.

Country	No. of infants screened	No. of cases detected	Rate
Austria	290 788	55	1:5287
Belgium	298 899	79	1:3784
Bulgaria	1 600	0	—
Czechoslavakia	42 836	9	1:4760
Denmark	268 685	74	1:3631
Finland	110 438	44	1:2510
France	2 229 236	590	1:3885
Germany, Dem. Rep.	20 278	7	1:2897
Germany, Fed. Rep.	1 380 394	475	1:2906
Greece	224 475	63	1:3563
Ireland	178 722	41	1:4359
Italy	684 016	207	1:3304
Luxembourg	13 819	6	1:2303
Netherlands	248 459	86	1:2889
Norway	142 143	39	1:3645
Spain	154 251	43	1:3587
Sweden	195 067	71	1:2747
Switzerland	357 657	83	1:4309
United Kingdom	855 354	233	1:3671
Yugoslavia	14 716	4	1:3679
Total	7 774 833	2209	1:3520[a]

Source: Delange *et al.* (1981); Alm *et al.* (1981); Illig *et al.* (1982).
[a] Illig *et al.* (1987), have recently calculated a rate of 1:3800 after screening 25 million.

cases: in Japan with a peak during summer months (Miyai *et al.* 1979) and in France with a peak during the first trimester of the year (Fariaux 1983). More research is needed to support these findings and relate them to possible environmental factors.

Finally, there is some evidence that maternal immunoglobulins influencing the TSH-induced processes of thyroid growth may play a part in the pathogenesis of CH. In a recent study from Quebec, such immunoglobulins were found in 15 out of 34 mothers of infants with CH and in 8 out of 16 postpartum infant blood samples (Van der Gaag *et al.* 1985).

Nature of intervention

Screening for CH was first established in Quebec in 1974 (Dussault *et al.* 1976) and shortly after, the New England Congenital Hypothyroidism

Collaborative (NECHC) was formed to begin a similar programme in 1976. In 1974 France and Belgium were the first countries in Europe to start screening programmes for CH. Other European countries followed soon after so that by 1979 most of them ran one or more programmes, some of which were covering their whole population (Delange *et al.* 1981; Alm *et al.* 1981).

Most European countries now run national screening programmes for CH (Table 14.3). In most European countries more than 90 per cent of newborns are covered by the screening programmes. In some countries it is between 50 and 70 per cent, whilst in others coverage is less than 20 per cent (Table 14.4) (Illig *et al.* 1987).

The screening procedure involves the collection of a blood spot on a filter paper (Guthrie card), although in a few cases screening is performed on umbilical blood serum (Illig *et al.* 1982). In most countries blood collection for screening for CH is performed in association with that for phenylketonuria.

There are two main approaches to the screening methodology, the advantages and disadvantages of which have been debated extensively. The first is to measure TSH as the primary screening test, and to regard elevated

Table 14.3 Year of initiation of screening for congenital hypothyroidism in European countries with screening programmes for congenital hypothyroidism.

Country	Year of initiation of screening
Austria	1976
Belgium	1974
Czechoslovakia	1981
Denmark	1977
Finland	1979
France	1974
Germany Dem. Rep.	1979
Germany, Fed. Rep.	1975
Greece	1979
Hungary	NS
Iceland	NS
Ireland	1979
Italy	1977
Luxembourg	1977
Netherlands	1978
Norway	1979
Poland	NS
Portugal	NS
Spain	1978
Sweden	1977
Switzerland	1975
United Kingdom	1979
Yugoslavia	1979

Source: Alm *et al.* (1981); Illig *et al.* (1982).
NS = not stated.

Table 14.4 European countries by coverage of newborns for neonatal thyroid screening in 1985.

Countries covering more than 90 per cent of newborns	Countries covering 50–75 per cent of newborns	Countries covering 10–20 per cent of newborns
Austria	Czechoslovakia	GDR
Belgium	Italy	Poland
Denmark	Portugal	
Finland	Yugoslavia	
France		
Germany, Fed. Rep.		
Greece		
Hungary		
Iceland		
Ireland		
Luxembourg		
The Netherlands		
Norway		
Spain		
Sweden		
Switzerland		
United Kingdom		

Source: Illig *et al.* (1987).

TSH values as abnormal (Figure 14.1). The second approach is first to measure T4 and, if the values are below a certain level, to carry out a TSH test as well (Figure 14.2). The first approach is used in most European countries and the second in the USA and Canada. An investigation by the European Society for Paediatric Endocrinology, conducted in 1983, showed that TSH was measured as the primary screening test in all but two of the 21 European countries considered (Illig 1983). In the same investigation it was shown that the finances for the screening programmes were covered by state funds in 19 countries, by health insurance in one, and by mixed sources in another.

Efficacy and effectiveness of screening

The availability of an effective treatment is essential if a screening programme is to be justified. In the case of CH, the major issue is whether thyroid hormone replacement therapy given to those diagnosed by screening can prevent the otherwise inevitable mental retardation. Recent evidence, and particularly evidence from the follow-up of children with CH identified by screening, confirms that intellectual development is normal if treatment is started early and continued in adequate therapeutic dosage.

Retrospective studies in the early 1970s showed an improvement of intellectual development with early treatment. It was reported that about 80 per cent of hypothyroid children reached an IQ of 85 if treated before the age of 3 months, compared with 45 per cent if treatment began after this age (Klein *et al.* 1972). On the basis of such evidence, the introduction of screening programmes was considered justified and the performance of randomized controlled trials unethical.

Children with CH identified in a 5-year period (1976-81) by the New England Congenital Hypothyroidism Collaborative screening programme were followed up and their mental development was assessed by the Bayley developmental scale in the first 2 years, the Stanford-Binet test at 3, 4, and 5 years, and the Wechsler Intelligence Scale as well as the Stanford Early School Achievement Tests at 6 years. The IQ of these children at all ages and the school achievement at 6 years was the same as that of normal control children. Moreover, a significant association was found between IQ scores and adequacy of treatment (NECHC 1981, 1984, 1985).

Similarly, the mean development and intelligence quotient of hypothyroid children identified by the screening programme in the North-West and North-East Thames Regions in England was above 100 at all ages. These children were assessed at 1 year of age by the Griffith's scale, at 3 years by the McCarthy Scales of children's abilities, and at 5 years by the Wechsler Intelligence scale. The hypothyroid children were, however, found to have a slightly but not significantly lower IQ at the age of 3 years, as well as a significantly lower performance on motor skills (Hulse et al. 1982; Murphy et al. 1986).

However, the mental development of hypothyroid children identified by the Quebec screening programme was found to be below that of normal control children, although it was within the normal range. These children were assessed by the Griffith's scales at the ages of 1, 1½, 3, 5, and 7 years. Their mean IQ was always above 100 but at the ages of 1, 1½, 3, and 5 years it was found to be significantly lower than that of normal control children. This was mainly the result of lower scores on performance scales as well as in hearing and speech (Glorieux et al. 1983, 1985). It has been suggested that the differences in the findings of these studies may be partly caused by the greater verbal loading of the Stanford-Binet test compared to the Griffiths test (Editorial 1986).

Despite the normal intellectual development of most hypothyroid children with early onset of treatment, there is evidence that they may have an increased risk of abnormal motor co-ordination, clumsiness, visual disorders, learning difficulties, or behavioural problems (MacFaul et al. 1978; Birrell et al. 1983; Glorieux et al. 1985; Murphy et al. 1986). More research into this field and longer follow-up of children into school age and adolescence are necessary in order to assess more fully the long-term effectiveness of the early diagnosis and treatment of CH.

The normal mental development of hypothyroid children who were identified by screening and started treatment early compares favourably with that observed following treatment after diagnosis on clinical grounds. Klein (1980) collected the available published information on the IQ of 651 hypothyroid children diagnosed before the introduction of screening and calculated that their mean IQ was about 76. In two retrospective studies of children who were diagnosed before the establishment of screening, using the Wechsler Scales of Intelligence, mean IQs of 79.5 and 83.9 were reported. These findings were based on the assessment of 99 hypothyroid children in the former (Hulse 1984) and 50 in the latter (Birrell et al. 1983).

Apart from both the age at start and the adequacy of substitution therapy, some other factors are known to affect the prognosis of children with CH in terms of their intellectual development. The first is the aetiology of CH. Klein (1980), reviewing the literature on hypothyroid children diagnosed before the introduction of screening, estimated that about 70 per cent of patients with ectopic thyroid gland reached an IQ of more than 80-90, whereas the same IQ was reached by about 48 per cent of patients with goitre or hypoplastic thyroid gland and by 26 per cent of athyrotic patients. Moreover, there is evidence that hypopituitarism, which is commonly associated with secondary hypothyroidism, may not lead to mental retardation despite delay in starting treatment (Illig 1980).

The duration and severity of intrauterine thyroid deficiency have long been shown to play an important role in determining the degree and potential reversibility of brain damage (Smith *et al.* 1957; Morreale de Escobar and Escobar del Rey 1980). This is usually estimated by the difference of bone age at the time of diagnosis from that expected by the length of gestation (Letarte *et al.* 1980), but measurement of alpha-fetoprotein has been proposed as a possible alternative (Larsson *et al.* 1983).

Finally, the parents' social class has been found to exert a major influence on the IQ of children with CH, which is independent of later presentation and beginning of treatment (Hulse 1984).

The benefit brought about by screening and the resulting early onset of treatment may thus prove to be different in the various groups of hypothyroid children mentioned previously.

Validity of screening tests

The validity of a screening test is determined by its sensitivity (that is, the proportion of the truly positive results that are correctly identified by the screening test) and its specificity (that is, the proportion of the truly negative results that are correctly identified by the screening test).

Sensitivity

A highly sensitive screening test is essential for CH because of the major consequences of an undiagnosed case. Both primary TSH measurement and primary T4 measurement with supplementary TSH determination (Figures 14.1 and 14.2) are very sensitive tests for primary hypothyroidism. No false-negative results are reported from various screening programmes (Illig 1980; Delange *et al.* 1980). These findings should of course be interpreted with great caution as it is very difficult for those running a screening programme to identify a missed case of CH that is then diagnosed subsequently. Nonetheless, the New England Congenital Hypothyroidism Collaborative, using T4 measurement as the primary test, has reported five missed cases because of false-negative test results in 700 000 screened newborns and 145 cases of CH correctly identified (NERSP and NECHC 1982)—that is, a test sensitivity of 96.7 per cent. A similar test sensitivity (97.5 per cent) was found in the screening programme in the North-West and North-East Thames Regions, in England, where TSH measurement was used as the primary test. Two missed cases from false-negative test results were identified after the screening of about 300 000 newborns and the correct diagnosis of 78 hypothyroid children (Murphy *et al.* 1986). It should be remembered that the identification of false-negatives may still be incomplete in both these programmes.

There are two categories of CH that are not detected by primary TSH measurement. The first is secondary and tertiary hypothyroidism in which serum TSH is low. However, as mentioned earlier, this is a very rare

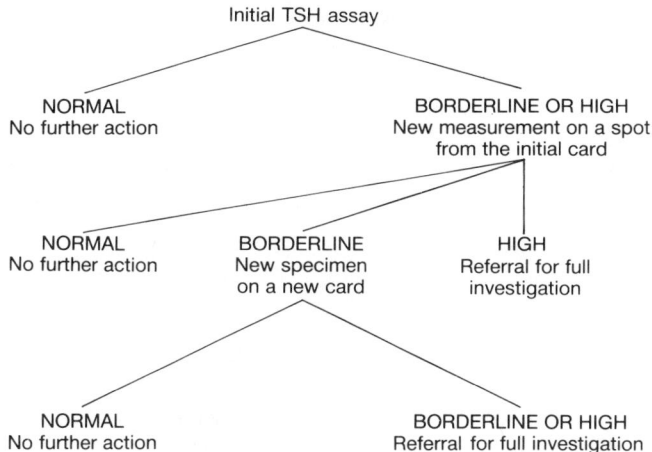

Fig. 14.1 Typical flow diagram of screening for congenital hypothyroidism using TSH measurement as the primary test. Adapted from Mengreli *et al.* (1983).

Note:
The cut-off points are different in the various screening programmes. Those between normal and borderline usually range from 20 to 40 mU/l and those between borderline and high from 50 to 80 mU/l.

condition with an incidence of about one in 100 000 newborns, and moreover most cases do not develop mental retardation even if treatment is delayed. It is also the case that, if a screening programme using serum T4 measurement supplemented by TSH determination, aims at the detection of secondary and tertiary hypothyroidism, a recall rate of about 1–2 per cent is necessary (Dussault *et al.* 1980a) and this is probably unacceptably high. The Second International Conference on Neonatal Thyroid Screening (held in Tokyo in 1982) recommended that screening for CH should be orientated to the detection of primary hypothyroidism (Fisher 1983).

The second category includes children with primary CH who have low serum T4 but normal TSH when the blood specimen is taken. Their serum TSH rises later on and is detected at follow-up. Few such cases have been described in New England (1 in 140 000 newborns screened) and Canada (2 in 93 000) and have been attributed to delay in maturation of feedback regulation of pituitary TSH secretion (Mitchell and Larsen 1980; Dussault and Morissette 1983). It has been suggested that the sooner after birth the blood specimen is obtained, the more common this finding is (Dussault and Morissette 1983). In North America, the source of this evidence, blood is usually taken around the third day of life, whereas in Europe where primary TSH measurement is mainly used, specimens are obtained at about the fifth to seventh day.

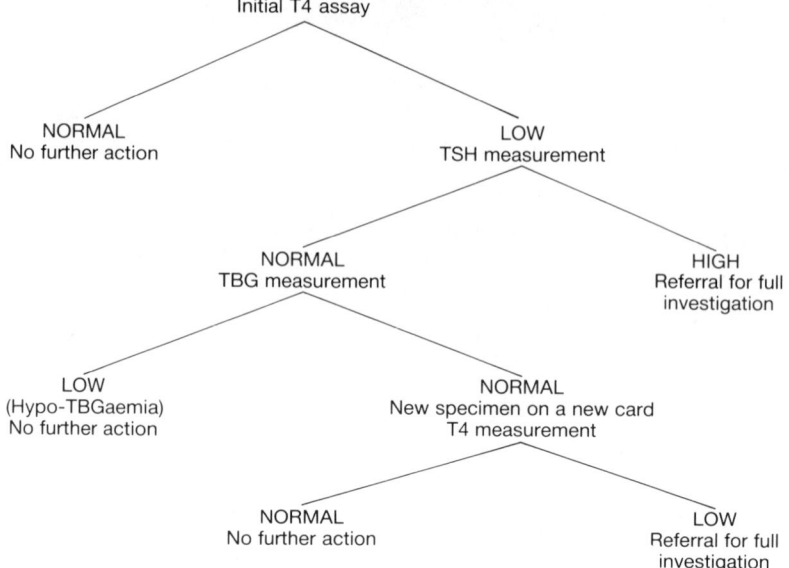

Fig. 14.2 Typical flow diagram of screening for congenital hypothyroidism using T4 measurement supplemented by TSH determination as the primary test. Adapted from Dussault et al. (1980b).

Note:
The T4 values of the initial measurement considered low vary among different screening programmes to include from 3 to 20 per cent of the infants screened.

Hypo-TBGaemia is a condition without clinical consequence and does not require treatment (TBG: thyroid binding globulin).

On the other hand, it has been found that some hypothyroid infants with ectopic thyroid gland escape detection on screening using serum T4 as the primary measurement as this may be in the normal range. Three such children were identified in North London after screening about 87 500 newborns (Hulse et al. 1980). This problem is caused by hyperstimulation of the residual thyroid tissue by the elevated TSH, resulting in compensatory secretion of T4, and it leads sooner or later to overt hypothyroidism (Kaplan et al. 1978; Delange et al. 1980). However, as has already been mentioned, hypothyroidism with ectopic thyroid gland has the best prognosis in terms of intellectual development (Klein 1980).

Specificity

The proportion of positive results—that is, the recall rate of the screening test—has been widely used as the measure of the specificity of the screening tests of CH. It is generally accepted that the recall rate of the TSH method is smaller than that of the T4—TSH approach (Barnes 1985). In Europe the former has been reported to range from 0.03 per cent to 0.85 per cent (weighted mean 0.3 per cent from 20 screening centres) and the latter from 0.13 per cent to 2.8 per cent (weighted mean 2.5 per cent from 4 centres) (Delange et al. 1980). The recall rate of the T4—TSH method in North America was reported to be 0.1 per cent to 1.1 per cent, with a weighted mean of 0.6 per cent derived from 3 screening centres (Dussault et al. 1980a). Various modifications of the laboratory methods and procedures have been reported to alter the recall rate (Morissette et al. 1980; Hummer et al. 1982).

It is not clear what proportion of the screening results presented as false-positive are caused by an inaccurate test result and what proportion by transient hypothyroxinaemia and transient hyperthyrotropinaemia (Fisher and Klein 1981). These transient conditions are more common in areas with iodine deficiency, and their identification can contribute to the reduction of the false-positive results in the screening for CH (see Chapter 8).

The problems caused by false-positive results should not be under-estimated. In a Swedish study of 102 families of infants with false-positive results on CH screening, anxiety regarding the child's health persisted in 18 families after a period of 6–12 months. However there was no comparison group in the study. It is suggested that this persistent anxiety may impair the parent–child relationship, and psychological support for the families of recalled infants should be considered (Bodegård et al. 1983).

The discussion on the validity of the screening tests brings forward the issue of cut-off points. The lower the cut-off point above which a TSH result is considered 'abnormal' (or the higher the cut-off point below which a T4 result is considered 'abnormal'), the greater the sensitivity and the smaller the specificity of the test and vice-versa. Available data are not conclusive on the optimal cut-off points. Each laboratory seems to use its own criteria, based on previous experience and particular techniques used.

Problems of the screening procedure

The screening procedure includes much more than just the laboratory tests themselves. The whole process, from taking blood from all newborns to actually meeting the recalled children for further clinical and laboratory examination at the appropriate centre, should be scrutinized.

Even in well organized screening centres, the false-negative results caused by human error outnumber those resulting from inaccurate test results. In an analysis of the false-negative results of the New England screening programme, after screening 700 000 infants, it was shown that 9 out of 14 false-negative results identified were related to human error (NERSP and NECHC 1982). The large amount of data dealt with in a laboratory, together with boredom and fatigue of laboratory staff performing repetitive work, were the main factors held responsible for those human errors.

Constraints in achieving elimination of CH

There is a dramatic decrease in the incidence of children who develop mental retardation as a result of CH. Nevertheless, the complete elimination of this condition does not seem possible with our present aetiopathological knowledge and available technology.

Neonatal screening cannot protect all the infants who are born with obvious signs and symptoms of hypothyroidism caused by intrauterine thyroid hormone deficiency and who represent 3-4 per cent of children with CH (NECHC 1981). Research to devise an effective prenatal screening test is currently being carried out (Dussault and Bernier 1985).

Present screening strategies do not aim to detect secondary and tertiary hypothyroidism. The rarity of these disorders, the good prognosis of a considerable number of these patients, even with late treatment, and the large recall rate necessary seem to justify the present strategy. Nevertheless, this should be kept under review as new, more discriminating tests become available.

The present screening practice in most European countries is based on taking a blood sample from the infant before discharge from the maternity hospital and looking primarily for TSH abnormality. A small number of hypothyroid children who have normal TSH values because of delay in the maturation of the feedback regulation of pituitary TSH secretion are likely to be missed by this type of screening. The number of these children could be reduced if blood were obtained a few days later in a home visit by health personnel. This cannot be recommended as a general approach, since it would require an extremely well organized network of services for home visits to ensure screening of all newborns at the appropriate time.

Recommendations

Screening for CH has proved extremely successful and is a totally justifiable practice. The cost of screening is relatively low and its cost-effectiveness has been documented (Layde *et al.* 1979; Laberge 1980). Both approaches to screening for CH—that is, TSH and T4-TSH—have their limitations. As there is no conclusive evidence about the superiority of either, it is recommended that laboratories generally remain with the method in which they are more experienced (Fisher 1983; Barnes 1985). It has been suggested that primary T4 measurement may be more discriminating when the blood specimen is obtained around the third day of life, and primary TSH screening when it is taken a few days later (Barnes 1985).

In view of the present state of the art, probably the most effective way to reduce mental retardation from CH in Europe is to achieve maximum coverage of newborns by screening. The European Society of Paediatric Endocrinology could continue to play an important advisory and co-ordinating role, in regions with established national screening programmes but with a coverage rate which has stabilized below 85–90 per cent. The coverage rate is likely to differ greatly within each country by geographical area (Mengreli, personal communication 1987) and socio-economic group, and to relate to the type and quality of the existing network of services. It is proposed that *ad hoc* studies should be performed in these areas to identify the particular reasons for the incomplete coverage and make recommendations for appropriate action.

Monitoring of the whole screening procedure is essential and should be built in routinely to its everyday structure. For the quality control of the tests themselves, a number of external programmes are in operation in Europe and most screening centres participate in one of them (Illig *et al*. 1982; Illig 1983). Nevertheless monitoring should include other parts of the screening process as well. Relevant guidelines should be issued by an expert European committee, which could also play some advisory and co-ordinating role.

Automation of data processing in the screening programmes should be encouraged. Computerization may be particularly useful in handling the large amount of data dealt with in a screening laboratory, not only to minimize human error and avoid misclassification of the infants screened, but also to perform statistical analyses and identify the appropriate cut-off points according to local data (Morissette *et al*. 1980).

Finally, physicians must continue to be aware of the early signs and symptoms and the consequences of untreated hypothyroidism as the condition becomes less common (Mengreli *et al*. 1981; Pantelakis *et al*. 1983). Despite the establishment of screening programmes, a few cases will remain undetected, and physicians must be alert to diagnose these clinically as early as possible.

Acknowledgements

I would like to thank Professor F. Delange, Departments de Pediatrie et de Radio-isotopes, Hôpital Universitaire Saint-Pierre, Brussels for the information he kindly provided, Dr C. Bartsokas, Dr S. Pantelakis, and Dr C. Mengreli, for their valuable assistance.

References

Alm, J., Larsson, A., and Zetterström, R. (1978). Congenital hypothyroidism in Sweden. Incidence and age at diagnosis. *Acta Paediat. Scand.* **67**, 1-3.

——, —— (1981). Report on the European Society for Paediatric Endocrinology Collaborative Study on Congenital Hypothyroidism, First Joint Meeting LWPES-ESPE, Geneva.

——, Hagenfeldt, L., Larsson, A., and Lundberg, K. (1984). Incidence of congenital hypothyroidism: retrospective study of neonatal laboratory screening versus clinical symptoms as indicators leading to diagnosis. *Br. Med. J.* **289**, 1171-5.

Barnes, N.D. (1985). Screening for congenital hypothyroidism: the first decade. *Arch. Dis. Child.* **60**, 587-92.

Birrell, J., Frost, G.J., and Parkin, J.M. (1983). The development of children with congenital hypothyroidism. *Dev. Med. Child Neurol.* **25**, 512-19.

Bodegård, G., Karin, F., and Larsson, A. (1983). Psychological reactions in 102 families with a newborn who has a false positive screening test for congenital hypothyroidism. *Acta Paediat. Scand. (Suppl.)* **304** 1-21.

De Jonge, E.A. (1976). Congenital hypothyroidism in the Netherlands. *Lancet* **2**, 143-4.

Delange, F., Beckers, C., Höfer, R., König, M.D., Monaco, F., and Varrone S., (1980). Progress report on neonatal screening for congenital hypothyroidism in Europe. In *Neonatal thyroid screening* (eds G.N. Burrow and J.H. Dussault). Raven Press, New York.

——, Illig, R., Rochiccioli, P., and Brock-Jacobsen, B. (1981). Progress report 1980 on neonatal thyroid screening in Europe. *Acta Paediat. Scand.* **70**, 1-2.

Dunger, D.B. and Grant, D.B. (1986). Endocrine disorders: diabetes mellitus, congenital hypothyroidism and congenital adrenal hyperplasia. *Br. Med. Bull.* **42**, 187-90.

Dussault, J.H. and Bernier, D. (1985). ^{125}I uptake by $FRTL_5$ cells: a screening test to detect pregnant women at risk of giving birth to hypothyroid infants. *Lancet* **2**, 1029-31.

——, Letarte, J., Guyda, H., and Laberge, C. (1976). Thyroid function in neonatal hypothyroidism. *J. Pediat.* **89**, 541-4.

——, Mitchell, M.L., La Franchi, S. and Murphey, W.H. (1980a). Regional screening for congenital hypothyroidism: results of screening one million North American infants with filter paper spot T4-TSH. In *Neonatal thyroid screening* (eds G.N. Burrow and J.H. Dussault). Raven Press, New York.

——, Letarte, J., and Guyda, H. (1980b). Screening for congenital hypothyroidism: four years of experience. In *Neonatal screening for inborn errors of metabolism* (eds H. Bickel, R. Guthrie, and G. Hammersen). Springer-Verlag, Berlin.

—— and Morissette, J. (1983). Higher sensitivity of primary thyrotropin in screening for congenital hypothyroidism: a myth?. *J. Clin. Endocrinol. Metab.* **56**, 849-52.

Editorial (1986). Outcome of screening for congenital hypothyroidism. *Lancet* **1**, 1130-1.

Fariaux, J.P. (1983). Dépistage néo-natal de l'hypothyroidie. Intérêt et limites. *La Presse Médicale* **12**, 1519-21.

Fisher, D.A. (1983). Second International Conference on Neonatal Thyroid Screening: progress report. *J. Pediat.* **102**, 653-4.
—— and Klein, A.H. (1981). Thyroid development and disorders of thyroid function in the newborn. *New Engl. J. Med.* **304**, 702-12.
Glorieux, J., Dussault, J.H., Letarte, J., Guyda, H., and Morissette, J. (1983). Preliminary results on the mental development of hypothyroid infants detected by the Quebec Screening Program. *J. Pediat.* **102**, 19-22.
——, Dussault, J.H., Morissette, J., Desjardins, M., Letarte, J., and Guyda, H. (1985). Follow-up at ages 5 and 7 years on mental development in children with hypothyroidism detected by Quebec Screening Program. *J. Pediat.* **107**, 913-5.
Hulse, J. (1984). Outcome for congenital hypothyroidism. *Arch. Dis. Child.* **59**, 23-9.
——, Grant, D.B., Clayton, B.E., Lilly, P., Jackson, D., Spracklan, A., Edwards, R.W.H., and Nurse, D. (1980). Population screening for congenital hypothyroidism. *Br. Med. J.* **280**, 675-8.
——, Grant, D.B., Jackson, D., and Clayton, B.E. (1982). Growth, development and reassessment of hypothyroid infants diagnosed by screening. *Br. Med. J.* **284**, 1435-7.
Hummer, L., Munkner, T., Sørensen, S.S., Brandt, N.J., and Jacobsen, B.B. (1982). Nationwide TSH screening with low recall rate. Laboratory results of a two-year study. *Scand. J. Clin. Lab. Invest.* **42**, 49-55.
Illig, R. (1980). Neonatal screening for hypothyroidism by TSH determination in dried blood. In *Neonatal screening for inborn errors of metabolism* (eds H. Bickel, R. Guthrie, and G. Hammersen). Springer-Verlag, Berlin.
Illig, R. (1983). Report on neonatal thyroid screening in Europe. 22nd Annual Meeting of ESPE, Budapest.
——, Larsson, A., and Rochiccioli, P. (1982). Report on the European Society for Pediatric Endocrinology Collaborative Study on Congenital Hypothyroidism, 21st Annual Meeting of the ESPE, Helsinki.
——, Largo, R.H., Qin, Q., Torresani, T. Rochiccioli, P., and Larsson, A. (1987). Mental development in congenital hypothyroidism after neonatal screening. *Arch. Dis Child.* **62**, 1050-5.
Kaplan, M., Kauli, R., Lubin, E., Grunebaum, M., and Laron, Z. (1978). Ectopic thyroid gland. A clinical study of 30 children and review. *J. Pediat.* **92**, 205-8.
Klein, R.Z. (1980). History of congenital hypothyroidism. In *Neonatal thyroid screening* (eds G.N. Burrow and J.H. Dussault). Raven Press, New York.
——, Meltzer, S., and Kenny, F.M. (1972). Improved prognosis of congenital hypothyroidism treated before three months. *J. Pediat.* **81**, 912-13.
Laberge, C. (1980). Organization and cost benefits of mass screening programs. In *Neonatal thyroid screening* (eds G.N. Burrow and J.H. Dussault). Raven Press, New York.
Larsson, A., Hagenfeldt, L., Blom, L., and Mortensson, W. (1983). Serum alpha-fetoprotein—a biochemical indicator of prenatal hypothyroidism. *Acta Paediat. Scand.* **72**, 481-4.
Layde, P. M., Von Allmen, S.D., and Oakley, G.P. (1979). Congenital hypothyroidism control programs. A cost-benefit analysis. *JAMA* **241**, 2290-2.
Letarte, J., Gudya, H., and Dussault, J.H. (1980). Clinical, biochemical and

radiological features of neonatal hypothyroid infants. In *Neonatal thyroid screening* (eds G.N. Burrow and J.H. Dussault). Raven Press, New York.

MacFaul, R., Dorner, S., Brett, E.M., and Grant, D.B. (1978). Neurological abnormalities in patients treated for hypothyroidism from early life. *Arch. Dis. Child.* **53**, 611–9.

Mengreli, C., Kassiou, K., Tsagaraki, S., and Pantelakis, S. (1981). Neonatal screening for hypothyroidism in Greece. *Eur. J. Pediat.* **137**, 185–7.

——, Pitoulis, S., and Pantelakis, S. (1983). Distribution of TSH levels on dried blood spots in 188 872 Greek newborns: incidence of primary congenital hypothyroidism. *Acta Endocrinol. (Suppl.)* **261**, 19–20.

Mitchell, M.L. and Larsen, P.R. (1980). Screening for congenital hypothyroidism in New England using the T4–TSH strategy. In *Neonatal thyroid screening* (eds G.N. Burrow and J.H. Dussault). Raven Press, New York.

Miyai, K., Ichihara. K., Amino, N., Nose, O., Yabuuchi, H., Tsuruhara, T., Oura, T., and Kurimura, T. (1979). Seasonality of birth in sporadic cretinism. *Early Human Development* **3**, 85–8.

Morissette, J., Fiset, J., Laberge, E., Dussault, J., and Laberge, C. (1980). Automation of data processing in screening program for neonatal hypothyroidism. In *Neonatal thyroid screening* (eds G.N. Burrow and J.H. Dussault). Raven Press, New York.

Morreale de Escobar, G. and Escobar del Rey, F. (1980). Brain damage and thyroid hormone. In *Neonatal thyroid screening* (eds G.N. Burrow and J.H. Dussault). Raven Press, New York.

Murphy, G., Hulse, J.A., Jackson, D., Tyrer, P., Glossop, J., Smith, I., and Grant, D. (1986). Early treated hypothyroidism: development at three years. *Arch. Dis. Child.* **61**, 761–5.

New England Regional Screening Program and New England Congenital Hypothyroidism Collaborative (1982). Pitfalls in screening for neonatal hypothyroidism. *Pediatrics* **70**, 16–20.

New England Congenital Hypothyroidism Collaborative (NECHC) (1981). Effects of neonatal screening for hypothyroidism: prevention of mental retardation by treatment before clinical manifestations. *Lancet* **2**, 1095–8.

—— (1984). Characteristics of infantile hypothyroidism discovered on neonatal screening. *J. Pediat.* **104** 539–44.

—— (1985). Neonatal hypothyroidism screening: status of patients at six years of age. *J. Pediat.* **107**, 915–9.

Osler, W. (1897). Sporadic cretinism in America. *Transactions of the Congress of American Physicians and Surgeons* **4**, 169–206.

Pantelakis, S., Lambadaridis, I., and Mengreli, C. (1983). Forty-eight cases of primary congenital hypothyroidism diagnosed with the neonatal screening programme. *Acta Endocrinol. (Suppl.)* **261**, 21–2.

Smith, D.W., Blizzard, R.M., and Wilkins, L. (1957). The mental prognosis in hypothyroidism of infancy and childhood. A review of 128 cases. *Pediatrics* **19**, 1011–22.

Van der Gaag, R.D., Drexhage, H.A., and Dussault, J.H. (1985). Role of maternal immunoglobulins blocking TSH-induced thyroid growth in sporadic forms of congenital hypothyroidism. *Lancet* **1**, 246–50.

15
Congenital hip dislocation

Christos Bartsocas

SUMMARY

Congenital dislocation of the hip (CDH) is not a preventable disorder. However, screening early in the neonatal period aims to detect the abnormality at a reversible stage in its natural history, with the objective that early therapeutic intervention will prevent subsequent handicap. Theoretically, the incidence of handicap from CDH in Europe could be eliminated at little cost, the screening test forming part of routine neonatal physical examination. In practice, the test is frequently inadequately carried out and monitoring is rare. Current screening methods are also associated with false-positive and false negative rates that lead to unnecessary interventions on the one hand and a failure to detect all cases at birth on the other. Routine evaluation of newborns should include a thorough examination for CDH. There is a need for greater education of both health professionals and parents to ensure that infants are adequately tested.

Defining the problem

Congenital dislocation of the hip (CDH) is a common birth defect. It is characterized by the displacement of the femoral head outside the acetabulum before or shortly after birth. It is frequently associated with acetabular dysplasia, this being the development of an abnormally shallow acetabulum without actual displacement.

Congenital dislocation of the hip in the newborn can be subdivided into two kinds of abnormal hips. In the first, the hips are dislocated probably as a result of acetabular dysplasia. In the second there is an obvious joint laxity which causes a reversible dislocation or subluxation of the femoral head anteriorly or posteriorly with the examiner's manipulations.

In the first category the pathological lesions are permanent and immediate treatment is therefore required. In the second category the primary lesion, the joint laxity, may regress in the absence of any harmful environmental factors and the patients become asymptomatic. Of course joint laxity and acetabular dysplasia may coexist.

If treatment for CDH is omitted or delayed, the condition causes severe handicap in the future. Untreated CDH can result in very limited abduction of the hips because of retraction of the adductors and can cause locomotor difficulties, particularly in women, leaping to limping, Trendelenburg gait, or waddling gait. An effect on the spinal column is evident in adults with degenerative lesions of the lumbar region (osteoarthritis). Ultimately if therapy is delayed or unsuccessful, or the condition is complicated by aseptic necrosis or osteochondritis, osteoarthritis of the hip will develop. Consequently a large percentage of osteoarthritis of the hip in adults is attributable to dysplastic or subluxated hips in childhood (Murray 1965).

Size of the problem

The true birth prevalence of CDH is still unclear and depends in part on the definition of a case. Studies carried out before the start of widespread screening procedures for early diagnosis reported an incidence of CDH in childhood ranging between 0.9 and 1.6 per 1000 (MacIntosh *et al.* 1954; Severin 1956, cited in Palmen 1961).

Since those early studies, a thorough routine examination of the hips in the neonatal period has produced much higher figures. Thus, data from North America and Europe suggested a birth prevalence in the range 4 to 20 per 1000 newborns (Theodorou 1980).

In a large series of 23 408 newborns, Arzt and co-workers (1975) reported 312 (13 per 1000) with unstable hips. After more detailed examination of 211 of these newborns, 174 (82 per cent) were found to have potentially dislocatable hips and only 37 (18 per cent) had actual dislocated hips. It should be stressed that the increased articular laxity in the first days of life associated with potentially dislocatable hips subsides in 75 per cent of those affected.

Results of a survey of several European screening centres in the Eurocat project are shown in Table 15.1. The rate of CDH ranged between 5.8 and 27.3 per 10 000 newborns. This variation might reflect differences in screening policy. For example, when screening is carried out early in neonatal life and includes unstable hips, it produces a high incidence of the condition. The incidence of CDH is much lower when screening is restricted to older children, in whom a reversible hip defect may have been corrected earlier wtih spontaneous resolution of the defect.

Although there is a variation of incidence of CDH, it is interesting to note that the mean age at diagnosis has dropped because of better awareness of the problem. Greek data showed a mean age of 5.1 months at diagnosis for the period 1966–70 and 4.3 months for the period 1976–80 ($p<0.001$) (Theodorou *et al.* 1984).

Table 15.1 Incidence of congenital hip dislocation in different areas of Europe.

Centre	Years of screening	Number of newborns screened	Rate per 10 000 births
Hainaut (Belgium)	1979–84	47 541	19.6
Odense (Denmark)	1979–83	23 666	24.1
Paris (France)	1981–84	15 7665	27.3
Umbria (Italy)	1979–84	34 485	5.8
Dublin (Ireland)	1980–84	121 066	22.3
Groningen (Netherlands)	1981–84	30 687	12.1
Glasgow (UK)	1979–84	78 696	18.6
Liverpool (UK)	1979–84	121 952	7.0
Belfast (UK)	1979–82	167 345	16.8

We are most grateful to the Eurocat centres involved for providing these figures for our survey. Centres participating in the Eurocat project register any congenital anomaly recorded in children born to women residing in geographically defined areas. The various centres may differ, however, in terms of methods and completeness of case-finding, particularly for conditions diagnosed after the neonatal period (De Wals et al. 1984).

Risk factors

Sixty per cent of cases of CDH occur in first-born infants. The condition is more common in breech deliveries and occurs less frequently in premature infants. It is much more common in caucasians, less so in orientals, and even rarer in black children. Females are affected four times more often than males.

The preponderance of CDH in females may be explained in part by their increased joint laxity. However, there must be other explanations for the sex difference for, although the majority of boys with CDH (70 per cent) have generalized joint laxity, such laxity is only present in a minority of affected girls (30 per cent). Joint laxity is inherited in 5 per cent of children as an autosomal dominant disorder, suggesting that there is a genetic predisposition for CDH (Carter and Wilkinson 1964). In addition the depth of the acetabulum is inherited as a polygenic trait. Interestingly, there are cases where one parent had joint laxity while the other presented acetabular dysplasia. Studies have shown that joint laxity of the hip is usually inherited as a dominant trait. Conversely acetabular dysplasia was found in CDH of late onset. One unexplained oddity is that the left hip is affected more often than the right (Bartsocas 1982).

Nature of intervention

The basis of intervention is early detection by screening with treatment when indicated to correct potentially disabling disease in later life. There are three approaches to diagnosis: clinical, radiological, and by ultrasound.

Clinical approach

Despite the fact that diagnosis of CDH is much easier in older children, effective treatment is difficult, and thus screening should aim at earlier diagnosis. Putti (1933) and Ortolani (1937) were the first supporters of the early approach. Their ideas and suggestions were applied by Palmen (1961) in Sweden, Barlow (1962) in England, and MacKenzie (1972) in Scotland, and several others. They were the first to apply screening to all newborns in an effort to diagnose and threat CDH early, so that prevention of subsequent disability would be feasible.

The most common clinical method for early diagnosis is the Ortolani technique which is very simple. Should CDH exist, during hip abduction, the examiner will feel the dislocated head of the femur 'jump' over the tip of the acetabulum in an attempt to enter it. A characteristic 'click' is elicited which is felt, seen, and heard. This click is reproduced when the limbs are brought back from the abducted to the neutral position.

Modifications of Palmen and Barlow are based on the fact that if the femurs are pressed backwards when they are in a limited abduction, the femoral head is dislocated posteriorly. Conversely, if the femoral head is in the abduction position and is pressed forward the dislocation occurs anteriorly. Eliciting a click requires only simple manipulations and it is considered the basic diagnostic test for CDH. Nevertheless, although a click may be elicited easily in the first weeks of life, it is much more difficult after the third month when there may be no click in spite of gross limitation of hip abduction.

Other clinical signs should also be considered when screening for CDH. The most important is limited abduction of hips, but, since 15–20 per cent of newborns have limited abduction, this sign is not always diagnostic. Limited hip abduction is also observed in congenital varus hip and in infants with cerebral palsy. Asymmetry of the skin folds of the limbs might also be taken into account, although, again, this sign is present in 33 per cent of normal infants (Palmen 1961). Another sign is shortening of the limb, when dislocation exists only on one side. The limb is slightly flexed and externally rotated. Shortening alone is not diagnostic and asymmetry of the knees should be sought for confirmation.

Radiological approach

Hip radiographs are useful in the diagnosis of CDH, particularly in older children. The radiological signs are clear. The femoral head lags in development, it is located outside the acetabulum, and Shenton's line is broken. The neck of the femur is in a varus position because of anteversion. The acetabulum is oblique and shallow.

Three abnormalities of the hip joint can also be distinguished radiographically: (1) hip dysplasia, (2) hip subluxation, and (3) hip dislocation. In hip dysplasia there is obliqueness of the acetabular roof and possibly hypoplasia of the ossification centre of the femoral head. Usually this condition regresses in subsequent months, even without treatment. In hip subluxation there is an acetabular dysplasia and the femoral head is displaced laterally, but it is not completely out of the acetabular limits as is the case with hip dislocation. Screening, using radiographs, has been advocated in some parts of Europe, such as France. However, apart from the cost, there are a number of other reasons for preferring clinical to radiological testing. First, the femoral head and a large part of the neck, as well as acetabulum are cartilaginous and are, therefore, not radiologically visible. Second, the radiograph may be misleading when the neonatal pelvis is in a slightly abnormal position. False results may be obtained in the presence of CDH even in the special projections (Andren and Von Rosen 1958) because the femoral head might be inserted in its normal position when the hips are abducted. Finally, unnecessary human irradiation should be avoided.

Ultrasound

The use of ultrasound in the diagnosis of CDH has been advocated (Berman and Klenerman 1986). This non-invasive technique might prove to be of importance as a harmless and simple screening procedure, but data are required to evaluate its accuracy and efficiency.

Evidence for efficacy of screening

Sensitivity

There have been few follow-up studies of screening negatives at birth to determine the sensitivity of screening. It is apparent, however, that even in countries where systematic screening for CDH has been carried out by specialized personnel, a significant number of cases may be missed. Indeed the figure might be as high as 50 per cent (Jones 1977).

Table 15.2 shows the false-negative rates obtained from screening various

Table 15.2 Missed early diagnosis of congenital hip dislocation.

Origin	Author	Incidence (per 10 000)
Aberdeen (Scotland)	McKenzie 1972	11.2
Norway	Bjekreim 1974	10.1
Birmingham (England)	Record and Edwards 1958	7.0
N. Ireland	Williamson 1972	6.0
Norwich (England)	Jones 1977	6.0
Edinburgh (Scotland)	Mitchell 1972	1.25
Malmo (Sweden)	Von Rosen 1968	0.7
Uppsala (Sweden)	Hiertonn and James 1968	4.0
		(0 after 6th month)
New Zealand	Smaill 1968	6.7
Scotland	McKenzie and Wilson 1981	11.2
Sweden	Fredensborg 1977	7.0
Greece	Peonides et al. 1982	6.9
Scotland	MacNicol et al. 1982	6.0

Source: Theodorou et al. 1984.

populations. The rates vary considerably from 0.7 to 11.2 per 10 000. It is also interesting to note that MacKenzie and Wilson (1981) reported that the percentage of children with delayed diagnosis was similar in the decades 1960–69 and 1970–79. In this study newborns were screened by specialized personnel twice within the first year of life, in the first and sixth months. There were more missed cases requiring surgery than before the introduction of screening.

Specificity

While it is possible to detect individuals with clinical subluxation or dislocation, screening has a low predictive value for future dislocation because the majority of newborns with abnormalities will recover completely without any treatment (Place et al. 1978). The specificity of the test is, therefore, far below 100 per cent. The wide variation in the reported occurrence of CDH probably, in part, reflects the extent of overdiagnosis in different surveys.

It is difficult to assess the true specificity, given the variation in conduct and interpretation of the screening method used. There are no quantitative data on the reproducibility of neonatal screening for CDH, but there seems to be considerable inter- and intra-observer variation (Hiertonn and James 1968; Williamson 1972). Therefore the test is considered to be largely subjective (Parkin 1981).

Results of treatment

Infants with any degree of dysplasia are treated for an average of 6 weeks or longer with double or triple diapers. If CDH persists after this treatment a kind of brace, splint, or harness is recommended. This brace can easily be removed for bathing and should be worn for an average of 3 months. There is controversy about the advisability of treating cases of CDH diagnosed at birth. It has been observed that 20 per cent of untreated unstable hips subsequently develop hip dysplasia or progress to full dislocation (Dunn 1969) and that the untreated unstable hip may develop serious structural pathology within a few weeks (Dunn et al. 1985). Frankenburg (1981) in a review of the available evidence concluded, however, that there was little to suggest that early treatment is more efficacious than later therapy and, further, the efficacy of therapy had not been demonstrated in clinical trials.

Evidence for population effectiveness

Current screening policies have made little impact. Yamamuro and Ishida (1984) report the Japanese experience of CDH screening. They felt that early screening methods were not reliable and that the remarkable reduction in the incidence of observed CDH was achieved by a campaign to avoid prolonged extension of the hips and knees in infants rather than from screening. Catford et al. (1982) published the results of neonatal screening for CDH in Southampton. They claimed that neonatal screening failed to make a substantial impact on morbidity from the condition and recommended more vigilance from all health professionals dealing with infants and an examination of hips at every opportunity. Such conclusions are not universal and screening can be effective particularly when applied to high-risk groups (Dunn et al. 1985).

Hitherto the most compelling evidence to support the effectiveness of screening was related to infants presenting by breech delivery. These infants are known to be at high risk for developing CDH and are therefore likely to be screened carefully.

Constraints in maximizing the effectiveness of screening

The problems in screening have already been discussed but were summarized by Leck (1986) who recognized four main problem areas in the field of neonatal screening for hip joint instability: (1) false-positives, (2) false-negatives, (3) treatment policies, and (4) outcome of early treatment. He noted that there were several unanswered questions in these four areas and recommended the establishment of randomized clinical trials to test ethical treatment policies. He felt that these trials should be designed to allow comparison between the costs and benefits of different neonatal screening and treatment policies.

Cheetham et al. (1983) claimed that hip examination at birth may actually cause the condition it is intended to detect. Although it is difficult to dismiss this possibility, Dunn et al. (1985) suggest that such cases are borderline abnormal and that instability may be provoked even by gentle manipulation. They argue also that, without treatment, the hips of these infants could eventually become unstable and, therefore, there is an advantage in their early recognition.

Costs

If hips of neonates and infants are checked repeatedly by physicians within routine medical check-ups, 'screening for CDH' can be carried out without a special programme and without any increased cost over and above normal infant care. The true costs of screening, however, include the medical costs of treating those infants with early joint laxity who would not progress to later dislocation. The benefits from screening may be considered by the savings obtained from a reduction in the relatively more expensive cost of therapy of missed cases. Fulton and Baber (1984) suggested that screening for CDH is cost-effective relative to no screening, when one deals with large numbers of newborn babies and very low false-negative rates. They concluded that an increase in the proportion of cases missed by screening from 0.25 to 0.8 per 1000 would increase the cost of screening up to the range of their baseline cost estimate for no screening.

Conclusions

Theoretically, neonatal screening for CDH should be able to eliminate later morbidity and disability at little cost. However, as Parkin (1981) and Frankenburg (1981) discuss, after reviewing the data, the evidence for the population effectiveness of widespread screening is slim. There is considerable lack of information, owing to a paucity of clinical trials, on the efficacy of early detection and therapy, and there are anxieties about unnecessary treatment of reversible conditions.

The question whether to screen or not has been debated by various authors. While many reports claim success, others report failures and suggest that screening efforts be stopped (Dunn et al. 1985).

On the basis of the information gathered, we do not feel that formal screening for CDH should be included in well-established neonatal screening programmes. We would prefer that a thorough physical examination of newborns by the paediatrician, general practitioner, or any appropriate health officer, should include testing for CDH. On the follow-up visit, examination for CDH should also be included. We do not feel that all newborns should be screened by one individual specially trained to recognize CDH or be X-rayed for this purpose.

Recently, a Working Party of the Standing Medical Advisory Committee and the Standing Nursing and Midwifery Advisory Committee reviewed guidelines and recommended good practice in screening for CDH to all health professionals who have responsibility for newborns and young children. Continuing surveillance until the child is seen to be walking normally is suggested (Special Report 1986).

Recommendations

We believe that there is still considerable morbidity in Europe from CDH and that this results from missed cases in the neonatal period. As there is little to support the introduction of a formal programme of intervention, our recommendations are directed towards the improvement of current clinical practice.

1. All newborns should be examined specifically for the existence of CDH, as part of a good complete physical examination. Health professionals should be more aware of the problem.
2. Special attention should be paid to newborns with a family history of CDH, those born by breech delivery, and those with fibroma of the sternocleidomastoid muscle.
3. Repeat examination on a 4–6 week follow-up visit to the general practitioner or paediatrician will help detect missed cases of CDH. All health professionals who come in contact with infants should examine their hips as a routine procedure. It is advisable to set up a specific system, such as a check point on a health booklet or record card which would be presented by the mother and on which it could be recorded that the child's hips were checked by a qualified individual.
4. Parents should be fully informed of the condition and its prognosis so that treatment will not be discontinued early and follow-up appointments will be kept.
5. Special training and continuing education should be given to health professionals to enable them to carry out a correct examination of hips.

6. Finally, although we do not recommend a special neonatal screening programme for CDH, we emphasize the importance of full awareness of the problem by health professionals and further studies to evaluate the efficacy and effectiveness of early diagnosis and treatment.

Acknowledgement

We are most grateful to Dr S. Theodorou for his assistance and advice in the preparation of this chapter.

References

Andren, L. and Von Rosen, S. (1958). The diagnosis of dislocation of the hip in the newborns and the primary results of immediate treatment. *Acta Radiol.* **49**, 89.

Arzt, D.T., Levine, B.D., Lim, N.W., Salvati, A.E., and Wilson, D.P. (1975). Neonatal diagnosis, treatment and related factors of congenital dislocation of the hip. *J. Bone Jt Surg. (Br.)* **44B**, 292.

Barlow, T.G. (1962). Early diagnosis and treatment of congenital dislocation of the hip. *J. Bone Jt Surg. (Br.)* **44**, 292–301.

Bartsocas, C.S. (1982). Genetics of congenital dislocation of the hip. *Hellin. Chirurg. Orthoped. Traumatol.* **33**, 170–1.

Berman, L. and Klenerman, L. (1986). Ultrasound screening for hip abnormalities: preliminary findings in 1001 neonates. *Br. Med. J.* **293**, 719–22.

Carter, C.O. and Wilkinson, J.A. (1964). Genetic and environmental factors in the aetiology of congenital dislocation of the hip. *Clin. Orthop.* **33**, 119.

Catford, J.C., Bennet, G.C., and Wilkinson, J.A. (1982). Congenital hip dislocation: and increasing and still uncontrolled disability? *Br. Med. J.* **285**, 1527–30.

Cheetham, C.H., Garrow, D.H., Tarin, P., and Medhurst A.W.J. (1983). Congenital dislocation of the hip. *Br. Med. J.* **286**, 227.

David, T.J., Parris, M.R., Poynor, M.U. et al. (1983). Reasons for late detection of the hip dislocation in childhood. *Lancet* **2**, 147–9.

De Wals, P., Mastroiacovo, P., Weatherall, J.A.C., and Lechat, M.F. (1984). *Eurocat guide 1 for the registration of congenital anomalies.* Catholic University of Louvain, Brussels.

Dunn, P.M. (1969). The influence of the intrauterine environment in the causation of congenital postural deformities, with special reference to congenital dislocation of the hip. MD thesis, Cambridge University, Cambridge.

——, Evans, R.E., Thearle, M.J., Griffiths, H.E.D., and Witherow, P.J. (1985). Congenital dislocation of the hip: early and late diagnosis and management compared. *Arch. Dis Child.* **60**, 497–514.

Frankenburg, W.K. (1981). To screen or not to screen: congenital dislocation of the hip (Editorial). *Am. J. Publ. Hlth* **71**, 1311–13.

Fulton, M.J. and Baber, M.L. (1984). Screening for congenital dislocation of the hip: an economic appraisal. *Can. Med. Assoc. J.* **130**, 1149–56.

Hiertonn, T. and James, U. (1968). Congenital dislocation of the hip: experiences of early diagnosis and treatment. *J. Bone Jt Surg. (Br.)* **50B**, 542–5.

Jones, D. (1977). An assessment of the value of examination of the hip in the newborn. *J. Bone Jt Surg. (Br.)* **59B**, 318–22.

Leck, I. (1986). An epidemiological assessment of neonatal screening for dislocation of the hip. *J.R. Coll. Physicians Lond.* **20**, 56–62.

MacIntosh, P., Merritt, K.K., Richards, M.R., Samuels, M.H., and Bellows, M.T. (1954). The incidence of congenital malformations: a study of 5964 pregnancies. *Pediatrics* **14**, 505.

MacKenzie, I.G. (1972). Congenital dislocation of the hip. The development of a regional service. *J. Bone Jt Surg. (Br.)* **54B**, 18.

—— and Wilson, J.G. (1981). Problems in the early diagnosis and management of congenital dislocation of the hip. *J. Bone Jt Surg. (Br.)* **63B**, 38.

Murray, R.O. (1985). The aetiology of primary osteoarthritis of the hip. *Br. J. Radiol.* **38**, 810.

Ortolani, M. (1937). Un segno poco noto e sua importanza per la diagnosi precose di prelussazione congenital dell' anca. *Pediatria (Napoli)* **45**, 129.

Palmen, K. (1961). Preluxation of the hip joint. *Acta Paediat. Scand.* **50**, 129.

Parkin, D.M. (1981). How successful is screening for congenital dislocation of the hip? *Am. J. Publ. Hlth* **71**, 1378–83.

Place, M., Parkin, D.M., and Fitton, J.M. (1978). Effectiveness of neonatal screening for congenital dislocation of the hip. *Lancet* **2**, 249–50.

Putti, V. (1933). Early treatment of congenital dislocation of the hip. *J. Bone Jt Surg. (Br.)* **15**, 16.

Special Report (1986). Screening for the detection of congenital dislocation of the hip. *Arch. Dis. Child.* **61**, 921–6.

Theodorou, S., Ierodiaconou, M., Zoumbopoulos, H., and Gerostathopoulos, N. (1984). Congenital dislocation of the hip. The evolution of early diagnosis (in Greek). *Paediatriki* **47**, 257–66.

Williamson, J. (1972). Difficulties of early diagnosis and treatment of congenital dislocation of the hip in Northern Ireland. *J. Bone Jt Surg.* **54B**, 13–17.

Yamamuro, T. and Ishida, K. (1984). Recent advances in the prevention, early diagnosis, and treatment of congenital dislocation of the hip in Japan. *Clin. Orthop.* **184**, 34–40.

Section III

Preventable fetal and infant loss

16
Perinatal mortality

Valerie Dowding

SUMMARY

A steady decline in both stillbirth and early neonatal mortality rates has occurred in Europe during the last 20 years. Among infants weighing less than 1500 g at birth, an increase in the rate of decline began in the late 1970s and is attributed to improvements in neonatal intensive care. Low birthweight, though strongly correlated with perinatal mortality, has shown no comparable decline. There are wide variations both between and within countries in mortality rates, and intervention programmes should aim to reduce these differentials. There are a number of possible strategies to achieve this aim. Primary prevention of high-risk births has probably contributed to the observed falls in perinatal mortality. Opportunities for medical involvement in primary prevention are limited, and in the antenatal period medical services are mainly involved with the provision of secondary prevention, in the form of screening and management of abnormalities. Recent advances in the sampling of fetal tissues allow the detection of abnormalities with a view to termination of pregnancy. Later in pregnancy and during labour new methods of fetal observation allow informed decisions about obstetric management but may cause increased intervention as a result of difficulties of interpretation. Major technological advances in neonatal intensive care, including mechanical ventilation and total parenteral nutrition, have improved the survival rates of extremely immature infants. Information relating to morbidity and handicap among survivors is, however, still inadequate. Nevertheless, the generally high levels of handicap, especially among infants weighing less than 1000 g, are the subject of debate in view of the magnitude of the social and financial costs involved.

Defining the problem

The perinatal period

The perinatal period ends with the seventh day after birth, but the beginning is less precisely defined. The notification of births is governed by laws, some of them very old, which vary from country to country. Most require notification when pregnancy reaches the stage of extrauterine viability, which, until recently, was judged to be around 28 weeks from the onset of the last menstrual period, or 26 weeks actual gestation. Notification based on the uncertain factor of gestational age has yielded data which are unreliable where the smallest infants are concerned. The ninth revision of the World Health Organization International Classification of Diseases (1978) recommended that national statistics for perinatal mortality (PNM) should include all fetuses weighing 1000 g or more at birth. Regrettably, it added that, when weight was not available, 28 weeks gestation or 35 cm crown/heel length may define the beginning of the perinatal period. As Chalmers (1980a) has pointed out, there is no good clinical reason for not weighing even the illest infant, and birthweight should be available for all births without exception.

The persistence of differences in the interpretation of the beginning of the perinatal period, and the late gestation at which notification has been required, are now proving to have serious implications. The dramatic increase in survival of very low birthweight infants (VLBW, <1500 g,) involves increasing numbers weighing <1000 g and born before 28 weeks. Most European countries have not recorded data for denominators or numerators and cannot assess trends in PNM for these tiny babies (Kiely et al. 1981; Sepkowitz 1983). Some who would previously have been neither resuscitated nor notified, especially where there was some doubt as to gestational age, now enter statistics as live births. In Norway notification of all births of 16 weeks gestation or more has been required since the 1960s, giving one of the few accurate records of numbers of VLBW babies (Hoffman et al. 1983). The World Health Organization (1978) recommended that international statistics be based on all infants weighing 500 g or more at birth (or 22 weeks or 25 cm crown/heel length). In the light of recent trends in survival there can be little doubt that birthweight of 500 g or more should be the sole criterion for notification.

Stillbirth and live birth

Confusion also surrounds the distinction between live and stillbirth and indeed the term 'perinatal' was introduced to deal with the problem. There

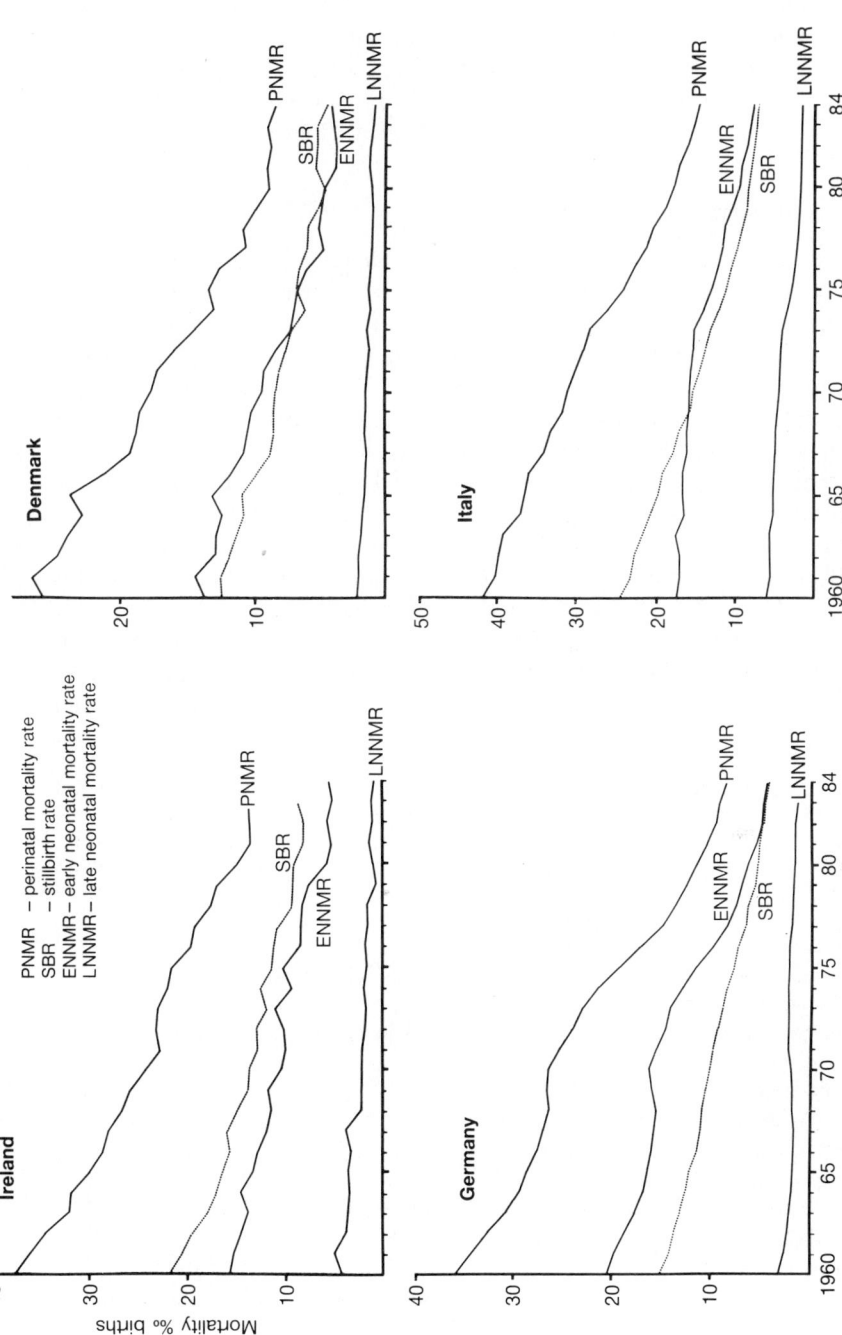

Fig. 16.1 Perinatal mortality, stillbirth, early neonatal mortality, and late neonatal mortality rates in Ireland, Germany, Denmark, and Italy 1960–84 (rates per 1000 births). Adapted from Eurostat (1986).

are religious and bureaucratic reasons for differing interpretations of 'live birth' and these contribute to regional and international differences. However, it is not clear to what extent these disagreements affect the puzzling differences between EEC countries in the proportions of PNM caused by stillbirths and early neonatal deaths (<7 days) (Figure 16.1).

Causes of perinatal mortality

Most perinatal deaths result from the coincidence of several adverse factors. Standardization of diagnosis of cause of death is therefore imperfect (Clarke 1982). The simple classification into four categories provided by Wigglesworth (1980) has proved valuable for perinatal audit. Comparison of the causes of perinatal deaths in 1968 and 1978 in England and Wales indicates that congenital malformations and prematurity were the two most important causes of death (Table 16.1). In practice most of the other causes are strongly associated with prematurity and the importance of this is therefore understated by these figures. The major decline in deaths from haemolytic disease, mostly because of Rhesus incompatibility, resulted from reduced family size and the use of anti-D therapy. This is a notable success of perinatal medicine. The decline in deaths attributed to difficult labour and birth injury is also encouraging, and may be the result of increased resort to Caesarian section for failure to advance in labour, or to improved growth and stature of mothers, or both. It is often impossible to distinguish maternal

Table 16.1 Causes of perinatal mortality in England and Wales.

Condition	P list code	Rate (%) 1968	Rate (%) 1978	Decline %
Malformation	68–80	4.3 (17.6)	3.5 (22.3)	19
Prematurity	36–7, 57, 61	3.8 (15.3)	2.3 (14.9)	39
Placental insufficiency	44–6, 67	2.8 (11.5)	1.8 (11.7)	36
Cord accidents and placental haemorrhage	42–3, 47–9	3.0 (12.1)	1.7 (11.0)	43
Anoxia (cause unspecified)	58–60	2.1 (8.6)	1.5 (9.5)	29
Difficult labour and birth injury	21–35, 50–2	2.1 (8.5)	0.9 (5.9)	57
Pre-eclampsia	13–15, 17	1.7 (6.7)	0.8 (4.9)	53
Multiple pregnancy	40	0.8 (3.2)	0.7 (4.2)	13
Haemolytic disease	53–6	0.9 (3.6)	0.2 (1.3)	78
Others		3.2 (13.0)	2.3 (14.5)	28
All		24.7 (100)	15.5 (100)	37

Adapted from Edouard and Alberman (1980).

from medical responsibility for improvements in perinatal results (Sunderland and Greenfield 1984). Reproductive efficiency is related to the mother's health and physique, which in turn is related to the quality of the environment in which she grew up (Baird 1985).

Current trends

All EEC countries have experienced a rapid and steady decline in both stillbirth and neonatal death rates (Figure 16.1). PNM rates in 1984 among EEC member countries fell into three groups: Denmark, Germany, and Luxembourg had rates below 9 per 1000 births, the Netherlands, the United Kingdom and France between 9 and 12, and the remaining five countries had rates above 13 (Table 16.2). There is an almost two-fold difference between the highest (Greece) and lowest (Denmark) rates. Explanation can be sought either in the delivery of medical care or with the mothers themselves.

PNM rates are only available for a minority of countries in the world (WHO 1985). Most Third World countries suffer much higher mortality than Western nations, but Savage (1986) recently warned against hasty interpretations of mortality rates in terms of quality of care, having observed the frequent practice of infanticide of unwanted, but usually healthy, infants in a Third World country. Some developing countries, such as Singapore (PNM rate: 13.4/1000,1980) and Hong Kong (PNM rate: 12.2/1000,1978), have

Table 16.2 Perinatal mortality, legal abortions, and fertility characteristics of European Community countries, 1984.

Country	PNM rate	Total fertility	Fecundity <20 yr	40–44 yr	Legal abortion	Abortion ratio
Denmark	8.4	1.40	10.1	2.3	<1960	40.0
Germany	8.6	1.33[a]	10.3[a]	3.4[a]	1976	14.6
Luxembourg	8.8	1.43	10.8	4.1		
The Netherlands	10.0	1.49	7.4	3.2	1971	11.5[a]
United Kingdom	10.2	1.77	27.8	4.6	1969	20.7
France[a]	11.4	1.79	13.9	5.4	1976	24.4
Belgium	13.2	1.61	17.3	3.0		
Ireland[a]	13.7	2.75	18.3	21.8		
Italy	14.5	1.53	13.5[a]	5.0	1980	38.9
Portugal	16.4	2.19[b]	40.6[b]	14.3[b]		
Greece	16.8	1.82	41.2	4.6		

Source: Eurostat (1986).
[a]1983
[b]1980
(No figures available for Spain from 1980).

mortality rates comparable with the best Western countries. Both have a low incidence of birthweight less than 1500 g (Lau and Fung 1984; Hughes 1985). They have not made the major investment in high technology that characterizes modern Western childbirth, but there has been little or no research in the West into the reasons for their success. Chalmers (1980b) reported a PNM rate of 16.5 per 1000 births during the period 1972–76 in a Shanghai hospital serving a population of 400 000 and admitting some high-risk cases from outside the area. The rate in Denmark in the same period was 15, in England and Wales it was 20, and only fell below 16.5 in 1978. The Shanghai mothers had fewer multiple pregnancies and hypertensive disorders, and fewer infants with congenital abnormalities, than mothers in Britain. The incidence of low birthweight was only 4.7 per cent. Unfortunately the percentage of VLBW infants was not available, so that the very low neonatal mortality rate for birthweights of less than 2500 g was difficult to interpret, but it was achieved without sophisticated neonatal intensive care.

Explanations for differences in rates

Birthweight

The importance of the association between low birthweight and PNM has long been known. Low birthweight results from premature delivery or intrauterine growth retardation, or both. A world-wide study showed that, in developed countries, where the incidence of low birthweight was low (< 10 per cent), premature delivery was the major component. The higher incidence of low birthweight in developing countries was found to be caused by intrauterine retardation while premature delivery remained almost unchanged (Villar and Belizan 1982). This latter factor is therefore very resistant to improvement.

Routine nationwide collection of birthweight data has been rare outside Scandinavia. Norway, Sweden, Iceland, and Denmark have well-established systems for nationwide medical registration of birth and perinatal death. A comprehensive range of data covers perinatal socio-demographic factors and medical details of pregnancy, birth, and the neonatal period. In Denmark linkage with deaths up to one year is achieved. In Ireland a medical registration system has recently reached full national coverage. Such systems are essential if full audit and surveillance of perinatal performance is to be achieved. In England and Wales births below 2500 g have been recorded since 1953, and those below 1000 g have been recorded separately since 1962 (MacFarlane and Mugford 1984; OPCS 1982,83,84). There was a steady decline in PNM rates in England and Wales throughout the period 1962 to 1984 in the birthweight ranges 1500–2000, 2001–2250 and 2250–2500 g, and, until 1977, among infants weighing under 1000 and 1000–1500 g (Figure

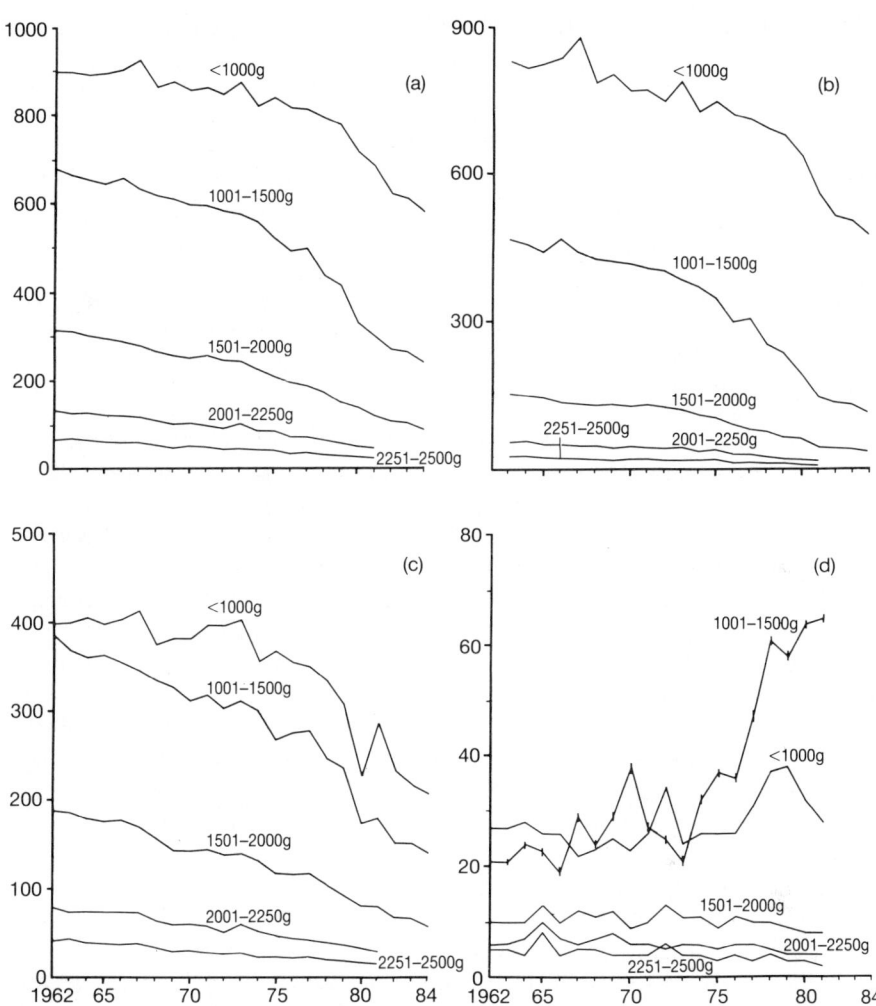

Fig. 16.2 Birthweight-specific mortality rates in England and Wales 1962–84.

(a) Total perinatal/1000 births
(b) Early neonatal/1000 live births
(c) Stillbirth/1000 births
(d) Late neonatal/1000 live births
(Adapted from MacFarlane and Mugford (1984); OPCS (1982–83), (1984a).)

16.2a). At this point the rate of decline among infants under 1500 g increased abruptly and remained elevated for about six years. In the three years, 1982–84, a return to the previous rate of decline in mortality among VLBW infants seems to have occurred.

Table 16.3 Cumulative percentages of total births and perinatal deaths (for which weight was known) by birthweight, England and Wales, 1984.

Birthweight (g)	Births	Perinatal deaths	Stillbirths	Early neonatal deaths
<1000	0.37	21.6	13.4	32.2
<1500	1.04	37.8	30.2	47.7
<2000	2.40	50.6	44.8	58.1
<2500	7.02	64.5	61.7	68.3

Source: OPCS (1984).

The relative importance of low birthweight for PNM has increased as mortality has declined in recent years. By 1984 in England and Wales 22 per cent of perinatal deaths were among 0.4 per cent of infants who weighed less than 1000 g, 38 per cent among the 1 per cent under 1500 g, and 65 per cent among those weighing 2500 g or less at birth (Table 16.3). Perinatal mortality rates in Sweden were similar to those in Britain for infants of low birthweight (less than 2500 g), but considerably lower for those of normal birthweight (Alberman 1980). It would therefore seem that the excess of low birthweights in England and Wales, 7 per cent, compared with Sweden's 4 per cent, together with the inferior outcome for normal birthweight infants, are important factors in the longstanding inferiority of Britain's PNM rates compared with those in Sweden. Britain also suffers more lethal congenital deformities than Sweden, although the prevalence of these is declining.

Low birthweight is always described as the most important cause of PNM. It is all the more remarkable that the universal steady decline in PNM in Europe has occurred in the absence of any comparable decline in the incidence in low birthweight. In Britain in the last 20 years there has been no change in the percentage of babies weighing less than 2500 g at birth. The percentage of live births weighing less than 1500 g rose from 0.75 per cent to 0.87 per cent of live births between 1970 and 1984, (MacFarlane and Mugford 1984; OPCS 1982, 1983, 1984). This increase is not fully explained by the decline in stillbirths (Gordan 1985). In Norway an average of 99.5 per cent of all birthweights were recorded between 1967 and 1980 (Hoffman et al. 1977). This coverage was only achieved in England and Wales in 1983. In the author's experience missing birthweights tend to include a large excess of low birthweight cases and of sick and dead infants. The figures from England and Wales (Figure 16.2) must therefore be interpreted with caution, especially in view of the very high proportion of perinatal deaths for which birthweight was not obtained (Table 16.4).

Table 16.4 Percentage of births and perinatal deaths for which weight was not recorded, England and Wales.

Year	Births	Perinatal deaths	Stillbirths	Early neonatal deaths
1981	4.6	12.1	9.1	15.9
1982	4.4	14.0	11.4	17.5
1983	0.14	3.2	1.4	7.1
1984	0.14	3.3	1.9	5.2

Source: OPCS (1981–84).

Table 16.5 Fertility rates among women aged 15–19 years in Europe.

Country	Year of highest fertility	PNM rate 1984	Highest fertility rate
Denmark	1966	8.4	49.6
Germany	1969	8.6	36.1
Luxembourg	1971	8.8	31.2
The Netherlands	1967	10.0	22.5
United Kingdom	1971	10.2	50.6
France	1972	11.4	29.4
Belgium	1971	13.2	32.3
Ireland	1980	13.7	23.0
Italy	1974	14.5	33.3
Portugal	1977	16.4	47.6
Greece	1979	16.8	52.9
Spain	1979		27.1

Source: Eurostat (1986).

Fertility

Total fertility, like PNM, has been declining in all member countries of the EEC but there are still considerable differences between them (Table 16.2). There is a clear tendency for countries with low fertility to have low PNM rates. Outside the West, it is interesting to note that Singapore and Shanghai, with their strikingly low PNM rates, are also characterized by low fertility. Low fecundity among age groups at high risk of PNM, the under 20 and the 40–45 years age groups, should reduce PNM. The average fecundity of these two age groups (Table 16.2) shows a strong positive correlation with national PNM rates in Europe. (Spearman's Rank correlation coefficient: $r_s = 0.88$, $n = 11$ ($p < 0.001$). There is thus a close parallel between the PNMR and the frequency with which women in these high-risk groups have babies in each of the 11 countries. All these countries experienced an increase in births to teenagers since the 1950s, but this trend seems now to have reversed. Table 16.5 shows the year in which the highest number of live births per 1000 women under 20 years of age occurred in each country. There is a close correlation between the duration of the decline in teenage fertility in each country and the present PNM rate (r_s = 0.88, p<0.001). This suggests that countries with long-established and effective sex education and high expectations of personal fertility control are likely to be those with low PNM rates. In England and Wales there was a decline of 19.4 births per year per 1000 women under the age of 20 between 1970 and 1979 (Francome 1983) (Table 16.6). This was achieved with an increase in abortion rate of only 7.5. Thus a fall in conceptions must have accounted for the rest of the decline in births (11.9 per 1000 women under 20). Between 1973 and 1977 abortion rates in this age group remained steady while numbers of births continued to decline. There was a sudden rise in both births and abortions in 1979 which has been attributed to the major publicity given to adverse effects of the contraceptive pill (Ashton 1983). The rise in births as well as abortions might indicate that there are still many, even in the youngest age groups, who will carry through an unwanted pregnancy rather than resort to abortion.

The ratio of terminations to live births in each age and parity group gives an indication of the degree of parental rejection of pregnancy at different stages of the life cycle (Table 16.7). It is interesting to see that the ratios mirror the PNM rates of the age and parity groups. There is an increasing awareness of many risk factors among the general public and the findings of major perinatal surveys have probably contributed to the fund of knowledge informing decisions about parenthood. Changes in age and parity are estimated to have accounted for 9 per cent of the fall in PNM rates in Sweden

Table 16.6 Births and abortions/1000 women aged 15–19 years, England and Wales, 1970–9.

Year	Births	Abortions
1970	50.4	9.1
1971	51.5	12.1
1972	48.7	14.4
1973	44.3	15.4
1974	36.8	15.7
1975	36.8	15.3
1976	32.7	14.8
1977	30.0	15.2
1978	30.1	15.4
1979	31.0	16.6

Adapted from Francome (1983).

Table 16.7 Ratio of induced abortions to live births compared with perinatal mortality (PNM) rate by age and parity, England and Wales, 1984.

Age (years)	<20	20–24	25–29	30–35	35+
Ratio	0.69	0.20	0.11	0.14	0.36
PNM rate	12.7	9.6	8.9	8.7	12.8
Birth order[a]	1	2	3	4+	
Ratio	0.37	0.10	0.29	0.35	
PNM rate	10.4	7.8	9.3	13.5	

[a]Statistics on birth order not collected for 'illegitimate' births.
Denominator: 'legitimate' live births
Numerator: all abortions to residents
Calculated from: OPCS (1984).

between 1953 and 1975 (Meirik et al. 1979), and 24 per cent between 1966 and 1976 in England and Wales (Hellier 1977). Significant age and parity changes have continued since these studies were published. Such estimates took no account of the fact that the reduction involved births that were not wanted by their potential parents. The absence of these births is likely to have had a disproportionately beneficial effect on PNM and morbidity, but we have no information on which to assess the size of this effect.

Social class and ethnic group

The British Registrar General's classification of five social classes, based on male occupation, provides a scale of socio-economic status which is related to health status. It has consistently produced a close correlation with PNM rates and birthweight in Britain (Butler and Bonham 1963; Chamberlain et al. 1975; MacFarlane and Mugford 1984). The author has found similar results in the Irish Republic for birthweight (Dowding 1981) and PNM. This social class scale is not in routine use in Europe outside Britain and potentially useful international comparisons cannot therefore be made. Results from England and Wales show a steady decline in PNM rates in all social classes between 1958 and 1980 (Table 16.8). There was a fall of 56–59 per cent in all three social class groups which involved a remarkable decrease of 22 deaths per 1000 births among social classes IV and V. During this time a major change occurred in the relative numbers of maternities in social classes I, II, and III while the proportion in IV and V remained static.

Disadvantage, in health terms, is not only related to social class. There are sizeable ethnic immigrant minorities in many European countries most of whom have PNM rates above those of the indigenous populations. For instance in England and Wales, in 1984, mothers born in Pakistan experienced a PNM rate of 16.9 while the rate among those born in the

Table 16.8 Perinatal mortality rates by social class 1958–80 in England and Wales[a].

Social class (husband)	1958 (Butler and Bonham 1963)	1970 (Chamberlain et al. 1978)	1980 (MacFarlane and Mugford 1984)	Improvement 1958–80 /1000 births	per cent
I and II	24.3	13.3	10.7	13.6	56
III (N and M)	30.7	19.6	12.7	18.0	59
IV and V	37.6	26.8	15.5	22.1	59
Difference between I/II and IV/V	13.3	13.5	4.8		

[a]'legitimate' births only.

United Kingdom was 9.7 per thousand births (OPCS 1984). Figures for low birthweight by country of origin were not published. Most of these groups include a high proportion of unskilled workers and, increasingly, of unemployed people. Late attendance for antenatal care was found to be very common among Asian mothers in Bradford, and there was no improvement between 1969 and 1978 (Lumb et al. 1981). It is important to take account of cultural rules and taboos in the design of antenatal care, especially for members of immigrant groups. Failure to do this may seriously discourage attendance.

Cigarette smoking

The effect of smoking in reducing birthweight and increasing PNM is well known. The social class gradient in prevalence of smoking has become very marked and may be a major factor in the continuing inferiority of pregnancy outcome among lower social classes (Simpson and Smith 1986). This effect is likely to be more important now that other adverse factors have declined, especially in communities with high proportions of smokers. Analysis of data from the British Births 1970 study cohort (Rush and Cassano 1983) showed that, while smoking was associated with reduced birthweight in all social classes, PNM was increased only among smokers in the lower social classes. Thus the adverse effect of smoking seems to be disproportionately high among the more disadvantaged mothers.

A correlation has been demonstrated between stress during pregnancy and poor outcome (Newton et al. 1979) and between low social class and stress levels, especially in relation to domestic events and circumstances (Oakley et al. 1982). Stress is likely to be important in relation to pregnancy but is poorly understood.

Intervention strategies to reduce perinatal mortality

There are numerous different approaches using health services to reduce PNM. The primary prevention of the causes of perinatal death by altering, for example, the social environment of the women most at risk is beyond the scope of this volume. Health services action can be directed at three stages of pregnancy: during the antenatal period, during delivery, and in the early neonatal period. The possibilities offered by each of these approaches are considered below.

Intervention during the antenatal period

Within the antenatal period there are three distinct approaches that can be applied. First, the screening for detection of specific disorders, both maternal and fetal, where intervention can alter the natural history. Second, there are aspects of antenatal care where interventions are applied to the total population. Third, there is the concept of antenatal *care* with the emphasis more on the total package of care, provided particularly to high-risk mothers, rather than the individual interventions mentioned above.

Antenatal screening

Screening for abnormalities is the main component of antenatal care for most women, the great majority of whom have no pregnancy complications. Screening begins at the first antenatal visit and intensifies as the end of pregnancy approaches. Screening includes blood pressure and urine protein measurements at every visit in the hope of detecting toxaemia in its early stages. This condition often develops very rapidly, escaping detection at antenatal clinics.

Ultrasound scanning for gestational age and fetal abnormality at the first visit has also rapidly become routine in many hospitals. The possibility of an adverse influence of ultrasound needs to be tested in larger controlled trials than have been conducted to date. It is unlikely at this stage that any major ill-effect has escaped notice, but it is still premature to assume that ultrasound is totally without danger, especially to the very early fetus. Selective use of the procedure to answer clearly defined and important questions in specific cases would seem the wisest course. The general use of a screening method, especially where interpretation requires advanced skills and experience, usually has the expensive and sometimes harmful effect of increasing investigations and admissions to hospital in the wake of false-positive diagnoses. Bakketeig and his colleagues in Norway (1984) estimated that, if associated costs such as extra hospital admissions were included, the cost of screening was US$ 250 per pregnancy.

The diagnostic sampling of amniotic fluid and, more recently, of fetal placental tissues are in common use to detect genetic and chromosomal defects with a view to terminating affected pregnancies. There is a known risk of spontaneous abortion associated with amniocentesis, but the possibility of more insidious, longer-term sequelae of this penetration of the fetal defences against infection requires investigation. A randomized controlled trial of genetic amniocentesis (Tabor et al. 1986) showed significantly raised incidence of respiratory distress syndrome and pneumonia among infants of mothers who had received amniocentesis at an average of 16 weeks gestation. However, there was a suggestive, but not significant, excess of VLBW infants in the study group which is likely to have contributed to the excess of respiratory problems.

Direct assessment of fetal hypoxia by sampling umbilical cord blood *in utero* has recently been reported (Nicolaides et al. 1986). In 29 growth-retarded pregnancies the results showed good correlation wtih the non-invasive Doppler ultrasound measurement of blood velocity in the fetal aorta (Soothill et al. 1986). This latter method may therefore assist obstetric judgements regarding elective early delivery (Beattie et al. 1987; Reuwer et al. 1987).

Hall and her colleagues (1982, 1985) examined the productivity of routine antenatal care. They concluded that expectations of what can be achieved were unrealistic, and that the frequent screening tests failed to detect or prevent many conditions severe enough to cause admission to hospital during pregnancy. A most important finding was that clinicians failed to recognize significant previous medical and obstetric history at first visits (Chng et al. 1980).

Routine interventions

Routine antenatal care frequently includes intervention of many forms which have not been rigorously evaluated—for example, iron and folate supplementation, limitation of weight gain, and bed rest.

The advisability of iron supplementation has recently been questioned following the finding of a strong association between high haemoglobin concentrations at first visit and increased PNM and low birthweight rates, as well as maternal hypertension (Murphy et al. 1986). The fall in haemoglobin, which occurs during pregnancy, is now understood to be a normal consequence of an essential expansion in maternal plasma volume rather than failure of maternal physiological adaptation.

Limitation of weight gain in pregnancy through dietary restrictions or the use of diuretic drugs has been popular in the belief that it reduces the incidence of pre-eclampsia. Diuretics have been justified for prevention of oedema which is now understood to be a normal concomitant of the increase in plasma volume in late pregnancy and of no clinical significance in the majority of cases.

The expensive treatment option of bed rest in hospital from 32 weeks gestation for the prevention of premature labour in twin pregnancies increased the incidence of premature delivery in a recent randomized controlled trial (Saunders *et al.* 1985).

General care

There is a difference between antenatal care and antenatal screening. Screening detects abnormalities which have already occurred, but care should be able to prevent some of them from occurring. One definition of antenatal care is the provision, through pregnancy, of a personal service of health education, social support, and readily accessible advice by a team who get to know their mothers as they work with them to promote a good outcome to their pregnancies.

The last opportunities for primary prevention are in the antenatal period, although this is largely left to mothers themselves. The marked differences in low birthweight and PNM between social classes and between geographic regions and ethnic subcultures are likely to result, to a major extent, from differences in the effectiveness of primary prevention as practised by mothers themselves. It is easy to identify groups of mothers who are disadvantaged by reason of their youth, lack of education, language problems, rejection of their pregnancy, chronic domestic difficulties, or social disadvantage in dealing with medical personnel. These groups, who contribute disproportionately to PNM, might be effectively helped in their practice of primary prevention by suitably designed antenatal care. This care should be delivered with the involvement of midwives and health visitors; consultant obstetricians are more suitably employed to investigate and manage abnormalities. It is difficult to provide this type of care in the traditional, large, hospital antenatal clinics. Small health care teams, such as the one at Sighthill in Edinburgh (McKee 1984) and many general practitioner primary health teams (Marsh 1985) are pioneering this sort of antenatal care in disadvantaged areas. The Edinburgh results suggest some success in reducing premature delivery and PNM, but the small numbers and lack of control subjects preclude demonstration of statistical significance.

Evaluation of antenatal care is even rarer than evaluation of antenatal screening. Indeed there has been little to evaluate and the few teams who are involved in delivering this type of care lack the resources for additional research. The deficiency in evaluation of this type of project is often taken as proof that the care it delivers is ineffective in improving pregnancy outcome. Chalmers (1984) has pointed out that reports of success in primary prevention, such as at Sighthill, have not been published in obstetric journals, and that different models of obstetric care have not been adequately discussed in the literature. The WHO Perinatal Study Group found health professionals uninterested in testing new models of antenatal care and recommended further evaluative research (WHO 1985; Inch, 1987).

Intra-partum care

Improvements in intra-partum monitoring may have decreased the number of fetal deaths in labour, but, as these latter were rare, this cannot fully account for the observed changes. Increasing success of intensive care in preventing early neonatal death may have encouraged a greater readiness to resuscitate infants previously classified as stillborn (Hack and Faneroff 1986), or to resort to elective delivery of very premature infants previously thought to be incapable of survival. Two methods of observation of the fetus during labour are commonly employed. Intermittent auscultation is generally used where risk status is low and there is no reason to suspect complications. Continuous electronic fetal monitoring (CEFM) is used, with varying frequency, for high-risk labours. The controversy over the value of CEFM for low-risk labours, which none the less produce an appreciable proportion of PNM and morbidity, has continued for over a decade. Most trials have shown an increase in operative delivery when CEFM has been extended to all labours (Sawers 1983).

The two most recent large trials of CEFM, both from single hospitals, have again produced conflicting results. The Dublin trial involved 12 964 women (MacDonald *et al.* 1985). Fewer neonatal convulsions occurred among the monitored group, but there were identical numbers of abnormal infants at one year among those who convulsed in monitored and control groups. The Texas trial involved 34 995 women and found no difference in the incidence of neonatal convulsions or in any other measure of outcome (Leveno *et al.* 1986). Monitoring was associated with an increase in Caesarian sections in Texas and in forceps deliveries in Dublin where there was a long-standing policy restricting the use of Caesarian section (Stronge 1986). More importantly, neither trial showed any difference in PNM. There were important differences in the design of the two trials, and indeed no two trials have yet been carried out to the same design. There is as yet no evidence that any possible benefits from monitoring low-risk deliveries outweigh the disadvantages. The benefits from CEFM in high-risk cases can be maximized by a high standard of clinical judgement as to who is at high risk. While major effort and expenditure goes into electronic fetal monitoring, much less attention has been given to simple, non-technical aspects of the process of labour. Klaus and his colleagues (1986) recently showed a highly significant decrease in perinatal complications associated with the simple measure of continuous social support in labour from a female companion.

Many reviews of perinatal deaths have attempted to identify 'avoidable' factors in the effort to improve future performance. They have tended to identify non-intervention as blameworthy, but, only rarely, intervention itself. Crowley (1982) considered that 'this fosters defensive obstetrics ... and operates to absolve a doctor who intervenes in a normal pregnancy. This places a premium on intervention as a personal insurance for the doctor.' The legal profession have compounded the problem by following the same approach.

There is much concern about the rising rates of delivery by Caesarian section with its attendant risk to the mother (Anderson and Lomas 1984; Editorial 1986). It has to be admitted that this has occurred at the same time as a steady fall in PNM, but there is no firm evidence of any causal connection. The relative advantage of delivery by section for infants with any particular indication will, of course, depend on the skill of the obstetric team in delivering such babies vaginally. Increased resort to delivery by section may reduce this skill from lack of practice (Russell 1982), so that the superiority of delivery by section will become a self-fulfilling prophecy. This problem is present in several areas of major intervention in the field of perinatal medicine.

Neonatal care

Prevention of neonatal mortality is dependent on resuscitation of asphyxiated infants at birth and the provision of intensive care. These are discussed in detail below. In general, the sharp downturn in PNM among VLBW babies coincided with the introduction of modern neonatal intensive care methods, including mechanical ventilation and total parenteral nutrition. These methods, which benefit very premature babies in particular, are generally accepted as the cause of the acceleration of the already established decline in early neonatal mortality (before 7 days) among VLBW infants (Figure 16.2b). It is not so easy to explain the appearance of a closely similar picture of weight-specific disparities in the rates of decline of stillbirths (Figure 16.2c).

Resuscitation

Delay in establishing spontaneous and regular respirations at birth is common. In the British births study it was found that 6 per cent of infants took longer than 3 minutes to establish spontaneous respiration (Chamberlain *et al.* 1975) and 7 per cent was recorded more recently (Thomas and Hey 1982). Few of these children become handicapped, but we have little knowledge of more minor impairments. Skill in providing rapid resuscitation at birth is clearly of primary importance in neonatal care and all births should be attended by a person with adequate training in resuscitation. It is not feasible at present that this should always be a neonatal paediatrician.

Neonatal intensive care (NIC)

Life-support technology for neonates entered a new phase in the late 1970s in Western countries with the widespread introduction without controlled trials of mechanical ventilation and total parenteral nutrition. These methods had been pioneered in advanced units. The accelerated decline in neonatal mortality has generally been attributed to these developments. Hazards of NIC include transfusion-mediated infection (Morfeldt-Manson 1984; Yaeger 1984) and mechanical ventilation carries the risk of pulmonary infection, pneumothorax, broncho-pulmonary dysplasia causing long-term respiratory disablement, and subglottal stenosis necessitating tracheostomy (Baum *et al.* 1977; Yu *et al.* 1979; Haas and Davies 1980). Current controversy (Maddock 1987; Cooke *et al.* 1988; Roberton 1988; Maddock *et al.* 1988) suggests that review of the indications for mechanical ventilation and of the balance between benefit and damage is now required. Three recent developments may reduce resort to mechanical ventilation, the need for drugs to paralyse infants on ventilators, and the severity of the ventilatory procedure when it must be used. These are percutaneous oxygen supplmentation for very premature infants (Cartlidge and Rutter 1988), patient-triggered ventilation (Mehta *et al.* 1986, Clifford *et al.* 1988), and administration of surfactant (Merritt *et al.* 1986). Regular review of established procedures is essential: for instance, most endotracheally-intubated babies in 242 neonatal units surveyed recently in Britain were receiving inspired gas of well below physiological humidity. This could contribute to several of the complications of artificial ventilation by inhibiting muco-ciliary clearance (Tarnow-Mordi *et al.* 1986). The value of minimizing disturbance and traumatic or stressful procedures for ill and premature babies has been described by Hughes Davies (1979).

Increased survival, childhood handicap, and morbidity

Several observers have noted that, even if the *proportion of survivors* who are handicapped does not increase, the substantial increase in survival of these tiny infants, with their high risk of handicap, will result in an increase in the *proportion of all children* who are handicapped, as well as an increase in the numbers of normal VLBW survivors (Chalmers and Mutch 1981; Paneth *et al.* 1981; McDonald 1981; Powell *et al.* 1986). There are no adequate data relating to the prevalence of handicap in children generally, nor among low birthweight survivors in particular, so that proper monitoring of the effects of the new intensive care is impossible. A large number of follow-up studies have been published by leading neonatal units. However, neonatal units differ in admission policies and in the social, racial, economic, and health status of the population they serve. Policies regarding the resuscitation and maintenance of profoundly ill infants vary. Their reports have differed in length of follow-up and even in definitions of health and handicap. Children classified as significantly handicapped by Kitchen and colleagues (1979) were classified as healthy by Stewart and her colleagues (1981). Reports from the few units which publish results cannot provide the information so urgently required. Inferior results are unlikely to be published.

Three reviews, published in 1981, examined the aggregated results from a number of hospital studies of VLBW infants born between the mid-1960s and the mid-1970s. Kiely and colleagues (1981) and McDonald (1981) reviewed many, widely differing hospital results. They found evidence of a decline in mortality but no evidence of a fall in the prevalence of handicap, neither could they exclude the possibility that handicap was increasing. Stewart and her team (1981) sounded a more optimistic note, but their review began with infants born in the late 1940s. They found no decrease in handicap among survivors born since 1965. The short follow-up of recent studies has precluded assessment of handicap which was less than moderate to severe. Three more recent reviews presented data on the prevalence of handicap among children born after the introduction of NIC (Table 16.9).

Geographically-based studies are more helpful, but have been rare in Europe outside the United Kingdom. Results from three recent studies are included in (Table 16.9). These were in Mansfield, 1963–71, with no intensive care (Steiner *et al.* 1980), in Wolverhampton 1975–9 (Lloyd 1984), and in Mersey 1979–81 (Powell *et al.* 1986). They show much closer agreement on levels of neurodevelopmental handicap than individual hospital follow-up studies have done. The only two with data relating to minor as well as major

Table 16.9 Mortality and impairment among infants of birthweight less than 1500 g.

Review (no. studies)	Birthweight (g) (cases)	Year of birth	Mortality: per cent of live births	Impairment: per cent of survivors	
				Moderate and severe	Minor
Hospital studies					
Lloyd 1984 (7)	<1500 (67)	1961–79	62	14	20
Hack and Faneroff 1986 (6)	500–800 (148)	1975–84	67	32	—
Yu *et al.* 1986 (3)	<28 weeks (460)	1977–84	42	18	—
Geographical studies; birthweight <1500 g					
Mansfield (131 cases) (Steiner *et al.* 1980)		1963–71	50	14	24
Wolverhampton (67 cases) Lloyd (1984)		1975–79	57	15	22
Mersey (322 cases) Powell *et al.* (1986)		1979–81	42	12	—

handicap found 37 per cent and 38 per cent of VLBW survivors were handicapped in Wolverhampton and Mansfield, respectively. Major handicap occurred in 14 per cent and 15 per cent, respectively, slightly more than the 12 per cent recorded later in the Mersey region. It has been customary to express outcome in terms of the percentage of live births who died or were handicapped. It is important to know the percentage of survivors who were handicapped, and this has therefore been calculated, where necessary, for Table 16.9. Little is known about the prevalence of the 'minor' disabilities of clumsiness, behavioural disorders, learning difficulties, and poor health among children not classified as handicapped, but there are indications that such problems are more common in survivors of NIC than in the population at large (D'Souza et al. 1981; Yu et al. 1986).

Cerebral palsy is the condition most commonly associated with low birthweight. The overall rate of cerebral palsy in VLBW survivors has been calculated from the 19 studies reviewed by Kiely and colleagues (1981) as 10 per cent of infants under 1000 g, and 8 per cent of those under 1500 g and born between 1963 and 1978. A geographically-based study in the Mersey region recently produced almost identical rates (Powell et al. 1986).

In Australia Stanley and Atkinson (1981) have reported a rise in prevalence of cerebral palsy among survivors of birthweight under 2000 g who were born between 1961 and 1975 from 26 to 32 per 1000. The total prevalence of spastic diplegia, the type of cerebral palsy most strongly associated with low birthweight, rose from 0.6/1000 born in 1970–75, to 1.3/1000 in 1976. Rates of diplegia (spastic and ataxic) also rose from 0.5/1000 in 1967–70 to 0.8/1000 in 1975–78 among the population of Gothenburg, with the highest rate in 1978 (Hagberg et al. 1984). Preliminary analysis of the author's large geographically-based study in Dublin shows a rise of one-third in diplegia between 1976–78 and 1979–81. The highest level occurred in children born in 1981 (Dowding 1987; Dowding unpublished).

Health problems in survivors of neonatal intensive care

Several reports have shown that very small babies who survive intensive care continue to have health problems. Survivors of VLBW born in the Liverpool maternity unit and discharged from the NIC unit in 1980–82 required 16 times more inpatient facilities in the year after term than a random selection of term infants. Many were seriously ill with lung disease and other problems (Morgan 1985). Morgan reviewed previous reports with similar findings. Recently Skeoch and colleagues (1987) found 46 per cent of VLBW survivors suffered severe morbidity in their first 15 months.

Although there have been many follow-up studies by individual neonatal units, there have been no randomized controlled trials of NIC with mechanical ventilation, as practised during the last decade. Such trials are extremely difficult to carry out for both practical and ethical reasons. A WHO working group meeting in Trieste in October 1986 have recommended that any technology used in postnatal care should be evaluated as to efficacy, safety, economic implications, and cultural acceptability before entering general use. This and other recommendations of the symposium group have been summarized (WHO 1986). Many new procedures and drugs have come into general use for tiny infants without proper trials, and it will be very difficult to trace the origins of adverse sequelae.

Little research has been reported into the views and experiences of parents of handicapped children. At a British hospital the parents of 47 out of 51 infants, who were judged by the NIC team to be virtually certain to suffer total incapacity, chose to have treatment withdrawn (Whitelaw 1986). Parents of American schoolchildren assessed some forms of dysfunction as worse than death (Boyle et al. 1983). Hey (1980) has reported that parents often told him that they dread severe handicap more than death itself. He showed that the contemporary risk of severe handicap among normally-formed infants over 1000 g was already greater than the risk of PNM in England and Wales. These observations highlight the urgency of the problem of accurate prognosis in NIC and inevitably raise difficult questions of priorities in the context of limited resources.

Prediction of outcome
It is now evident that improvements in PNM can no longer be judged without consideration of the prevalence of handicap in the survivors. In the light of the high levels of impairment among VLBW, compared with other children, the outcome of all these infants should be monitored on a national basis by independent monitoring teams.

Research is currently directed toward better prediction of the long-term outcome for sick neonates in intensive care. A number of technologies are available for observation of the occurrence and development of haemorrhage or ischaemic lesions in the brain. At present the most reliable predictor of severe handicap in survivors appears to be the diagnosis, possible with the most recent ultrasound imaging equipment, of extensive leucomalacia in the brain. This condition usually arises by the end of the first week of extra-uterine life and later progresses to the formation of fluid-filled cysts as the affected nervous tissue breaks down. Stewart and her colleagues (1987) identified leucomalacia before 1 week of age in nine infants from a series of 342 survivors born at 33 weeks gestation or less. At 1 year of age all nine were handicapped, eight severely. The combined results of two other studies of preterm infants who survived to assessment at 9 months or older showed cystic leucomalacia in 18. All these infants were severely handicapped (Weindling et al. 1985; de Vries et al. 1985; De Vries and Dubowitz 1985).

Cooke (1985) reported handicap in 20 out of 21 infants with bilateral cystic leucomalacia and in 18 out of 29 in whom the cysts were restricted to one side of the brain. Multiple cysts in the occipital region are ominous (Graham et al. 1987).

Haemorrhage is common in the brains of very premature infants; for instance; almost half of the 219 infants in a series born at 32 weeks or less had brain haemorrhages (Sinha et al. 1985). Haemorrhage occurs, on average, before the appearance of the much rarer condition of leucomalacia, but its value as a predictor of handicap is much more limited. Even severe haemorrhage does not reliably predict severe handicap. De Vries and his colleagues (1985) found nine out of 18 survivors of severe brain haemorrhage were handicapped, five severely so.

The condition of the brain of the newborn can also be investigated with other non-invasive methods. Karch and colleagues (1984) found that electrical recording of brain activity of infants on assisted ventilation provided significant correlations with psychomotor development at 1 year, and the prognostic value was better than that of clinical neurological examination of infants carried out at the same time.

Phosphorus nuclear magnetic resonance spectroscopy can detect areas of abnormal metabolism (Hamilton et al. 1986) and Doppler ultrasonography, abnormal blood flow in the anterior cerebral arteries (Archer et al. 1986). Both methods provided 100 per cent sensitivity for severe handicap or death, and specifities of around 80 per cent. Doppler studies *in utero* on small (<2000 g) growth-retarded infants give promise of very early prognosis of neonatal death or severe illness (Hackett 1987). Near infrared spectrophotometry (Wyatt et al. 1986) has been reported to give good monitoring of changes in cerebral blood flow of neonates and this may prove valuable for informing clinical management and prognosis. Combined use of these non-invasive methods on the same set of infants in a research context may help to improve sensitivity in prognosis still further and to devise a realistic and effective protocol for general use in neonatal units.

Cost of neonatal intensive care

Some estimates of the cost of NIC are given in Table 16.10. The total national cost of NIC in the USA, excluding the cost of any subsequent morbidity or handicap, was estimated at US$ 1500 million in 1980 (Johnstone 1982). From 1972 to 1982 increasing length of stay and changing clinical procedures more than doubled the cost (in 1982 US$) of neonatal care for an infant with respiratory distress syndrome in San Francisco (Showstack 1985) to US$ 50 000. Brooten and her colleagues (1986) carried out a randomized controlled trial of discharge at 2000 g instead of the customary 2200 g for the infants who were well. Mothers were given full home support after discharge of the infants. Costs were reduced, with no detectable adverse effect on outcome, from US$ 64 940 to US$ 47 520 per child discharged.

Table 16.10 Costs of neonatal intensive care for very low birthweight infants (<1500 g).

Category	Region (source)	Birthweight (g)	Year/currency	Cost per infant
Survivor	Paris (1)	<1500	1981/FE	200 356
Live birth	Canada (2)	1000–1499	1978/Can$	14 200
		500– 999		13 600
Survivor to discharge		1000–1499		18 442
		500– 999		61 818
Survivor	UK (3)	1000–1499	1984/Stg	5 500
		500– 999		10 000
Non-Survivor		<1500		<1000
Survivor	UK (4)	<1500	1984/Stg	4 490
Non-Survivor				3 346
Survivor	USA (5)	500– 999	1974/US$	40 287
Non-Survivor				14 236
Normal Survivor				88 058
Survivor	USA (6)	500– 750	1982–5/US$	158 800
Survivor	Australia (7)	<800	1982/Aust$	39 845
(adjusted[a])		801–1000		14 137
		1001–1500		4 782
Estimated lifetime cost/survivor	USA (8)	900– 999	1982/US$	40 647
		600– 699		362 992
Estimated lifetime earnings/survivor		900– 999		77 084
		600– 699		0

Sources: 1—Monset-Couchard 1984. 2—Boyle *et al.* 1983.
3—Newns *et al.* 1984. 4—Sandhu *et al.* 1986.
5—Pomerance *et al.* 1978. 6—Hack *et al.* 1986.
7—John *et al.* 1983. 8—Walker *et al.* 1984.

[a]cost adjusted for expenditure on non-survivors.

Recommendations

There are three areas where progress is desirable.

1. Routine data collection. International harmonization of perinatal data collection should be encouraged to include fetuses weighing 500 g or more at birth. Definition of the perinatal period by length of gestation should be discontinued. National handicap registers, preferably on an internationally agreed protocol, are needed for perinatal audit, for monitoring of trends, and to provide a basis for investigation of the origins of handicap.

Continuation of our present ignorance of the prevalence of handicap is unacceptable.

2. Research. Recent developments in NIC, which have increased survival of very low birthweight infants, should be matched by research into improved prognostic capabilities for very sick neonates. Increased investment in the search for causes of premature delivery and the origins of handicap is urgently needed.

3. Primary prevention. Much of the continuing difference between social classes and ethnic groups in the incidence of PNM and low birthweight represents preventable mortality and morbidity. New initiatives in primary prevention among easily identified disadvantaged groups should be financed and evaluated.

References

Alberman, E. (1980). Prospects for better perinatal health. *Lancet* **1**, 189–91.
Anderson, G.M. and Lomas, J. (1984). Determinants of the increasing Caesarean birth rate. *New Engl. J. Med.* **311**, 887–92.
Archer, L.N.J., Levene, M.I., and Evans, D.H. (1986). Cerebral artery Doppler ultrasonography for prediction of outcome after perinatal asphyxia. *Lancet* **2**, 1116–17.
Ashton, J.R. (1983). Trends in induced abortion in England and Wales. *Br. Med. J.* **287**, 1001–2.
Baird, D. (1985). Changing problems and priorities in obstetrics. *Br. J. Obstet. Gynaecol.* **92**, 115–21.
Bakketeig, L.S., Eik-nes, S.H., Jacobsen, G., Ulstein, M.K., Brodtkorb, C.J., Balstad, P., Eriksen, B.C., and Jorgensen, N.P. (1984). Randomised controlled trial of ultrasonographic screening in pregnancy. *Lancet* **2**, 207–10.
Baum, D., MacFarlane, A., and Tizard, P., (1977). The benefits and hazards of neonatology. In *Benefits and hazards of the new obstetrics* (eds T. Chard and M. Richards). Heinemann Medical for Spastic International Medical Publications, London.
Beattie, R.B., Dornan, J.C., and Thompson, W. (1987). Intrauterine growth retardation: prediction of perinatal distress by Doppler ultrasound. *Lancet* **2**, 974.
Boyle, M.H., Torrance, G.W., Sinclair, J.C., and Horwood, S.P. (1983). Economic evaluation of neonatal intensive care of very-low-birth weight infants. *New Engl. J. Med.* **308**, 1330–7.
Brooten, D., Kumar, S., Brown, L.P., Butts, P., Finkler, S.A., Bakewell-Sachs, S., Gibbons, A., and Delivoria-Papadopoulos, M. (1986). A randomised clinical trial of early hospital discharge and home follow-up of very-low-birth weight infants. *New Engl. J. Med.* **315**, 936–8.
Butler, N.R. and Bonham, D.G. (1963). *Perinatal mortality*. First report of the 1958 British perinatal mortality survey. Livingstone, Edinburgh.
Cartlidge, P.H.T. and Rutter, N. (1988). Percutaneous oxygen delivery to the preterm infant. *Lancet* **2**, 315–17.

Chalmers, I.G. (1980a). An introduction to perinatal audit and surveillance. In *Perinatal audit and surveillance* (eds I.G. Chalmers and G. McIlwaine). Royal College of Obstetricians and Gynaecologists, London.
—— (1980b). Shanghai. *Lancet* 1, 137-9.
—— (1984). In *Pregnancy care for the 1980s* (eds L. Zander and G. Chamberlain). MacMillan Press and Royal Society of Medicine, London.
Chalmers, I. and Mutch, L., (1981). Are current trends in perinatal practice associated with an increase or a decrease in handicapping conditions? *Lancet* 1, 1415.
Chamberlain, R., Chamberlain, G., Howlett, B., and Claireaux, A. (1975). *British births 1970. Vol 1. The first week of life.* Heinemann Medical Books, London.
Chng, P.K., Hall, M.H., and MacGillivray, I. (1980). An audit of antenatal care: the value of the first antenatal visit. *Br. Med. J.* 281, 1184.
Clarke, M. (1982). Perinatal audit: a tried and tested epidemiological method. *Comm. Med.* 4, 104-7.
Clifford, R.D., Whincup, G., and Thomas, R. (1988). Patient-triggered ventilation prevents pneumothorax in premature babies. *Lancet* 1, 529-30.
Cooke, R.W.I. (1985). Neonatal cranial ultrasound and neurological development at follow up. *Lancet* 2, 494-5.
——, Powell, T.G., and Pharoah, P.O.D. (1988). Mechanical ventilation for the newborn. *Lancet* 1, 178.
Crowley, P. (1982). Inquiring into perinatal deaths. *Lancet* 1, 675.
D'Souza, S.W., McCartney, E., Nolan, M., and Taylor, I.G. (1981). Hearing, speech and language survivors of severe perinatal asphyxia. *Arch. Dis. Child.* 56, 245-52.
De Vries, L.S. and Dubowitz, L.M.S. (1985). Cystic leucomalacia in preterm infant: site of lesion in relation to prognosis. *Lancet* 2, 1075-6.
——, ——, Dubowitz, V., Kaiser, A., Lary, S., Silverman, M., Whitelaw, A., and Wigglesworth, J.S. (1985). Predictive value of cranial ultrasound in the newborn baby: a reappraisal. *Lancet* 2, 137-40.
Dowding, V.M. (1981). New assessment of the effects of birth order and socio-economic status on birth weight. *Br. Med. J.* 282, 683-6.
—— and Barry, C. (1987). Cerebral palsy in the Eastern Health Board area. *Irish J. Med. Science* 156, 79.
Editorial (1986). More Caesarean sections in England and Wales. *Lancet* 1, 569-70.
Edouard, L. and Alberman, E.D. (1980). National trends in the certified causes of perinatal mortality, 1968-78. *Br. J. Obstet. Gynaecol.* 87, 833-8.
Eurostat Demographic Statistics (1985). Series C. Luxembourg: Office des Publications Officielles des Communautés Européennes, 1986.
Francome, C. (1983). Unwanted pregnancies amongst teenagers. *J. Biosoc. Sci.* 15, 139-43.
Gordon, R.R. (1985). Numbers of immature births. *Br. Med. J.* 291, 55.
Graham, M., Levene, M.I., Trounce, J.Q., and Rutter, N. (1987). Prediction of cerebral palsy in very low birthweight infants: prospective ultrasound study. *Lancet* 2, 593-6.
Haas, R. and Davies, P. (1980). Iatrogenic hazards in the newborn intensive care unit. In *Topics in perinatal medicine* (ed. B.A. Wharton). Pitman Medical, London.

Hack, M. and Fanaroff, A.A. (1986). Changes in the delivery room care of the extremely small infant (<750 g). Effects on morbidity and outcome. *New Engl. J. Med.* **314**, 660–4.

Hagberg, B., Hagberg, G., and Olow, I. (1984). The changing panorama of cerebral palsy in Sweden. *Acta Paedia. Scand.* **73**, 433–40.

Hall, M.H. and Chng, P.K. (1982). In *Effectiveness and satisfaction in antenatal care* (eds. M. Enkin and I. Chalmers). Spastics International Medical Publications. Heinemann Medical Books, London; Philadelphia.

——, ——, and MacGillivray, I. (1980). Is routine antenatal care worth while? *Lancet* **2**, 78–80.

——, MacIntyre, S., and Porter, M. (1985). *Antenatal care assessed*. Aberdeen University Press, Aberdeen.

Hamilton, P.A., Hope, P.L., Cady, E.B., Delpy, D.T., Wyatt, J.S., and Reynolds, E.O.R. (1986). Impaired energy metabolism in brains of newborn infants with increased cerebral echodensities. *Lancet* **1**, 1242–6.

Hellier, J. (1977). *Population trends*. **10**, 13. OPCS (Office of Population Censuses and Surveys), London.

Hey, E. (1980). Retrolental fibroplasia as one index of perinatally acquired handicap. In *Perintal audit and surveillance* (eds I. Chalmers, G. McIllwaine). Royal College of Obstetricians and Gynaecologists, London.

Hoffman, H.J., Lundin, F.E., Bakketeig, L.S., and Harley, E.E. (1977). Classification of births by weight and gestational age for future studies of prematurity. In *Epidemiology of prematurity* (eds D.M. Reed and F.J. Stanley). Urban and Schwarzenberg, Baltimore.

——, Meirik, O., and Bakketeig, L.S. (1983). Analysis of perinatal mortality rates through time and in relation to weight or maturity at birth. In *Perinatal epidemiology* (ed. M.B. Bracken). Oxford University Press, Oxford.

Hughes, K. (1985). Comparison of birthweight and infant mortality between Singapore and England and Wales, 1980. *J. Epid. Comm. Hlth.* **539**, 135–40.

Hughes-Davies, H. (1979). Conservative care of the newborn baby. *Arch. Dis. Child.* **54**, 59–61.

Inch, S. (1987). Having a baby in the United Kingdom. *Lancet* **1**, 989–90.

John, E., Lee, K., and Li, G.M. (1983). Cost of neonatal intensive care. *Austr. Paediat. J.* **19**, 152–6.

Johnstone, T. (1982). Primary prevention and low birthweight. *Lancet* **1**, 805.

Karch, D., Rohmer, K., and Lemborg, P. (1984). Polygraphic recording in newborn infants. *Dev. Med. Child Neurol.* **26**, 358–68.

Kenepp, N.B., Kumar, S., Shelley, W.C., Stanley, C.A., Gabbe, S.G., and Gutsche, B.B. (1982). Fetal and neonatal hazards of maternal hydration with 5% dextrose before Caesarean section. *Lancet* **1**, 1150.

Kiely, J.L., Paneth, N., Stein, Z., and Susser, M. (1981). Cerebral palsy and newborn care. II: Mortality and neurological impairment in low-birthweight infants. *Dev. Med. Child Neurol.* **23**, 650–9.

Kitchen, W.H., Rickards, A., Ryan, M.M., McDougall, A.B., Billson, F.A., Keir, E.H., and Naylor, F.D. (1979). A longitudinal study of very low-birthweight-infants. II: results of controlled trial of intensive care and incidence of handicaps. *Dev. Med. Child Neurol.* **21**, 582–9.

Klaus, M.H., Kennell, J.H., Robertson, S.S., and Sosa, R. (1986). Effects of social support during parturition on maternal and infant morbidity. *Br. Med. J.* **293**, 585–7.
Knudson, L.B. and Kristensen, F.B. (1986). Monitoring perinatal mortality and perinatal care with a national register: Content and usage of the Danish Medical Birth Register. *Comm. Med.* **8**, 29–36.
Lau, S.P. and Fung, K.P. (1984). Ethnic variables in perinatal mortality rates. *Lancet* **2**, 402.
Leveno, K.J., Cunningham, F.G., Nelson, S., Roarke, M., Williams, M.L., Guzick, D., Dowling, S., Rosenfeld, C.R., and Buckley, A. (1986). A prospective comparison of selective and universal electronic fetal monitoring in 34,995 pregnancies. *New Engl. J. Med.* **315**, 615–9.
Lloyd, B.W. (1984). Outcome of very-low-birthweight babies from Wolverhampton. *Lancet* **2**, 739–41.
Lumb, K.M., Congdon, P.J., and Lealman, G.T. (1981). A comparative review of Asian and British-born maternity patients in Bradford, 1974–8. *J. Epidemiol. Comm. Hlth* **35**, 106–9.
MacDonald, D., Grant, A., Sheridan-Pereira, M., Boylan, P., and Chalmers, I. (1985). The Dublin randomised controlled trial of intrapartum fetal heart rate monitoring. *Am. J. Obstet. Gynecol.* **152**, 524–39.
MacFarlane, A., and Mugford, M. (1984). *Birth counts: statistics of pregnancy and childbirth.* Vol II. HMSO (Her Majesty's Stationery Office), London.
Maddock, C.R. (1987). A population-based evaluation of sustained mechanical ventilation of newborn babies. *Lancet* **2**, 1254–8.
——, Carpenter, R.G., and Gardner A. (1988). Mechanical ventilation for the newborn, *Lancet* **1**, 707.
Marsh, G.N. (1985). New programme of antenatal care in general practice. *Br. Med. J.* **291**, 646–8.
McDonald, A.D. (1981). Survival and handicap in infants of very low birthweight. *Lancet* **2**, 194.
McKee, I.H. (1984). Community antenatal care: the Sighthill community antenatal scheme. In *Pregnancy care for the 1980s* (eds L. Zander and G. Chamberlain). MacMillan Press, London.
Mehta, A., Wright, B.M., Callan, K., and Stacey, T.E. (1986). Patient-triggered ventilation in the newborn. *Lancet* **1**, 17–19.
Meirik, O., Smedby, B., and Ericson, A. (1979). Impact of changing age and parity distributions of mothers on perinatal mortality in Sweden, 1953–1975. *Int. J. Epidemiol.* **8**, 361–4.
Merritt, T.A., Hallman, M., Bloom, B.T., Berry, C., Benirschke, K., Sahn, D., Key, T., Edwards, D., Jarvenpaa, A-L., Pohjavouri, M., Kankaanpaa, K., Kunnas, M., Paatero, H., Rapoli, J., and Jaaskelainen, J. (1986). Prophylactic treatment of very premature infants with human surfactant. *New Engl. J. Med.* **315**, 785–90.
Monset-Couchard, M., Jaspar, M.L., De Bethmann, O., and Relier, J.P. (1984). Cout de la prise en charge initiale des enfants de poids de naissance inférieur ou égal a 1500 g en 1981. *Arch. Fr. Pédiatr.* **41**, 579–85.

Morfeldt-Manson, O. (1984). Transfusion-induced AIDS in four premature babies. *Lancet* **2**, 1346.

Morgan, M.E.I. (1985). Late morbidity of very low birthweight infants. *Br. Med. J.* **291**, 171-3.

Murphy, J.F., O'Riordan, J., Newcombe, R.G., Coles, E.C., and Pearson, J.F. (1986). Relation of haemoglobin levels in first and second trimesters to outcome of pregnancy. *Lancet* **1**, 992-4.

Newns, B., Drummond, M.F., Durbin, G.M., and Culley, P. (1984). Costs and outcomes in a regional neonatal intensive care unit. *Arch. Dis. Child.* **59**, 1064-7.

Newton, R.W., Webster, P.A.C., Binu, P.S., Maskrey, N., and Phillips, A.B. (1979). Psychosocial stress in pregnancy and its relation to the onset of premature labour. *Br. Med. J.* **2**, 411-13.

Nicolaides, K.H., Soothill, P.W., Rodeck, C.H., and Campbell, S. (1986). Ultrasound-guided sampling of umbilical cord and placental blood to assess fetal well-being: *Lancet* **1**, 1065-7.

Oakley, A., Macfarlane, A., and Chalmers, I. (1982). Social class, stress and reproduction. In *Disease and the environment* (eds A.R. Rees and H.J. Purcell). Proceedings of the Inaugural Conference of the Society for Environmental Therapy 1981. John Wiley and Sons Ltd, Chichester.

Office of Populations Censuses and surveys (OPCS) mortality statistics. Perinatal and infant; social and biological factors. Series Dh3. nos. 13(1981), 14(1982), 15(1983), 17 (1984).

—— abortion statistics. (1984a) General and demographic. Series AB no. 11, Department of Health and Social Security, London.

Paneth, N., Kiely, J.L., Stein, Z., and Susser, M. (1981). Cerebral palsy and newborn care. III: Estimated prevalence rates of cerebral palsy under differing rates of mortality and impairment of low-birthweight infants. *Dev. Med. Child Neurol.* **23**, 801-17.

Pomerance, J.J., Ukrainski, C.T., Ukra, T., Henderson, D.H., Nash, A.H., and Meredith, J.L. (1978). Cost of living for infants weighing 1000 grams or less at birth. *Pediatrics* **61**, 908-10.

Powell, T.G., Pharoah, P.O.D., and Cooke, R.W.I. (1986). Survival and morbidity in a geographically defined population of low birthweight infants. *Lancet* **1**, 539-43.

Reuwer, P.J.H.M., Sijmons, E.A., Rietman, G.W., van Tiel, M.W.M., and Bruinse, H.W. (1987) Intrauterine growth retardation: prediction of perinatal distress by Doppler ultrasound. *Lancet* **2**, 415-19.

Robertson, N.R.C. (1988). Mechanical ventilation for the newborn. *Lancet* **1**, 178.

Rush, D. and Cassano, P. (1983). Relationship of cigarette smoking and social class to birth weight and perinatal mortality among all births in Britain, 5-11 April 1970. *J. Epidemiol. Comm. Hlth* **37**, 249-55.

Russell, J.K. (1982). Breech: vaginal delivery or caesarean section? *Br. Med. J.* **285**, 830-1.

Sandhu, B., Stevenson, R.C., Cooke, R.W., and Pharoah, P.O. (1986). Cost of neonatal intensive care for very-low-birthweight infants. *Lancet* **1**, 600-3.

Saunders, M.C., Dick, J.S., Brown, I.M., McPherson, K., and Chalmers, I. (1985).

The effects of hospital admission for bed rest on the duration of twin pregnancy: a randomised trial. *Lancet* **2**, 793–5.

Savage, A. (1986). Perinatal mortality—a suitable index of health worldwide? *Lancet* **2**, 1209–10.

Sawers, R.S. (1983). Fetal monitoring during labour. *Br. Med. J.* **287**, 1649–50.

Sepkowitz, S. (1983). Intensive care of low-birth-weight infants. *New Engl. J. Med.* **309**, 1058–9.

Showstack, J.A., Hughes Stone, M., and Schroeder, S.A. (1985). The role of changing clinical practices in the rising costs of hospital care. *New Engl. J. Med.* **313**, 1201–7.

Simpson, R.J. and Smith, N.G.A. (1986). Maternal smoking and low birthweight: implications for antenatal care. *J. Epidemiol. Comm. Hlth.* **40**, 223–7.

Sinha, S.K., Davies, J.M., Sims, D.G., and Chiswick, M.L. (1985). Relation between periventricular haemorrhage and ischaemic brain lesions diagnosed by ultrasound in very preterm infants. *Lancet* **2**, 1154–5.

Skeoch, C., Rosenberg, K., Turner, T., Skeoch, H., and McIlwaine, G. (1987). Very low birthweight survivors: illness and readmission to hospital in the first 15 months of life. *Br. Med. J.* **295**, 579–80.

Soothill, P.W., Nicolaides, K.H., Bilardo, C.M., and Campbell, S. (1986). Relation of fetal hypoxia in growth retardation to mean blood velocity in the fetal aorta. *Lancet* **2**, 1118–9.

Stanley, F.J. and Atkinson, S. (1981). Impact of neonatal intensive care on cerebral palsy in infants of low birthweight. *Lancet* **2**, 1162.

Steiner, E.S., Sanders, E.M., Phillips, E.C.K., and Maddock, C.R. (1980). Very low birth weight children at school age: comparison of neonatal management methods. *Br. Med. J.* **281**, 1237–1240.

Stewart, A.L., Reynolds, E.O.R., and Lipscomb, A.P. (1981). Outcome for infants of very low birthweight: survey of world literature. *Lancet* **1**, 1038–40.

Stewart, A.L., Reynolds, E.O.R., Hope, P.L., Hamilton, P.A., Baudin, J., Costello, A.M.D., Bradford, B.C., and Wyatt, J.S. (1987). *Dev. Med. Child Neurol.* **29**, 3–11.

Stronge, J.M. (1985). *Clinical report for the year 1985*. National Maternity Hospital, Dublin.

Sunderland, R. and Greenfield, A.A. (1984). Declining mortality in the immature: medical or biological effect? *J. Epidemiol. Comm. Hlth* **28**, 326–30.

Tabor, A., Madsen, M., Obel, E.B., Philip, J., Bang, J., and Norgaard-Pedersen, B. (1986). Randomised controlled trial of genetic amniocentesis in 4606 low-risk women. *Lancet* **1**, 1287–92.

Tarnow-Mordi, W.O., Fletcher, M., Sutton, P., and Wilkinson, A.R. (1986). Evidence of inadequate humidification of inspired gas during artificial ventilation of newborn babies in the British Isles. *Lancet* **2**, 909–13.

Thomas, S.S. and Hey, E.N. (1982). Special newborn care nursing. *Lancet* **1**, 674–5.

Villar, J. and Belizan, J.M. (1982). The relative contribution of prematurity and fetal growth retardation to low birthweight in developing and developed societies. *Am. J. Obstet. Gynecol.* **143**, 793–9.

Walker, D.J., Feldman, A., Vohr, B.R., and Oh, W. (1984). Cost–benefit analysis of neonatal intensive care for infants weighing less than 1000 grams at birth. *Pediatrics* **74**, 20–5.

Weindling, A.M., Rochefort, M.J., Calvert, S.A., Fok, T., and Wilkinson, A. (1985). Development of cerebral palsy after ultrasonographic detection of periventricular cysts in the newborn. *Dev. Med. Child Neurol.* **27**, 800–806.

Whitelaw, A. (1986). Death as an option in neonatal intensive care. *Lancet* **2**, 328–31.

World Health Organization (1978). International Classification of Diseases, Ninth Revision, WHO, Geneva.

—— (1985). Annual Statistical Report.

—— (1986). Appropriate technology following birth (report). *Lancet* **2**, 1387–8.

Wigglesworth, J. (1980). Monitoring perinatal mortality—a pathophysiological approach. *Lancet* **1**, 684.

Wyatt, J.S., Cope, M., Delpy, D.T., Wray, S., and Reynolds, E.O.R. (1986). Quantification of cerebral oxygenation and haemodynamics in sick newborn infants by near infrared spectrophotometry. *Lancet* **2**, 1063–5.

Yaeger, A.S. (1984). Transfusion-acquired CMV infection in newborn infants. *Am. J. Dis. Child.* **128**, 478.

Yu, V.Y.H., Hewson, P.H., and Hollingsworth, E. (1979). Iatrogenic hazards of neonatal intensive care in extremely low birthweight infants. *Austr. Paediat. J.* **15**, 233–7.

——, Loke, H.L., Szymonowicz, W., Orgill, A.A., and Astbury, J. (1986). Prognosis for infants born at 23 to 28 weeks' gestation. *Br. Med. J.* **293**, 1200–3.

17
Post-neonatal mortality

Elizabeth Watson

'Infant mortality is the most sensitive index we possess of social welfare and of sanitary administration under urban conditions' (Sir Arthur Newsholme 1910)

SUMMARY
The post-neonatal death rate (deaths from 28 days to less than 1 year from birth) has declined dramatically in Western European countries during the last 50 years, although the rate of decline has slowed down over the last two decades. The main factor in this decrease has been the gradual reduction in deaths from infection, particularly of gastrointestinal and respiratory origin. Since 1960, in most EEC countries there has, however, been a sharp increase in post-neonatal deaths recorded as 'sudden death cause unknown'. This is partly the result of changes in diagnosis recorded on death certificates. Some of these deaths are considered avoidable and intervention has been based on trying to identify high-risk children on whom to concentrate child health services. Risk scoring systems have been developed and have had some success in reducing the death rate in a target population in the United Kingdom. Whether such intervention will be effective elsewhere remains to be demonstrated. It is essential, however, that particular districts or communities devise their own risk factor scores specific to the needs of their particular population. Routinely available data on infant deaths should be used as a tool for planning and monitoring of child health services and for increasing professional and parental awareness of the problem.

Definition

It is customary to divide infant mortality into the *neonatal period*, that is deaths in the first 28 days of life, and the *post-neonatal period*, from 28 completed days to less than 1 year from birth, that is, up to and including 364 days. The neonatal period is further divided more precisely into early and late. The much longer time span of the post-neonatal period is not sub-divided, possibly because until recently it has attracted less attention. This is probably because of the complexities of the environmental factors which mainly contribute to death in this period. The factors affecting the post-neonatal rate are predominantly social—a disproportionate number of these deaths occur among the lower social classes, in large families, especially if the mother is young (Morris 1979). The infant death rate is affected by varying factors at different stages of infancy, as was observed over a century ago (Farr 1868) and discussed more recently (Pharoah and Morris 1979). The post-neonatal death rate is a good indicator of a country's socio-economic development while the neonatal death rate is more dependent on the standing of health care at or around the time of birth.

Routine publication of post-neonatal mortality rates is more recent than that of neonatal mortality, and data on the former have appeared in the World Health Organization statistics only since 1971 (World Health Statistics, Annual).

The causes of death during the post-neonatal period are more varied than in the neonatal period where 90 per cent of deaths are caused by conditions originating in the perinatal period or from congenital anomalies. In the post-neonatal period congenital anomalies usually account for 25 to 35 per cent of mortality, and symptoms and ill-defined conditions, including the *sudden infant death syndrome*, account for a similar percentage, except in a small proportion of countries where the syndrome is not recognized. Deaths from respiratory disease and accidents are the other two most common causes of death in the post-neonatal period. In this period deaths are conveniently divided into two categories 'avoidable'—for example, respiratory and infectious disease—and 'unavoidable'—for example, life-threatening congenital anomalies.

Trends

During the last 50 years there have been dramatic falls in the infant mortality rates of Western European countries. The predominant feature over the earlier years has been a particularly steep decline in discernible post-neonatal deaths followed by relative stability over the last two decades. This has caused some commentators to speculate whether we are now approaching an irreducible minimum (Pharoah and Morris 1979). In the European Community between 1960 and 1980 the post-neonatal infant mortality rate fell from 11.4 to 4.1 per 1000 live births. This fall occurred despite evidence that babies who would formerly have died during the neonatal period may be surviving to die in the post-neonatal period (Hack *et al.* 1980; Pharoah and MacFarlane 1982). The post-neonatal mortality rate for babies with a gestational age of less than 32 weeks or birthweight of less than 1500 g or

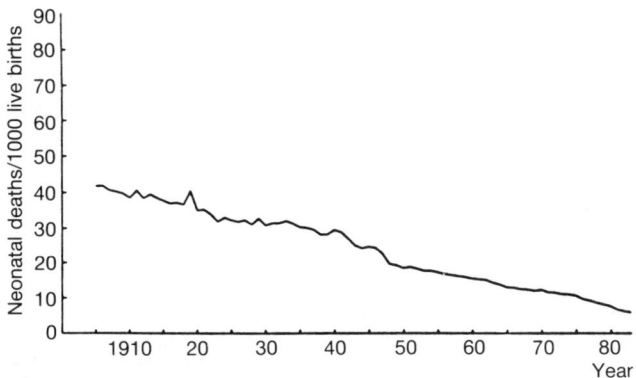

Fig. 17.1 Neonatal mortality, England and Wales 1905-83. (Source: OPCS Mortality Statistics. Series DH3.)

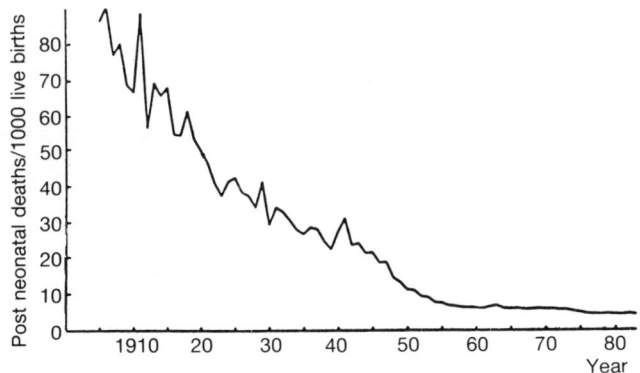

Fig. 17.2 Post-neonatal mortality, England and Wales 1905-83. (Source: OPCS Mortality Statistics. Series DH3.)

both has been shown to be significantly higher than that for other infants (Starfield *et al.* 1982).

In the United Kingdom, post-neonatal mortality rates have shown a much sharper decrease than neonatal rates and have contributed the major portion of the improvements in infant mortality from the beginning of the century (Figures 17.1 and 17.2).

Direct international comparisons must be treated with some caution, however, because of variations between countries in birth and death registration practice within Europe.

The European figures for the post-neonatal mortality rate are similar for most countries (Figure 17.3). Greece and Italy, however, show remarkable falls between 1960 and 1980 (from over 20 to less than 5 per 1000 livebirths).

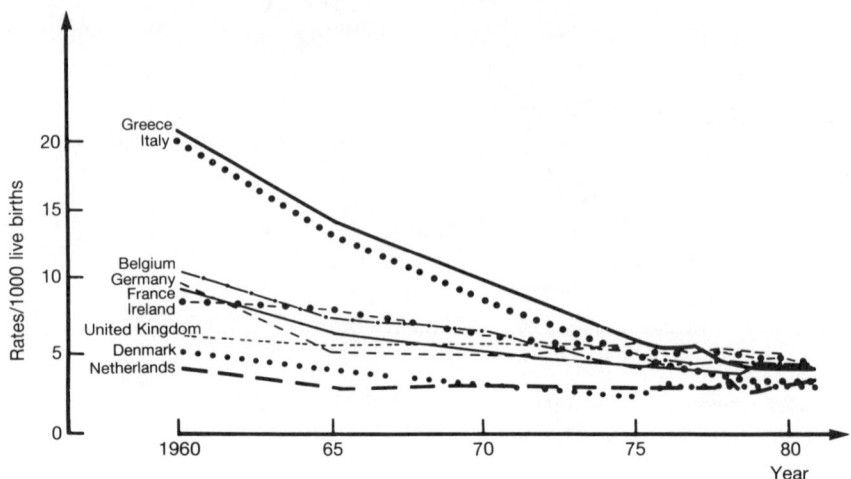

Fig. 17.3 Post-neonatal mortality rates in EEC countries 1960–80 (per 1000 live births). (Adapted from Kaminski and Blondel (1985).)

Table 17.1 Post-neonatal mortality rates in EEC countries 1960–80.

Country	Rate per 1000 live births			Decline
	1960	1970	1980	1960–80[a]
FRG	9.9	5.3	4.8	48
France	9.7	5.5	4.3	44
Italy	19.9	9.0	3.3	16
Netherlands	4.6	3.3	2.9	64
Belgium	10.8	6.8	4.5	43
United Kingdom	6.0	5.4	3.3	68
Republic of Ireland	8.9	6.7	4.4	48
Denmark	5.4	3.2	2.9	54
Greece	20.6	10.0	4.0	20

Source: Eurostat Demographic Statistics 1986, Theme 3, Series C.
[a]Post-neonatal mortality in 1980 as a percentage of the 1960 rate (Kaminski and Blondel 1985).

Denmark and Holland had the lowest rates throughout this period (Table 17.1), with Germany having the highest rate in 1980. The United Kingdom showed the smallest decline in the post-neonatal rate in the EEC countries judged by the 1980 rate as a proportion of the 1960 rate.

The Nordic countries have led the field in lower rates of infant mortality, both perinatal and post-neonatal, since the last war. The leading position of Sweden now seems to be challenged by Finland (Figure 17.4). One

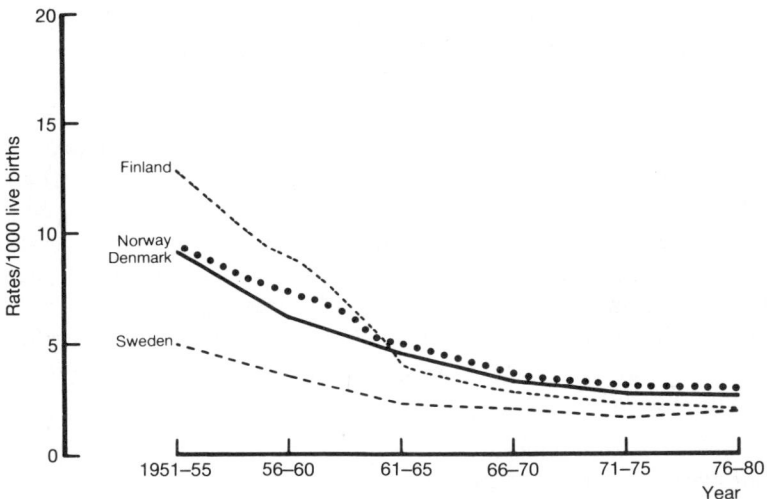

Fig. 17.4 Post-neonatal mortality rates in four Nordic countries 1951-80 (per 1000 live births). (Adapted from Bolander (1984).)

explanation for this is that the large proportion of infants born to immigrant parents in Sweden, especially from Southern Europe and Asia, may run a higher risk of dying in the post-neonatal than in the neonatal period when they are more supervised and therefore receive the same protection from the health care system as the Swedish babies (Bolander 1984).

The organizational pattern of services obviously varies from country to country, but the central impression to emerge is that the countries which have made the greatest advances in reducing mortality in children are those in which the health of children stands higher in the scale of social priorities. For example, compared to the United Kingdom, most other European countries place much greater emphasis on regular supervision of all children throughout childhood, especially in the pre-school years (Wynn and Wynn 1974).

It is unquestionable, however, that the differences in the rate and timing of improvement in post-neonatal mortality in various countries suggest an impact of factors other than the availability of specific medical technologies. The period of maximum improvements seemed to coincide with national changes in the organization of health services or the access to contraception and abortion. Far more significant, however, is the degree of economic prosperity of the relative countries. The dramatic fall in Greece's post-neonatal mortality rate, for example, coincided with the upsurge of industrialization which began in the 1960s when Greece first formed links with the EEC. This process has taken place earlier in the cases of many of the EEC countries which had relatively lower rates of post-neonatal mortality at the beginning of the period. Low socio-economic status is a high risk factor at all ages, but highest for post-neonatal deaths (Alberman 1985).

Most countries, and in particular the United Kingdom have marked regional differences in post-neonatal death rates, and it is often difficult to disentangle the effects of local health services and the relative prosperity of an area in determining the reasons for differing local rates. In the United Kingdom, the general trend has been for mortality in the more prosperous South of England to be much lower than in the more socially disadvantaged North and in Scotland, for both adults and children, although recently there has been a levelling out between regions. The overall picture is of a narrowing of regional differentials so that declines in the regions with the highest rates contributed most to the fall in England and Wales between 1970 and 1980 (Pharoah and MacFarlane 1982).

Reasons for lack of recent progress

Various investigations have been undertaken to study why so little improvement has been achieved in lowering the post-neonatal mortality rate in recent years. A confidential enquiry was set up in the 1960s in Great Britain to investigate the relatively poor post-neonatal rate figures, to establish avoidable factors contributing to the deaths, and to provide a base for an effective preventive inquiry (Department of Health and Social Security 1970). The enquiry established that in about half of all cases the child died without ever reaching hospital, a quarter (predominantly very premature infants and those with congenital malformations) had remained in hospital from birth, and only a quarter were admitted as a result of their terminal illness. This report had no obvious impact on the post-neonatal mortality rate. There have been two more recent studies of the problem, widened to include post-perinatal deaths. One was undertaken in nine areas of Southern England of all cases of unexpected perinatal deaths reported to the coroner (Watson *et al.* 1981) and the other in eight urban centres (Knowelden *et al.* 1984) with the aims of establishing possibly avoidable factors in the deaths and assisting in the planning of child health services. Both had very similar findings. Underestimation of the severity of illness by medical attendants or parents, or both, occurred in a proportion of cases, and the use of medical services, particularly in the inner city, was less 'appropriate' than for matched live control subjects. In the 1960s enquiry only 23 per cent of the avoidable factors were attributed to medical services while 71 per cent were social or parental in origin. The parental factors listed were incompetence or inadequacy, neglect, failure to summon medical aid or to appreciate the seriousness of the situation, and mental subnormality or low intelligence. In the two more recent enquiries, 20% and 25%, respectively, of the infants' parents had acted 'inappropriately', not realizing their child was ill or failing to summon help sufficiently quickly. As Pharoah (1986) has pointed out, failure to use medical services is a recurring theme in studies on post-neonatal deaths, and half the children involved do not reach hospital.

Can reports of this nature affect the post-neonatal mortality rate? During the period of the study in Southern England, there was an unexpected fall in infant deaths in the inner city, although no specific intervention strategies were adopted, apart from alerting the health care professionals to the potentially preventable nature of some of the deaths. It is certainly true that reports of this nature generate enormous interest in the subject of the infant death rate at particular ages as the recent large fall in perinatal mortality testified. The Short Report in the United Kingdom (Second Report from the Social Services Committee 1980) and its sequel (Third Report from the Social Services Committee 1984) and the series of confidential enquiries into perinatal mortality (McIlwaine et al. 1979; Mersey Region Working Party on Perinatal Mortality 1982; Mutch and Elbourne 1983; Northern Regional Health Authority 1984) may well be responsible for some of this fall by highlighting medical shortcomings (Lancet 1985). It is, however, far easier to study avoidable factors in perinatal deaths where the sins of omission and commission are mainly medical in nature and can be corrected, than in the less definable areas of social and environmental factors which characterize post-neonatal deaths.

Risk factors for post-neonatal mortality

Social class

The main risk factor for post-neonatal mortality in the United Kingdom is social class which is officially determined by father's occupation. The social class V/social class I differential in post-neonatal mortality is greater than in any other age-specific group (Office of Population, Censuses and Surveys 1978). Antonosky and Bernstein (1977) showed that the social class differential for neonatal mortality at worst can be about two-fold whereas the differential for post-neonatal mortality can be as much as eight-fold. As much as 85–90 per cent of neonatal deaths occur during the infant's first week of life with relatively little class differential. It can be speculated that the reason for the relatively small class differences found for first week mortality, in contrast to relatively high differentials for late neonatal and post-neonatal mortality, is that most births occur in hospital, so that the exposure of infants to detrimental home environments is minimized.

The post-neonatal class differential has persisted since data were first available in 1911, although there is some indication that the social class gap narrowed in the 1970s (Table 17.2). As social class is determined in England

Table 17.2 Post-neonatal mortality rates by social class of father and cause.

Social class of father		Diarrhoea and enteritis (ICD 008, 009)	Pneumonia (ICD 480–6)	Other infections (ICD 000–7 010–136 320, 360 381–3 460 465 470–4 510, 511 680–6)	Congenital anomalies (ICD 740–59)	Sudden death unknown (ICD 795)	Other causes	All causes
I	1970–72	0.12	0.56	0.19	0.90	0.11	1.02	2.90
	1975–76	0.04	0.36	0.11	0.77	0.76	0.79	2.83
	1977–78	0.05	0.37	0.11	0.65	0.77	0.98	2.93
II	1970–72	0.15	0.72	0.21	1.00	0.20	1.39	3.67
	1975–76	0.09	0.45	0.18	0.77	0.60	1.05	3.14
	1977–78	0.09	0.45	0.12	0.73	0.74	0.93	3.07
III Non-manual	1970–72	0.16	0.78	0.23	1.10	0.19	1.40	3.86
	1975–76	0.10	0.56	0.19	0.76	0.81	0.97	3.39
	1977–78	0.05	0.40	0.14	0.75	0.28	1.12	3.24
III Manual	1970–72	0.34	1.31	0.41	1.20	0.28	2.07	5.61
	1975–76	0.15	0.72	0.32	0.98	0.81	1.43	4.41
	1977–78	0.11	0.49	0.27	0.93	0.94	1.24	3.96
IV	1970–72	0.44	1.69	0.52	1.30	0.35	2.36	6.66
	1975–76	0.21	0.91	0.41	1.09	1.14	1.82	5.58
	1977–78	0.14	0.69	0.24	0.93	1.24	1.43	4.67
V	1970–72	0.86	3.55	0.98	2.00	0.65	5.09	13.13
	1975–76	0.39	1.74	0.80	1.59	1.64	2.79	8.95
	1977–78	0.22	1.25	0.61	1.58	1.80	2.47	7.57

Source: Pharoah and MacFarlane 1982.

and Wales by father's occupation, which is subject to change in classification and recently by the problem of unemployment across all sections of society, there are problems in interpreting these trends, although the adverse impact of unemployment and low economic status on post-neonatal mortality has been demonstrated in a number of countries. Brenner's analysis of post-neonatal mortality in the United States suggested a statistical association between it and the unemployment rate 4 years earlier (Brenner 1973). Brenner's unconfirmed hypothesis is that it takes time for the effect of unemployment to become evident.

An early paper by Winter showed that post-neonatal mortality improved in the United Kingdom during the First World War and linked this with the employment of women and better nutrition (Winter 1977). Wilkinson (1986) has suggested that increased female earnings may have contributed to the recent narrowing of social class differentials in post-neonatal mortality. It is true to say that, while low social class as presently recorded does not *cause* high post-neonatal mortality, it is a powerful indicator of risk.

The social class differential in mortality becomes even more apparent when certain diseases are examined. Mortality from respiratory and gastro-intestinal infections is about six to nine times as high in social class V as in social class I and these two conditions account for almost all the difference observable between industrialized countries (Pharoah 1986). In contrast, the social class differential in post-neonatal mortality from congenital anomalies is only about 2:1 and international rates do not differ significantly, at least for Denmark, the United Kingdom, Norway, and Sweden (Pharoah and Morris 1979).

Sex

Throughout the post-neonatal period, as throughout the first year of life, sex is a powerful risk factor. In all European countries the level of infant mortality among males is some 20 to 40 per cent higher than among females. The one exception to this is for congenital anomalies, where in the post-neonatal period more girls die. Certain malformations are more common in girls than in boys—for example, there is a higher incidence of spina bifida in girls, particularly marked in the Republic of Ireland (Kaminksi and Blondel 1985).

Low birthweight

In the post-neonatal period, low birthweight infants remain at increased risk of death. However, post-neonatal mortality is not as closely related as neonatal mortality to birthweight (McCormick 1985). Low birthweight infants are five times more likely to die later in the first years and account for

20 per cent of all post-neonatal deaths (Shapiro *et al.* 1980). Some infants who would formerly have died within the first week of life are now surviving into the post-neonatal period. As suggested by earlier reports Shapiro *et al.* 1968; Pharoah and Morris 1979) the impact of birthweight on post-neonatal mortality is affected by socio-economic factors (Shah and Abbey 1971).

Age of mothers and parity

Infants of young mothers, particularly when combined with high parity in the latter, are at increased risk of post-neonatal death (Shah and Abbey 1971), but, again, this increase is less than for perinatal or neonatal death (Office of Population, Censuses and Survey 1982).

Causes of post-neonatal mortality

Throughout this century the main factor in the falling post-neonatal mortality rate has been the gradual decline in deaths from infections, particularly gastrointestinal (diarrhoea and enteritis) and respiratory (influenza, bronchitis, and pneumonia) infections. Countries with the lowest post-neonatal mortality rates show few such deaths, although mortality associated with disease of the respiratory system, infective and parasitic diseases, and symptoms and ill-defined conditions varies widely between countries (Shapiro 1976).

The distribution of the main causes of post-neonatal death in Europe is shown in Table 17.3. Rates of post-neonatal deaths associated with congenital anomalies in the EEC countries in 1980 contributed some 25 to 30 per cent of all deaths, and represented the principal cause of death during this period in Italy, Belgium, and Greece. Respiratory disease is responsible for a large number of deaths, particularly in the Republic of Ireland (46 per cent) and to a lesser extent in the United Kingdom and Greece. Infections and parasitic disease are of minor importance except in Greece and Italy where they represent 9 to 15 per cent of deaths. Mortality from accidents varies from country to country, ranging from around 22 per cent in Belgium to 6 per cent in the United Kingdom. In England the accident rate has fallen considerably since 1965 (about 5 per cent of deaths in 1980) while there has been a significant increase in Belgium, France, and Greece in the same period. In Belgium the rate now stands at over 20 per cent of post-neonatal deaths. These differences in part reflect differences in classification of suffocation or obstruction as causes of death recorded as accidents. Certain confusions and dangers exist, therefore, in comparing data in the respective countries. If deaths from suffocation or obstruction are excluded,

Table 17.3 Distribution of main causes of post-neonatal deaths (%) in EEC countries in 1980.

Cause		FRG	France	Italy[a]	Netherlands[b]	Belgium[a]	UK	Ireland[a]	Denmark	Greece
790–779	Certain conditions originating in the perinatal period	10	8	12	6	3	4	2[c]	5[c]	0
740–759	Congenital anomalies	25	22	32	31	30	20	37	22	41
780–790	Signs, symptoms, and ill-defined conditions	24	29	4	34	18	32	0[d]	39	2[c]
460–519	Diseases of the respiratory system	10	5	—	4	11	24	46	12[c]	17
001–139	Infections and parasitic illnesses	6	5	12	3	7	4	8[c]	3[c]	9
001–799	Other illnesses	11	13	—	—	11	12	—	9[c]	16
E800–E999	Accidents	15	20	4	—	22	6	—	10[c]	15
001–E99	All causes	100	100	100	100	100	100	100	100	100

[a]Last year available: 1978.
[b]Last year available: 1979.
[c]Number of deaths less than 15.
[d]This figure is not in agreement with Republic of Ireland Vital Statistics 1980.

Source: Adapted from Table in *Principales causes de mortalité infantile* Chap IV. Beatric Blondel, Monique Kaminski et Pierre Darchy. In: Kaminski, M.H., Bouriver-Colle, E., Blondel, B. 1985 Mortalité des jeunes dans les pays de la Communauté europeene (de la naissance à 24 ans) Paris, Coedition Doin/INSERM.

there is little variation between countries in death rates as a result of accidents (Blondel et al. 1985).

Sudden infant death syndrome

Between 1960 and 1980 in most of the EEC countries there has been a large increase in post-neonatal deaths recorded as 'sudden death cause unknown' (International Classification of Diseases (ICD) 795 Eighth revision). This increase is particularly striking as infant mortality has decreased for all other causes. In 1980 the proportion of deaths caused by the sudden infant death syndrome in the Federal German Republic, France, the Netherlands, the United Kingdom, Ireland, and Denmark was 8 to 20 per cent of all infant deaths, but as much as 20 to 40 per cent of post-neonatal deaths. According to one published analysis (Kaminski and Blondel 1985), the rate of sudden infant death was virtually zero in Italy and in Greece (Table 17.4). This is highly unlikely to be the case and probably results from difference in recording causes of death in individual countries.

Table 17.4 Mortality from sudden infant death syndrome in EEC countries in 1980.

Country	Rates per 100 000 live births		Sudden infant deaths as percentage of all causes of infant deaths	
	M	F	M	F
FRG[a]	121	94	9	8
France[a]	130	74	11	9
Italy[b]	0	0	0	0
Netherlands[a]	118	66	12	9
Belgium[b,c]	38	12	3	1
United Kingdom[a]	180	125	13	12
Republic of Ireland[d]	181	205	15	20
Denmark[b]	140	100	15	13
Greece[e]	18	10	1	1

[a] 9th revision, code 798.
[b] 8th revision, code 795.
[c] Last year available 1978.
[d] Republic of Ireland Vital Statistics 1980.
[e] Assembled from the category 'Symptoms, signs, and ill-defined conditions' (780–799).
Source: As Table 17.3 (Chapter V).

The increase in sudden infant deaths has not been continuous, but striking changes have followed as interest in this condition has grown in the last 20 years in certain countries, very notably the United Kingdom. It has gained respectability internationally since 1979 when it was entered in the World Health Organization's International Classification of Diseases. It is probable that there has not been a true increase in the incidence of 'sudden deaths', any increase being a consequence of change in the diagnosis given on the death certificate (Gardner 1982). These deaths, which are often referred to as 'cot deaths', would probably in the past have been attributed to, for example, acute respiratory or gastrointestinal infection. Since 1971 when they were accepted by the Registrar General as natural registrable causes of death in the United Kingdom, they are more likely to be certified as 'sudden death cause unknown'. This change in certification appears to be more marked in social classes I and II (Adelstein et al. 1982) than in similar deaths in families with fathers in manual occupations.

Sudden unexpected death has been recognized since biblical times. The most famous case was reported in the Old Testament—'this woman's child died in the night; because she overlaid it' (*1 Kings* Chapter 3, verse 19). Overlaying by an adult was the usually attributed cause of these deaths throughout the centuries (Paré 1841). In the 1890s Templeman reviewed 258 cases of alleged asphyxiated infants and concluded that overlaying was the main cause of death (Templeman 1891). During the nineteenth century, an enlarged thymus gland was often reported to be the cause (Paultauf 1889), and this theory gained currency for several decades.

A standardized international terminology was agreed at a Seattle Conference in 1969 that cot death was 'the sudden death of any infant which is unexpected by history and in which a thorough post-mortem fails to demonstrate an adequate cause of death'. This definition serves to focus research, but it is a definition of *exclusion* and raises several questions, not least among them what is an 'adequate' post-mortem and who decides the historical antecedents to the death.

Characteristics of the condition identified include a higher winter incidence, death occurring particularly during the seasonal increase in respiratory disease; a male preponderance; a higher incidence in cities than in rural areas; a characteristic age distribution with three-quarters of the cases occurring between 4 weeks and 6 months and few outside these limits; an increased incidence in twins (Gardner and Carpenter 1974); in babies of low birthweight (Protestas et al. 1973); among offspring of young parents who have several children (Steele and Langworth 1966); in poor living conditions; and in bottle-fed babies (Carpenter and Shaddick 1965). Most fatalities seem to occur during the night with the babies being found dead in the morning (Froggatt et al. 1971). Many of the affected infants had a history of mild illness, especially of the respiratory tract and to a lesser degree of the gastrointestinal tract, during the last week or two of life (Cameron and Watson 1975). Most recent reports have highlighted non-specific behavioural symptoms as being prognostic of unexpected infant death (Stanton *et al.* 1978; Watson *et al.* 1981). Many of the features described above are common to other causes of infant death, but the age distribution with a pronounced peak between 2 and 4 months is peculiar to cot death.

The precise aetiology of cot death remains obscure, but various theories have been put foward to explain the epidemiological factors in the syndrome. Among these are an inadequate immune mechanism (Gunther 1975), a hypersensitivity to cow's milk protein (Coombs and McLaughlan 1975), or house dust mites (Turner *et al.* 1975) or other antigens, an overwhelming virus infection (Scott *et al.* 1978), respiratory cause including sleep apnoea (Steinschneider 1974), obligatory infant nose breathing with obstruction (Cross 1972; Tonkin 1974), and infant botulism (Arnon *et al.* 1978).

Other studies have concentrated on sociological factors and have examined, retrospectively, health care delivery to the affected infant by parents and medical attendants to search for 'avoidable' factors (Watson *et al.* 1981; Taylor and Emery 1982). In addition, attempts have been made to establish at-risk predictive factors which make a child more likely to die from a cot death, ideally before the child is born (Carpenter *et al.* 1979) and updated after birth to include social factors (Carpenter *et al.* 1977). The original study on this, centred on Sheffield, has been used as a model in several other areas in the United Kingdom.

Interventions

One way of attempting to lower the incidence of post-neonatal mortality is by identifying at-risk groups in the population and adopting policies of positive discrimination. In the United States the improvement in post-neonatal mortality after 1965 coincided with the federal 'Great Society' legislation of the 1960s, particularly the federal programmes for the poor, such as the Children and Youth Projects. Although evaluation of the project in New York City could find no evidence that post-neonatal rates in project areas improved differentially and penetration of the at-risk child population was less than 40 per cent, infant mortality rates did fall in the project areas and eliminated the differences between areas and the city as a whole (McNamara *et al.* 1978).

The use of community nurses visiting infants at home might be related to the low mortality rates in Finland. The Finnish system places great emphasis on the Public Health nurse who has a long-term relationship with the whole family. She starts visiting, at her discretion, with the registration of the child at a Child Health Centre where each child is seen 10 to 11 times in the first year (twice by a doctor), and there are also financial incentives to bring the child for surveillance. France also has a highly organized follow-up programme for non-attenders to child health clinics, a policy which might be associated with its substantial decline in mortality.

In the United Kingdom, intervention trials involving the concentration of resources on at-risk groups in the population have been aimed at preventing deaths in the post-neonatal period, in particular cot deaths. Studies of unexpected infant deaths in Sheffield have generated a scoring system based on the measurement of certain factors at birth and again at 1 month of age (Carpenter 1983). This system has been extended to other centres (Knowelden *et al*. 1984). Infants rated as at increased risk of dying unexpectedly from 'possible preventable causes' (including sudden deaths, pneumonia, meningitis, and a few accidents, but excluding congenital abnormalities) were identified at birth and their status confirmed after a month. Special health care attention was given to babies with a high-risk score in the form of an increased number of home visits by health visitors, during which detailed attention was paid to the babies' weight gain, general health and progress, and feeding. Over the 7-year period of the intervention study the unexpected post-perinatal infant death rate fell in Sheffield from 5.2 to 1.9 per 1000 live births. A recent analysis of the factors contributing to this reduction estimated that 12 per cent was associated with a fall in the birth rate, 24 per cent with increased breast feeding, 9 per cent with changes in obstetric practice, and 15 per cent with increased care of high-risk infants. The remaining 40 per cent was attributed to other factors such as heightened awareness of the problem (Carpenter 1983). The scoring system appears to be more successful in identifying deaths in which possible preventable factors are found than the wholly unexplained deaths (Taylor *et al*. 1983).

The benefits of medical intervention to prevent sudden infant deaths using the Sheffield scoring system have been estimated by a health economist as a 'good buy' for the health services in terms of cost per quality-adjusted life years (Conference Report 1985). It was calculated that the mean cost of a death avoided would be £8000. This calculation was based on the assumption that each child scored as at-risk would receive six extra visits by a health visitor to improve infant care and identify early symptoms of illness. Using the same Sheffield data, other researchers (Roberts *et al*. 1985) have estimated that it costs £14 000 to prevent an unexpected infant death, and conclude that this is a service which can be afforded by the United Kingdom National Health Service.

However, the cost-benefit of the scoring and intervention scheme would depend on the accuracy of the predictive factors selected and on the commitment of the community health staff to extra home visiting. What is actually done by health visitors at these additional visits which prevents deaths is difficult to determine. The Sheffield multicentre study (Knowelden *et al.* 1984) found that, although the risk score distinguished between children who died and their controls, none of the centres in the study achieved high levels of sensitivity and specificity. As the score did not discriminate between those at risk of sudden unexpected death and those at risk of dying from other causes, it was not recommended that the risk-scoring system should be universally adopted.

Madeley (1985) has also pointed out that the highly significant fall in the post-neonatal mortality rate in Sheffield measured between 1968 and 1981 took place mostly in the period 1970–75—that is, it started 3 years before the introduction of the Birth Scoring System, the most significant factor at the time being the dramatic fall in the birth rate. It has been suggested that the most beneficial effect of the scheme in the long term is its function in generating up-to-date local data for educational purposes. There is a need, however, for an objective method of identifying deprived, high-risk children and communities, and it is suggested that statistical scoring systems provide this objectivity (Sunderland *et al.* 1986) and those that take account of daily clinical practice have increased the delivery of care to all children (Powell 1984). It is universally recognized (World Health Organization 1978) that risk strategy is a managerial tool for the organization of health services, in particular for mothers and children. Although the principles of health care delivery may be similar for each country, the risk score needs to be developed individually by each. Different strategies may be necessary too for different areas within countries.

Other strategies for helping to lower the incidence of unexpected post-neonatal deaths involve alerting health care professionals and parents to the preventability of many of the deaths in the post-neonatal period and, particularly, to the importance of symptoms in young children. This is especially important in countries such as Ireland and the United Kingdom where the incidence of respiratory deaths is high. The nine areas study in Southern England adopted this approach and during the period of study the rate of unexpected infant deaths fell from 5 to 2.5 per 1000 live births (Watson *et al.* 1981).

Recommendations

Various health authorities are now routinely collecting available data on infant deaths as a vehicle for monitoring, planning, and improvement of services and the education of professionals (Taylor and Emery 1982; Madeley *et al.* 1986).

Heightening professional awareness by this form of audit is an economic and readily available method of helping to improve the post-neonatal rates where there are avoidable factors. Obviously, in the case of unavoidable post-neonatal deaths, such strategies are less appropriate, and further reductions in these deaths will depend on skilled medical techniques, in particular improved screening before birth to detect anomalies and provide genetic counselling.

The most important step in the lowering of child deaths in the post-neonatal period, however, lies in the prevention of child poverty (Black Report 1982). In countries, such as Finland and France, where governments have made substantial child benefits available and there is a rigorous follow-up procedure for clinic non-attenders to increase systematically the coverage of the health of the child population, major improvements in the infant mortality rates have occurred most rapidly.

Although there is little data on the reasons for international differences in post-neonatal mortality rates, it has been suggested that these might well be attributed, at least in part, to variations in the organization and financing of child health services (Hein 1982). With present knowledge it is impossible to specify the relative contributions of socio-economic change and improvements in health services to the reduction in post-neonatal mortality in specific countries other than to observe that historically the two go hand in hand. Although the evidence is largely speculative, it seems feasible that, with increased prosperity and improved organization of child health services, the low rate of post-neonatal mortality of Holland and Denmark could be achieved by the rest of the European community by the end of the century.

References

Adelstein, A.M., McDonald Davies, I., Weatherall, J.A.C., and White, G.C. (1982). *Sudden infant deaths: social and biological factors*. Studies on Medical and Population Subjects No 45, HMSO (Her Majesty's Stationery Office), London.

Alberman, E. (1985). The needs of Special Client Groups: Children. In *Oxford textbook of public health, specific applications* (eds W.W. Holland, R. Detels, and G. Knox **4**, 325-37. Oxford University Press, Oxford.

Antonovsky, A., and Bernstein, J. (1977). Social class and infant mortality. *Soc. Sci. Med.* **11**, 453-70.

Arnon, S.S., Midura, T.F., Damus, F., Wood, R.M., and Chin, J. (1978). Intestinal infection and toxin production by clostridium botulinum as one cause of sudden infant death syndrome. *Lancet* **2**, 1277-8.

Black Report. (1982). Inequalities in health. Report of a research working group. DHSS (Department of Health and Social Security), London.

Blondel, B., Kaminski, M., and Darchy, P. (1985). Principales causes de mortalite infantile. In *La mortalite des jeunes dans les pays de la CEE: de la naissance a 24 ans* (eds M. Kaminksi, M.H. Bouvier-Colle, and B. Blondel). INSERM/Doin, Paris.

Bolander, A-M. (1984). Trends of perinatal and infant mortality in Sweden and in other Nordic countries and their association with demographic and socio-economic variables. Statistics Sweden, Stockholm, Socio-economic Differential Mortality in Industrialised Societies, World Health Organization, Geneva.

Brenner, M.H. (1973). Fetal, infant and maternal mortality during periods of economic instability. *Int. J. Health Serv.* **3**, 145-59.

Cameron, J.M. and Watson, E. (1975). Sudden death in infancy in Inner North London. *J. Pathol.* **117**, 55-61.

Carpenter, R.G. (1983). Prevention of unexpected infant death. *Lancet* **1**, 723-7.

—— (1983). Scoring to provide risk-related primary health care: evaluation and updating during use. *J. R. Stat. Soc. Series A* **146**, 1-32.

——, Gardner, A., McWeeny, P.M., and Emery, J.L. (1977). Multistage scoring system for identifying infants at risk of unexpected death. *Arch. Dis. Child.* **528**, 606-12.

——, ——, Pursall, E., McWeeny, P.M., and Emery, J.L. (1979). Identification of some infants at immediate risk of dying unexpectedly and justifying intensive study. *Lancet* **2**, 343-6.

Carpenter, R.G. and Shaddick, C.W. (1965). Role of infection, suffocation and bottle feeding in cot death. *Br. J. Prev. Soc. Med.* **19**, 1-7.

Conference Report (1985). Sudden infant death. *Lancet* **1**, 591.

Coombs, R.R.A., and McLaughlan, P. (1982). The enigma of cot death: is the modified anaphylaxis hypothesis an explanation for some cases. *Lancet* **1**, 1388-9.

Cross, K.W. (1972). Airway obstruction. Sudden and unexpected deaths in infancy (cot deaths). In *Proceedings of the Sir S. Bedson Symposium* (eds F.E. Camps and R.G. Carpenter) pp 57-66. Foundation for the Study of Infant Deaths, London.

Department of Health and Social Security (1970). *Confidential enquiry into post-neonatal deaths 1964-1966*. Report of a Public Health Medical Study, No 125. DHSS (Department of Health and Social Security), London.

Farr, W. (1868). *Registrar General's twenty fifth annual report*. London.

Froggatt, P., Lynas, M.A., and Marshall, T.K. (1971). Sudden unexpected death in infancy (cot death). *Br. J. Prev. Soc. Med.* **25**, 119-34.

Gardner, A. (1982). An attempt to identify cases of the sudden infant death syndrome (cot death) from death certificates and hence determine the incidence. In *Studies in sudden infant deaths*. Studies on Medical Population Subjects No. 45, 33-38. HMSO, London.

—— and Carpenter, R.G. (1974). Recent trends in unexpected infant deaths in England and Wales. SIDS 1974. In *Proceedings of the Francis E. Camps International Symposium on Sudden and Unexpected Deaths in Infancy*, pp. 143-6. Canadian Foundation for the Study of Infant Deaths.

Gunther, M. (1975). The neonate's immunity gap, breast feeding and cot death. *Lancet* **1**, 441-2.

Hack, M.B., Merkatz, I.R., Jones, P.I.C., and Fanaroff, A.A. (1980). Changing trends of neonatal and postneonatal deaths in very low birthweight infants. *Am. J. Obstet. Gynecol.* **137**, 797-800.

Hein, H. (1982). Secrets from Sweden. *JAMA* **247**, 986-7.

Islam, M., Rahaman, M., Aziz, K., Rahman, M., Munshi, M., and Petwari, Y. (1982). Infant mortality in rural Bangladesh: an analysis of causes during neonatal and postneonatal periods. *J. Trop. Pediat.* **28**, 294–7.

Kaminski, M., and Blondel, B. (1985). Mortalité des enfants de moins de 1 an. In *Mortalité des jeunes dans les pays de la Communauté Europeene de la naissance at 24 ans* (eds M. Kaminski, M.H. Bouvier-Colle, and B. Blondel). INSERM/Doin, Paris.

Knowelden, J., Keeling, J., and Nicholl, J.P. (1984). *A multicentre study of postneonatal mortality*. Medical care Research Unit, University of Sheffield.

Lancet (1985). Postneonatal mortality in the UK. *Lancet* **1**, 322.

Madeley, R. J. (1985). A study of postneonatal mortality in Nottingham 1974–1981. D.M. Thesis. University of Nottingham.

Madeley, R.J., Hull, D., and Holland, T. (1986). Prevention of postneonatal mortality. *Arch. Dis. Child.* **61**, 459–63.

McIllwaine, G.M., Howat, R.C.L., Dunn, F., and MacNaughton, M.C. (1979). The Scottish Perinatal Mortality Survey. *Br. Med. J.* **2**, 1103–6.

McNamara, J.J., Blumental, S., and Landers, C. (1978). Trends in infant mortality in New York City health areas served by Children and youth projects. *Bull. NY Acad. Med.* **54**, 484–98.

McCormick, M.C. (1985). The contribution of low birthweight to infant mortality and childhood morbidity. *New Engl. J. Med.* **312**, 82–90.

Mersey Region Working Party on Perinatal Mortality (1982). Confidential enquiry into perinatal deaths in the Mersey Region. *Lancet* **1**, 491–4.

Morris, J.N. (1979). *Uses of epidemiology*. Livingstone, Edinburgh.

Mutch, L., and Elbourne, E. (1983). *Archive of locally based perinatal surveys*. National Perinatal Epidemiology Unit, Oxford.

Northern Regional Health Authority (1984). *Collaborative survey of perinatal mortality report*. Newcastle upon Tyne.

Office of Population Censuses and Surveys. (1982). *Infant and perinatal mortality*. Series 84/6. HMSO (Her Majesty's Stationery Office), London.

Office of Population Censuses and Surveys. (1978). *Occupational mortality*. 1970–72. Decennial supplement. HMSO (Her Majesty's Stationery Office), London.

Paré, A. (1841). *Oeuvres completes d'Ambroise Paré*. J.R. Malgaigne (ed. J.B. Balliere) **3**, p. 658. Paris.

Paultauf, A. (1889). Uber die Beziehung der Thymus Zur plotzlichen Tod. *Wein. Klin. Wochenschr.* **2**, 877.

Pharoah, P.O.D. (1986). Perspective and patterns. In *Childhood epidemiology* (eds E.D. Alberman and C.A. Peckham). *Br. Med. Bull.* **42**, 119–26.

—— and MacFarlane, A. (1982). *Recent trends in postneonatal mortality*. Office of Population Censuses and Surveys Studies in Medical Population Subjects, SMPS No 45. HMSO, London.

—— and Morris, J.N. (1979). Postneonatal mortality. *Epidemiol. Rev.* **1**, 170–83.

Powell, J. (1984). Cot deaths—can they be prevented? *Maternity Action* **14**.

Project on preterm and small for gestational age infants in the Netherlands (1983). Unpublished report. Academish Ziekenhius, Leiden.

Prostestos, C.D., Carpenter, R.G., McWeeny, P.M., and Emery, J.L. (1973).

Obstetric and perinatal histories of children who died unexpectedly (cot deaths). *Arch. Dis. Child.* **48**, 835–41.

Roberts, C.J., Farrow, S.C., and Charny, M.C. (1985). How much can the NHS afford to spend to save a life or avoid a severe disability? *Lancet* **1**, 89–91.

Scott, D.J., Gardner, P.S., McQuillan, J., Stanton, A.M., Downham, M.A. (1978). Respiratory viruses and cot death. *Br. Med. J.* **2**, 12–13.

Second Report from the Social Services Committee. (1980). *Perinatal and neonatal mortality.* HMSO (Her Majesty's Stationery Office), London.

Shah, F.K., and Abbey, H. (1971). Effects of some factors on neonatal and postneonatal mortality: analysis by a binary variable multiple regression method. *Milbank Mem. Fund Quart.* **49**, 33–37.

Shapiro, S. (1976). A perspective of infant and fetal mortality in the developed countries 1950–1970. *World Hlth Stat. Rep.* **29**, 96–116.

——, McCormick, M.C., Starfield, B.H., Krischer, J.P., and Bross, D. (1980). Relevance of correlates of infant deaths for significant morbidity at 1 year of age. *Am. J. Obstet. Gynecol.* **136**, 363–73.

——, Schlesinger, E.R., and Nesbitt, R.E.L. (1968). *Infant, perinatal, maternal, and childhood mortality in the United States.* Harvard University Press, Cambridge, Mass.

Stanton, A.N., Downham, M.A.P.S., Oakley, J.R., Emery, J.L., and Knowleden, J. (1978). Terminal symptoms in children dying suddenly and unexpectedly at home. *Br. Med. J.* **2**, 1249–51.

Starfield, B., Shapiro, S., McCormick, M., and Bross, D. (1982). Mortality and morbidity in infants with intrauterine growth retardation. *J. Pediat.* **101**, 979–83.

Steele, R. and Langworth, J.T. (1966). The relationship of antenatal and postnatal factors to sudden unexpected deaths in infancy. *Can. Med. Assoc. J.* **94**, 1165.

Steinschneider, A. (1974). The concept of sleep apnoea as related to SIDS. In *Proceedings of the Francis E. Camps International Symposium on Sudden and Unexpected Deaths in Infancy*, pp 177–190. Canadian Foundation for the Study of Infant Deaths.

Sunderland, R., Gardner, A., and Gordon, R.R. (1986). Why did postperinatal mortality rates fall in the 1970's? *J. Epidemiol. Comm. Hlth* **40**, 228–31.

Taylor, E.M., and Emery, J.L. (1982). Two-year study of the causes of postperinatal deaths classified in terms of preventability. *Arch. Dis. Child.* **57**, 668.

——, ——, and Carpenter, R.G. (1983). Identification of children at risk of unexpected death. *Lancet* **2**, 1033–4.

Templeman, C. (1891). Two hundred and fifty eight cases of suffocation in infants. *Edinburgh Med. J.* **38**, 322–9.

Third Report from the Social Services Committee. (1984). *Perinatal and neonatal mortality report: a follow-up.* HMSO, (Her Majesty's Stationery Office), London.

Tonkin, S. (1974). Epidemiology of SIDS in Auckland, New Zealand. In *Proceedings of the Francis E. Camps International Symposium on Sudden and Expected Deaths in Infancy*, pp 169–175. Canadian Foundation for the Study of Infant Deaths.

Turner, K.J., Baldo, B.A., and Hilton, J.M. (1975). IgE antibodies to dermatophagoides pteronyssinus. *Br. Med. J.* **1**, 357–60.

Watson, E., Carpenter, R.G., and Gardner, A. (1981). An epidemiological and sociological study of unexpected death in infancy in nine areas of southern England I.

Epidemiology, II. Symptoms and patterns of Care. *Med. Sci. Law* **21**, 78–98.

Wilkinson, R.G., (1986). Income and mortality. In *Class and health* (ed. R.G. Wilkinson). Tavistock Publications, London.

Winter, J.M. (1977). The impact of the First World War on civilian health in Britain. *Econ. Hist. Rev.* 487–508.

World Health Statistics. Annual (various years). WHO (World Health Organization), Geneva.

World Health Organization Offset Publication No 39. (1978). *Risk approach for maternal and child health care*. WHO (World Health Organization), Geneva.

Wynn, A. and Wynn, M. (1974). *The right of every child to health care*. Council for Children's Welfare, London.

Section IV

Screening to reduce morbidity and mortality from cancer

18
Cervical cancer

Franco Berrino

SUMMARY

For women living within the EEC, the lifetime probability of getting an invasive cancer of the cervix uteri is about 1.5 per cent. It varies from 0.5 to 2.5 per cent among different populations. The incidence increases up to about the age of the menopause when it usually reaches a plateau. The cumulative incidence by 35 years of age is only about 1 per 1000. Conversely, most cases of cervical intraepithelial neoplasia occur by this age, but only a minority will surface as clinical illness. The incidence of cervical cancer is diminishing in almost all developed countries. Early detection and treatment of pre-invasive lesions through cytological screening have helped this trend. In England and Wales, however, mortality from cervical cancer is increasing in the youngest birth cohorts, despite these being the most extensively screened. Observational studies have provided strong evidence that the vast majority of cervical cancers (theoretically up to 90 per cent) could be prevented if all women were offered and complied with high quality cytological screening programmes. A screening programme starting at age 25 years, and with re-screening every third year, will achieve close to the maximum achievable benefit. The risks associated with cervical cancer screening are not easy to quantify. The major one is probably overtreatment, mainly hysterectomy for intraepithelial neoplasia in young women. In any case the implementation of screening programmes should be backed by quality control systems, the monitoring of efficacy and side-effects, health education, and the international standardization of diagnostic and therapeutic protocols.

Size of the problem

Cervical cancer is the most frequent cancer in women in many developing countries (Peto 1986). It was probably the second most frequent cause of cancer death in Europe up to a few decades ago, second only to stomach cancer. According to Rigoni-Stern (1841) cancer of the uterus was the leading cause of cancer death from 1760 to 1839 in Verona. Under 65 years of age it still ranked first in Italian cancer mortality statistics in 1950; it was surpassed by breast cancer only in the 1960s (Berrino 1982). At that time it was not possible to distinguish between mortality from cancer of the corpus and cancer of the cervix. It is reasonable to assume, however, that most deaths under the age of 65 years were caused by cancer of the cervix (Peto 1986). As for incidence, in the oldest European cancer registry (Denmark 1943–47) the cervix was the third most frequent cancer site, after breast and stomach (Clemmesen 1964). In the 1970s (Waterhouse *et al.* 1982), in most EEC cancer registries it ranked among the five or six most frequent cancer sites.

Within the EEC, the incidence of invasive cancer of the cervix, based on notifications to cancer registries, varies greatly, being four to five times higher in Denmark and in Northern Germany than in Spain. Table 18.1 shows the cumulative incidence rates for various age intervals in 11 EEC populations (Waterhouse *et al.* 1982); each value expresses the probability of developing invasive cancer of the cervix within the indicated age interval (conditional upon not dying from other causes). The cumulative incidence up to 35 years of age is about 1 per 1000, while the lifetime cumulative incidence (0–74 years) is about 1.5 per cent.

Table 18.1 Invasive cancer of the cervix: cumulative incidence per 1000 women, by decennial age intervals, in 11 EEC populations, 1973–77.

Cancer Registry	a	Age groups (yrs)						
		0–24	25–34	35–44	45–54	55–64	65–74	0–74
FRG, Saarland	(3)	0.17	1.4	3.6	5.0	7.9	5.7	23.8
Denmark	(4)	0.11	1.7	5.1	5.8	6.1	4.9	23.6
FRG, Hamburg	(4)	0.08	1.3	3.3	4.6	5.8	4.8	19.8
France, Bas Rhin	(3)	0.05	1.0	2.4	5.0	6.3	4.8	19.5
France, Doubs	(3)	0.00	0.3	1.1	6.1	5.6	6.0	19.2
UK, East Scotland	(5)	0.22	2.8	3.1	3.1	4.6	2.8	16.6
Italy, Varese	(6)	0.00	0.7	1.5	2.7	4.8	3.1	12.8
UK, Birmingham	(5)	0.05	1.0	1.9	3.3	3.7	2.6	12.6
UK, South Thames	(6)	0.06	0.7	1.3	2.3	2.8	2.2	9.3
Spain, Zaragoza	(8)	0.00	0.1	0.9	1.4	2.0	1.3	5.7
Spain, Navarra	(10)	0.00	0.0	0.4	1.1	1.8	1.2	4.4

[a]Rank among ICD-8 3 digit cancer sites.
Calculated from Waterhouse *et al.* (1982). Each figure in the table expresses the probability of getting the illness within the indicated age interval for a woman who enters the interval free of the illness and who survives other causes of death up to the end of the interval.

Higher lifetime rates (over 3 per cent) have been registered in South America, China, and India. Spanish rates are among the lowest in the world, at the same level as those for Israel. Among the United Kingdom Cancer Registries, Table 18.1 shows only those with the highest, the lowest, and the median cumulative rate. Overall they show intermediate values, but the rates for young women are relatively high.

Time trends

With a few exceptions, the incidence of and mortality from cervical cancer in developed countries began to decrease well before the introduction of mass screening programmes. In general, mass screening began in the 1950s in North America and in the 1960s in Europe, but a 10 to 30 per cent decrease in mortality from cancer of the uterus was already apparent in most European countries in the period 1950–60 (Peto 1986). Again the available rates refer to all parts of the uterus, but, if one assumes that endometrial cancer death rates are lower than those for the cervix and are not decreasing, then the decrease in cervix cancer mortality will be even more favourable. This 'natural' decrease of cervical cancer has presented a challenge to the interpretation of the effect of screening on the time trend of the illness.

The Scandinavian countries were the most notable exception to this decreasing trend. The Nordic Cancer Registries show that the incidence of invasive carcinoma of the cervix remained stable or increased slightly up to a few years after the introduction of mass screening. The subsequent decrease was related closely to the intensity of the organized mass screening (Hakama 1982; Hakama 1986). Another exception to the world-wide pattern of decrease in cervical cancer are young women in Britain, where two waves of increase in mortality rates can be seen. The first wave concerns women who were in their 20s at about the time of the Second World War. The second is more recent and still increasing; it concerns women who are now under 40–45 years of age (Peto 1986). An interruption of the decreasing trend occurred also in Canadian women aged 20–34 years (Canadian Task Force 1982) and in Australia. No similar increase, however, has been observed in other European countries or in the United States of America. Table 18.2 shows the age-specific mortality rates for cancer of the uterus among young women in England and Wales, France, and Italy (Decarli and La Vecchia 1984; Peto 1986; Hill in press). The increase in young British women is particularly surprising because the age-group involved includes those who have apparently been more intensively screened. The underlying changes in the causes of the disease, therefore, may be even more important. This has resulted in considerable debate on the optimal age for screening.

For a number of reasons, however, care must be taken in making

Table 18.2 Trends in uterine cancer death certification rates in young women in three EEC countries (per one million women-years).

| | Age group (yrs) | | | | | |
Time period	20–24	25–29	30–34	35–39	40–44	Country
1951–1955	1	10	30[a]	58	93	England and Wales
1956–1960	1	9	37	74[a]	119	Cervical cancer
1961–1965	1	5	18	66	134[a]	(Peto 1986)
1966–1970	2	7[a]	15	44	105	
1971–1975	3	10[a]	22[a]	38	67	
1976–1980	3	15[a]	32[a]	52[a]	59	
1981–1984	3	22[a]	42[a]	53[a]	77[a]	
1950–1953	3	16	46	93	166	France
1954–1958	2	13	43	98	165	Uterine cancer (cervix
1959–1963	2	7	33	86	157	plus corpus and
1964–1968	2	8	19	61	131	unspecified) (Hill, in
1969–1973	1	7	19	47	96	press)
1974–1978	2	7	18	43	79	
1979–1983	2	5	15	36	59	
1955–1958	3	13	46	120	195	Italy
1959–1963	4	13	36	105	156	(cervix plus corpus and
1964–1968	4	8	26	72	160	unspecified) (Decarli
1969–1973	3	8	21	53	90	1984)
1974–1978	2	7	19	41	80	

[a]Waves of increased mortality.

geographical and temporal comparisons. Cervical cancer is a disease whose definition, frequency, and perhaps also fatality have been influenced by screening. In principle, cancer registries include only new cases of invasive cervical cancer. Most registries, however, also include micro-invasive, clinically occult, carcinomas, whose incidence depends on the intensity of screening. About 10 to 15 per cent of cervical cancers are adenocarcinomas, adenosquamous carcinomas, or other minor morphological types. Their causes and their susceptibility to prevention by screening are quite different from the more frequent squamous cell carcinoma. Their relative frequency, therefore, may increase with the decreasing trend of squamous cancer. A further problem concerns the denominator for cervical cancer occurrence which is based on women-years of observation instead of uteri-years, and is therefore increasingly affected by hysterectomies for other conditions, at least at older ages. Problems concerning the quality of death certification may explain some of the patterns, but the secular trends and the international differences are probably too large to be explained by such biases.

Cervical intraepithelial neoplasia

There are much greater problems in interpreting the incidence of the so-called cervical intraepithelial neoplasia (CIN), probably an essential precursor of invasive cancer. These lesions are detectable, in practice, only through screening. The term carcinoma *in situ* (CIS) refers to lesions characterized by full-thickness replacement of the epithelium with undifferentiated neoplastic cells, but with no stromal invasion. Dysplasia refers to mild, moderate, or severe abnormalities of differentiation in a mucosa which otherwise retains some of its normal structural characteristics. The histological criteria for grading these lesions are not altogether clear. The old terminology is being progressively replaced by the terms CIN I (mild), CIN II (moderate), and CIN III (severe dysplasia or CIS). These terms suggest that at least part of these lesions may belong to a continuum, rather than being distinct entities.

The incidence of CIN is not known. Prevalence figures of CIN III vary from 1 to 5 per 1000 women. Its modal age range is 25 to 35 years, some 20 to 30 years earlier than the peak incidence of invasive cancer. Mild and moderate dysplasia are more frequent, especially in young women. Both regression and recurrence of CIN are probably common phenomena; their rates are not known, but may be of the order of 30 to 60 per cent (Canadian Task Force 1976).

In British Columbia (Canadian Task Force 1976) and in the United States (Cramer 1982), the incidence of CIS has been tentatively estimated from rescreening data of women with previous negative cytology. The results were quite consistent, showing a peak incidence of 120 per 100 000 women-years at about age 30 years. The bulk of disease extended from 20 to 50 years. It is noteworthy that this peak is over four times higher than the subsequent peak of invasive cancer. The lifetime cumulative incidence of CIS in British Columbia in 1960 was about 3 per cent—that is, 2.5 times higher than the corresponding cumulative incidence of invasive cancer in 1973–77. This suggests that about 60 per cent of CIS do not progress towards invasion.

Risk factors

No specific aetiological factor of cancer of the cervix has yet been identified. It has long been appreciated that the risk of cervical cancer increases with decreasing social class. The diminishing trend of the illness, therefore, is likely to be connected with socio-economic improvements and decreasing poverty. Poverty in turn is associated with poor housing, poor hygiene (in particular, lack of facilities for sexual hygiene), poor nutrition, dirty jobs, less uptake of health services, higher number of children, earlier age of marriage, and, perhaps, higher sexual promiscuity.

Sexual practice

This last is certainly the risk factor most consistently associated with cervical cancer. It emerges as the independent factor when other variables are controlled for. Women who had multiple sexual partners (Rotkin 1967; Terris *et al.* 1967; Cramer 1982; Brinton 1986; La Vecchia *et al.* 1986; Peters *et al.* 1986) or whose husbands have had multiple sexual partners (Buckley *et al.* 1981) have significantly elevated rates of cervical cancer. The same holds for the wives of men with penile cancer and the wives of men who had been previously married to women with cervical cancer (Smith *et al.* 1980; Brinton 1986). The risk of cervical cancer increases with the number of sexual contacts, the risk of women with five or more direct or indirect partners being 2.5 to 10 times that of women with a single partner. These findings on sexual behaviour strongly support the hypothesis of sexually transmitted infectious agent(s) (Knox 1984; Brinton 1986).

Most of the attention formerly focused on herpes virus type 2 (HSV2). The first case-control results showing a positive association between HSV2 antibodies and cervical cancer or pre-cancerous lesions aroused a great deal of interest (Cramer 1982). Further studies, however, could not confirm the results, and one prospective study showed no effect of antibodies to HSV2 on the risk of cervical abnormalities after adjustment for sexual variables (Vonka *et al.* 1984). In the last decade the advocates of a viral aetiology have concentrated on human papilloma viruses (HPV). A great deal of additional work is required, though, before their precise role is firmly documented (Koss, 1987).

Whether the HPV hypothesis will eventually be confirmed or not, the infection hypothesis relies on such a consistent pattern of observations that it is most unlikely to be dismissed. If the relationship with sexual behaviour were mediated only through a non-transmissible agent—whether physical, chemical, or otherwise biological—the risk would be associated with the sexual behaviour of females, but not to the independent behaviour of males (Knox 1984).

A number of other aetiological hypotheses have been formulated. Early age at first intercourse is associated with a fairly high risk of cervical cancer or CIN, relative risks increasing up to 4 or 5 with decreasing age (Rotkin 1967; Terris *et al.* 1967; Cramer 1982; Brinton 1986; La Vecchia *et al.* 1986; Peters *et al.* 1986). This has been interpreted as an indication of the susceptibility of the adolescent cervix to an oncogenic factor; but the effects of age at first coitus disappeared (Harris *et al.* 1980; Reves *et al*; 1985), or were substantially reduced (Brinton 1986), when social class and number of partners were controlled for.

The hypothesis of repeated obstetrical trauma has produced inconsistent findings (Cramer 1982), suggesting that multiparity was only a correlate of other risk factors.

A number of studies have found a slightly increased risk of cervical neoplasia with long-term oral contraceptive use (Vessey 1986). In some of the studies the increased risk persisted after controlling for sexual behaviour, but in this field it is always difficult to exclude all possible confounding variables. The observed effect may reflect, at least partly, a protection conferred by other types of contraception, namely barrier methods, rather than a true oncogenicity of oral contraceptives. Most studies on oral contraceptives, moreover, have focused on CIN; the observed effect, therefore, may depend also on an increased incidence of CIN resulting from the cytological surveillance of women taking oral contraceptives. The protection shown by barrier contraceptives (Cramer 1982; Peters *et al.* 1986), on the other hand, is quite compatible with the infection hypothesis.

A review of the epidemiological data shows that there is no basis as yet for scientifically based and socially acceptable primary prevention of cervical cancer. Until we can identify a specific aetiological agent, however, the improvement of sexual hygiene appears a reasonable goal of health education. Even in the absence of sound evidence of its effectiveness in preventing cervical cancer, it is an ethically acceptable intervention which will prevent other sexually transmitted diseases. Epidemiological studies on the potential effectiveness of improved hygiene are desirable. Their planning, however, requires extremely close attention to the major determinants of cervical cancer, namely sexual behaviour, social variables, and, today even more important, frequency of screening. Besides the number of sexual partners, the major risk factor so far documented, both in terms of magnitude of relative risk and of resistance to the control of social or sexual confounding, is the time interval since the last screening smear (Hakama 1986; Hakama *et al.* 1986).

Efficacy and effectiveness of screening

The efficacy of screening for cervical cancer has never been studied experimentally. The evidence of its efficacy has long been disputed. The first claim of efficacy was actually based on wrong arguments. Excellent reviews of the numerous pitfalls in screening evaluation are available (Cole and Morrison 1980; Morrison 1985). The presumption of screening efficacy, the simplicity of the procedure, coupled with the dedication of many cytologists and with the political appeal of promoting relatively cheap preventive programmes, made the practice of screening so widespread that large amounts of observational data became available for non-experimental research. Fortunately, sound evidence of the efficacy of cytological screening in preventing the occurrence of invasive cancer of the cervix could then be reached. Theoretically, about 90 per cent of invasive incidence could be prevented if all adult women were offered and complied with cervical cytology screening with optimal conditions of quality and frequency (Hakama 1986; Hakama *et al.* 1986). In practice, in Iceland, with a population compliance of 80 per cent, a fall in mortality of 80 per cent was observed between 1965 and 1982 (Larra *et al.* 1987). This fall cannot be totally attributed to screening as it may also represent changing trends in incidence and case fatality.

Screening strategies

If the basis for starting mass screening programmes was largely presumptive, the practical details such as the target age range, the frequency of screening, and the choice of personal invitations and reminders or merely opening screening centres and waiting for women to come in, were even more empirical.

In general, short intervals and wide age ranges were preferred by private or local institutions, while longer intervals and stricter age ranges were chosen where screening was organized within a national health service frame. In North America, for example, many authorities recommended, and still recommend, yearly intervals, while in Northern European countries the prescribed interval between successive negative examinations was 2–5 years. Table 18.3, which contains a summary of the recommendations of national and international agencies over the last 30 years, illustrates this controversy.

The original rule of screening every year had no scientific basis and no justification whatsoever, except, perhaps, for being easy to remember. In 1976, the Canadian Task Force for cervical cancer realized that the frequency of examination had to be decided on the basis of the available knowledge on the natural history of the pre-clinical illness, in particular on the length of the detectable pre-clinical phase (DPCP—that is, the interval between the time in which the illness first becomes detectable and the time at which symptoms arise). At that time it was appreciated that the mean length of DPCP could be of the order of a few decades. The shape of the DPCP distribution, however, was not known. It seemed reasonable, therefore, to relax the prescribed interval, within prudent limits. The Canadian Task Force decided to recommend a 3-year interval up to 35 years of age and 5 years thereafter up to the age of 60 years. The choice of a shorter interval for younger women is concerned with the priority of detecting intraepithelial lesions, whose frequency is highest in the 20s. A major drawback of this policy is that a large number of lesions will be detected that would not progress to clinical disease.

The British Society for Clinical Cytology subsequently chose an age policy that was the exact opposite. They recommended a 5-year interval with the possibility of reducing it to 3 years after the age of 35 years. Apparently they

Table 18.3 Ten official recommendations on cervical screening frequency.

Organization	Frequency
American Cancer Society, 1957	Every year
American College of Obstetricians and and Gynecologists, 1975	Every year
Canadian Task Force, Dept. Nat. Health and Welfare, 1976	Every 3 years from 18 to 35 years Every 5 years from 35 to 60 years
British Society for Clinical Cytology, 1977	Every 5 years from 25 to 35 years Every 5 or 3 years from 35 to 70 years
International Academy of Cytology, 1977	Every year
American Cancer Society, 1980	Every 3 years
American College of Obstetricians and Gynecologists, 1980	Every year
Consensus Conference, U.S. National Institutes of Health, 1981	Every 1 or 3 years
Canadian Task Force, Dept. Nat. Health and Welfare, 1982	Every year from 18 to 35 years Every 5 years from 35 to 60 years
UICC/IARC, 1986	Every 3 years from 25 to 60 years

realized that the greater problem is invasive cancer, and that it is more cost-effective to detect pre-clinical lesions at about the ages at which the incidence of invasive cancer is higher (Spriggs and Husain 1977).

More recently, the first information about the relatively beneficial effect of screening every 2–5 years on the time trend of cervical cancer in Nordic Countries became available. When, eventually, the American Cancer Society had the courage to change its policy from 1 to 3 years (American Cancer Society 1980), the American College of Obstetricians and Gynecologists took up a defensive position, strongly reaffirming the need for annual screening to prevent the risk of false-negative results. The National Cancer Institute then held a Consensus Conference which recommended regular screening every 1 or 3 years.

In 1982, the Canadian Task Force changed its policy to one of examinations once a year under the age of 35 years. This decision was based on a number of factors, ranging from a presumed greater sexual promiscuity in younger women, to the uncritical acceptance of mathematical models, to the dissatisfaction expressed by physicians with the previous recommendations.

Outcome of screening programmes

Beginning with the case-control study of Clarke and Anderson (1979) in Toronto in the late 1970s, a number of analytical studies were carried out in Switzerland (Raymond *et al.* 1984), Italy (La Vecchia *et al.* 1984; Berrino *et* al. 1986), Scotland (Macgregor et al. 1985), Iceland, Sweden, Denmark, Manitoba (Hakama et al. 1986), Colombia (Aristizabal et al. 1984), and the United States (Peters 1986), that eventually proved beyond any reasonable doubt the great preventive potential of cervical screening. All the studies that could control for sexual or social factors showed that these variables have only minor, if any, confounding effect (Clarke and Anderson 1979; La Vecchia et al. 1984; Berrino et al. 1986; Peters et al. 1986). Sexual behaviour did not prove to be associated with compliance and the association of some social determinants with cervical cancer tends to vanish when screening itself is controlled for (Berrino et al. 1986). Through international co-operation (IARC), the results of most of these studies were amalgamated. This allowed a quantitative interpretation of the protection achievable with different screening intervals and age ranges (Hakama et al. 1986). Table 18.4 shows the risk of invasive cancer, relative to unscreened women, by time interval since the last negative screening (among women with at least two negative smears). These relative risk figures can be interpreted also as cumulative frequencies of the detectable pre-clinical phase length distribution: only about 8 per cent of the invasive cases behave as if they had a detectable pre-clinical phase lasting less than 2 years, 13 per cent a detectable pre-clinical phase less than 3 years, and so on.

Table 18.5 shows the expected efficacy of screening with different intervals at different ages. The potential preventive effects in Table 18.5 are, perhaps over-optimistic. They are calculated from the results summarized in Table 18.4, based on the follow-up of asymptomatic women with negative tests. A negative test *per se*, however, does not confer protection. The low incidence after negative screening is determined by the removal from observation

Table 18.4 Risk of cervical cancer among women with at least two negative screening tests (and no positive ones), by interval since the last negative examination.

Months since last negative smear	Relative risk (number of cases in parentheses)
0–11	0.07 (25)
12–23	0.08 (23)
24–35	0.13 (25)
36–47	0.19 (30)
48–59	0.36 (30)
60–71	0.28 (16)
72–119	0.63 (6)
120+	1.25 (7)
Never screened	1.00

Source: modified from Hakama (1986).

Table 18.5 Effect of different screening policies assuming Western European type incidence rates.

Screening schedule	Cumulative rate 20–64 per 100 000	Percentage reduction in rate	Number of tests	Number of cases prevented per 100 000 tests
1. No screening	1575			
2. Screening every 5 years 20–64	258.6	83.6	9	146.3
2a. Screening every 5 years 25–64	287.8	81.7	8	160.9
2b. Screening every 5 years 35–64	480.9	69.5	6	182.4
2c. Screening every year 20–34 then every 5 years 35–64	233.4	85.2	21	63.9
2d. Screening age 25, 26, 30 then every 5 years	275.4	82.6	9	144.4
3. Screening every 3 years 20–64	138.9	91.2	15	95.7
3a. Screening every 3 years 25–64	161.8	89.7	13	108.7
3b. Screening every 3 years 35–64	354.9	77.5	10	122.0
3c. Screening every year 20–34 then every 5 years 35–64	132.0	91.6	25	59.4
3d. Screening age 25, 26, 29 then every 3 years	157.4	90.0	14	101.3
4. Screening every year, 20–64	105.2	93.3	45	32.7

Source: Hakama (1986).

(through detection by screening of pre-clinical lesions) of women destined to develop clinical cancer. The preventive potential shown in Tables 18.4 and 18.5, therefore, represents the true preventive effect only if all pre-clinical cases detected at screening are successfully treated. It is well known, however, that a minority of cervical neoplasia detected by screening will not be cured, but under optimal conditions of clinical management of positive women, the frequency of treatment failures would be so low that the figures in Table 18.4 and 18.5 can be considered realistic.

Problems in maximizing effectiveness in populations

The issue of why some screening programmes fail to control the disease has been reviewed by Chamberlain (1986). She identified five main reasons of failure: 'Firstly, the programme may fail to reach the entire population at risk; secondly the test may fail to detect all cases; thirdly the frequency with which the test is repeated may miss some fast-growing cases; fourthly there may be a failure to act upon abnormalities detected by screening; and lastly the treatment may not cure all cases'.

Population compliance

The failure to reach the women in the age ranges at which the incidence of cervical cancer is highest and women who belong to lower socio-economic groups, has been considered by the classical studies of Wakefield and Sanson (1966) and has been repeatedly confirmed in different populations (Berrino 1979; Chamberlain 1986). In England and Wales, for example, only 46 per cent of smears are taken from women aged over 35 years, among whom 85 per cent of invasive cancers occur. In Switzerland over 50 per cent of cases occur among women over 60 years, who are much less frequently screened than younger ones (Riotton 1985). The age differences in compliance are even greater when the overall compliance is low. The difference persists with personal invitation and re-invitation of non-compliant women. A call–recall mechanism, however, is essential to increase the compliance of the lower socio-economic groups. The low compliance of high-risk women is mainly the result of lack of motivation and of knowledge of the service (Berrino 1979). Hence invitations to screening need to be backed up by appropriate education. The continuing search for better strategies of information to increase compliance is the highest research priority today.

The compliance of the target population is a component of the overall sensitivity of the screening programme (Hakama 1984, 1986; Hakama *et al.* 1986). Further components are the sensitivity of the test, the frequency of examination with respect to the duration of the detectable pre-clinical phase, and the diagnostic confirmation of positive results. This last component, in turn, depends on the accurate identification of screened subjects, on the compliance of positive cases with diagnostic procedures, and on the reliability of such procedures.

Test sensitivity

The basic way to increase the sensitivity is the quality control of the performance of both the test—that is, proper collection and reading of smears—and the programme. Cervical screening consists of the collection of cells from the surface of the cervix and of the external os. Smears prepared from cells exfoliated from the cervix reflect the underlying histology. Cells exfoliated from abnormal epithelium show nuclei that are abnormal in their staining properties, size, and shape. Standards for proper collection of smears and for the operation of cytopathology laboratories have been published (Canadian Task Force 1976). Guidelines for the quality control of the overall performance of screening programmes and for information requirements are also available (Draper 1986). It is sufficient here to remember the recommendation of the second Canadian Task Force report on cervical cancer screening: 'it is inappropriate to establish the recommended screening frequencies as formal policy in the absence of established systems to monitor the frequencies and to issue reminders to attend at the recommended intervals in the absence of proper quality control systems' (Canadian Task Force 1982).

A method of minimizing the risk of false-negative results which has been frequently recommended (Canadian Task Force 1976; American Cancer Society 1980), is to repeat screening at a short interval after the first screen. This procedure, however, may be challenged on grounds of cost-effectiveness. Assuming that 80 per cent of the eligible population is screened with a 75 per cent sensitivity, 60 per cent of the prevalent pre-clinical cases will be detected at first screening. Re-screening the same women within a short interval would detect 75 per cent of the false-negatives from the first test. The alternative strategies to detect the remaining 40 per cent of prevalent cases are to re-screen the 80 per cent of the total population who attended and were negative to detect the false negatives or to attempt to screen the 20 per cent who were non-attenders. In this model both these groups would contain the same *number* of cases (equivalent to 20 per cent of the total prevalent pre-clinical cases), but given the larger size of the re-screened population, the detection of each false-negative case in that group would require four times as many examinations as the detection of each case in the originally unscreened group. The same economic investment would be justified to increase the sensitivity of the test to 94 per cent (= 75/80). If the sensitivity of the test were already about 94 per cent it would be reasonable to invest up to 16 times more to reach never screened women than to re-screen negative ones at very short intervals. Obviously the lower the risk of the population, the greater the waste involved in short-term re-examinations. There would be almost no advantage in re-screening, at age 19 years, a girl first screened at 18. On the contrary, if resources were still available after having tried to reach never screened women, it might be worthwhile re-screening at age 41 years a woman screened for the first time at 40 years.

Optimal age for screening

The advocates of frequent screening at younger ages argue that 'it is the younger women who have the highest rates of positive smears and of premalignant disease of the cervix which is, after all, the stage which we wish to detect' (Soutter et al. 1984). It may help here to remember that what we are truly interested in is not the sensitivity of the programme towards any lesion that would be diagnosed histologically as a CIN, but only towards the fraction of these lesions that, if left untreated, would surface as clinically invasive cancer. Theoretically, therefore, the best way to increase cost-effectiveness and to reduce overtreatment would be to detect CIN just before the onset of invasive cancer. This goal will be better approached by a policy that gives priority to reaching never screened older women than to re-screen younger ones.

The increasing mortality rates in young women, where they exist, do not imply that young women should be screened more frequently. It implies, on the contrary, that the reasons for and characteristics of such an increase must be understood. Were these young women who died from cervical cancer screened and, if so, with what frequency? What kind of cancer was it and would the usual cytological screening be the best solution? Is there any evidence that the detectable pre-clinical phase is shorter than for older women? If not, there would be no biological reason to increase frequency of screening.

Ethical considerations

The issue of overtreatment has not been emphasized in published reports. The days of hysterectomy and even, in some instances, radiotherapy, for CIN have mostly given way to less radical treatments (Chamberlain 1986). There is still some anecdotal evidence, however, that a number of young women are undergoing hysterectomy for intraepithelial lesions. This has been arguably the worst side-effect of cervical cancer prevention. Overtreatment for non-neoplastic conditions, however, should be prevented too. One must remember that the ethical implications of screening healthy people are more serious than those of treating sick people who require assistance. The monitoring of screening programmes must also consider these ethical issues, and the health education of the population must be coupled with adequate information given to doctors and other health professionals through the dissemination of agreed treatment protocols.

Recommendations

The 1986 UICC recommendation, the first based on sound analytical data, provides the basis for appropriate action. This comprises a screening programme starting at age 25 years and with re-screening every third year which will achieve close to the maximum possible reduction in the incidence of invasive cancer of the cervix (Hakama 1986). More frequent screening would result in considerably higher costs and in only a marginal effect on the risk. Low compliance is the reason why the protection actually conferred by screening programmes up to now has been less than effective. Major efforts should be made to decrease the proportion of never screened women and also to increase the sensitivity of the test itself. Available evidence does not suggest that women of different ages need differential screening frequencies, but further monitoring of ongoing programmes is recommended. To increase cost-effectiveness and to reduce overtreatment, priority should be given to reaching never screened older women rather than to re-screening younger ones. And to counteract the increasing mortality rates in young women, research is required into possibilities for primary prevention.

References

American Cancer Society (1980). Guidelines for the cancer-related checkup: recommendations and rationale. *Cancer J.* **30**, 193–240.

Aristizabal, N., Cuella, C., Correa, P., Conazos, T., and Haenszel, W. (1984). The impact of vaginal cytology on cervical cancer risk in Cali, Columbia. *Int. J. Cancer.* **34**, 5–9.

Berrino, F. (1982). Epidemiologia e prevenzione del cancro in Italia. *Practitioner* (Italian edition) **49**, 32–46.

—— , Chiappa, L., Oliverio, S., Todeschin, P., Turolla E., and Vegetti, P. (1979). Study of women who did not respond to screening for cervical cancer. *Tumori* **65**, 143–55.

—— , Gatta, G., D'Alto, M., Crosignani, P., and Riboli, E. (1986). Efficacy of screening in preventing invasive cervical cancer. A case-control study carried out in Milan, Italy. In *Screening for cancer of the uterine cervix* (eds M. Hakama, A.B. Miller, and N.E. Day). IARC Scientific Publications No. 76. IARC, Lyon.

Brinton, L.A. (1986). Current epidemiological studies—emerging hypotheses. In *Viral etiology of cervical cancer* (eds R. Peto and H. Zur Hausen). Banbury Report No 21. Cold Spring Harbor Laboratory.

Buckley, J.D., Harris, R.W.C., Doll, R., Vessey, M.P., and Williams, P.T. (1981). Case-control study of the husbands of women with dysplasia or carcinoma of the cervix uteri. *Lancet* **2**, 1010–4.

Canadian Task Force on Screening. (1976). Cervical cancer screening programs. *Can. Med. Assoc. J.* **114**, 1003–33.

—— (1982). Cervical cancer screening programs: summary of the 1982 Canadian task force report. *Can. Med. Assoc. J.* **127**, 581-2.

Chamberlain, J. (1986). Reasons why some screening programmes fail to control cervical cancer. In *Screening for cancer of the uterine cervix* (eds M. Hakama, A.B. Miller, and N.R. Day). IARC Scientific Publication No. 76. IARC, Lyon.

Clarke, E.A. and Anderson, T.W. (1979). Does screening by 'PAP' smears help prevent cervical cancer? A case control study. *Lancet* **2**, 1-4.

Clemmesen, J. (1964). *Statistical studies in the aetiology of malignant neoplasms*. Munksgaard, Copenhagen.

Cole, P. and Morrison, A.S. (1980). Basic issues in population screening for cancer. *J. Nat. Cancer Inst.* **64**, 1253-72.

Cramer, D.W. (1982). Uterine cervix. In *Cancer epidemiology and prevention* (eds D. Schottenfield and J.F. Fraumeni). Saunders, Philadelphia.

Decarli, A. and La Vecchia, C. (1984). Cancer mortality in Italy 1955-78. *Tumori* **70**, Supplement.

Draper, G.J. (1986). Screening for cancer of the cervix. Information requirement for screening programmes. In *Screening for cancer of the uterine cervix* (eds M. Hakama, A.B. Miller, and N.E. Day). IARC Scientific Publication No. 76. IARC, Lyon.

Hakama, M. (1982). Trends in the incidence of cervical cancer in the Nordic countries. In *Trends in cancer incidence* (ed K. Magnus). Hemisphere, Washington.

—— (1984). Selective screening by risk groups. In *Screening for cancer. General principles on evaluation of screening for cancer for lung, bladder and oral cancer* (eds P.C. Prorok and A.B. Miller). UICC Technical Report Series, 78. UICC, Geneva.

—— (1986). Efficacy of screening for cervical cancer. In *Viral etiology of cervical cancer* (eds R. Peto and H. Zur Hausen). Banbury Report No. 21. Cold Spring Harbor Laboratory.

——, Miller, A.B., and Day N.E. (eds). (1986). *Screening for cancer of the uterine cervix*. IARC Scientific Publication No. 76. IARC, Lyon.

Harris, R.W.C., Brinton, L.A., Cowdell, R.H., Skegg, D.C.G., Smith, P.G., Vessey, M.P., and Doll, R. (1980). Characteristics of women with dysplasia or carcinoma *in situ* of the cervix. *Br. J. Cancer* **42**, 359-69.

Hill, C., Benhamou, E., and Flamant, R. *Evolution de la mortalité par cancer en France*. In press. INSERM, Paris.

Knox, E.G. (1984). Epidemic cancer of the cervix? In *Hormones and sexual factors in human cancer aetiology*. (eds. J.P. Wolff and J.S. Scott). Elsevier.

Koss, L.G. (1987). Cytologic and histologic manifestations of human papillomavirus infection of the female genital tract and their clinical significance. *Cancer* **60**, 1942-50.

Larra, E., Day, N.E., and Hakama, M. (1987). Trends in mortality from cervical cancer in the Nordic countries: association with organized screening programmes. *Lancet* **1**, 1247-9.

La Vecchia, C., Franceschi, S., Decarli, A., Fasoli, M., Gentile, A., Parazzini, F., and Regallo, M. (1986). Sexual factors, venereal diseases, and the risk of intra-epithelial and invasive cervical neoplasia. *Cancer* **58**, 935-41.

——, ——, ——, ——, ——, and Tognoni, G. (1984). 'Pap' smear and the risk of cervical neoplasia: quantitative estimates from a case-control study. *Lancet* **2**, 779-782.

Macgregor, J.E., Moss, S.M., Parkin, D.M., and Day, N.E. (1985). A case-control study of cervical cancer screening in north east Scotland. *Br. Med. J.* **290**, 1543–48.
Morrison, A.S. (1985). *Screening in chronic disease.* Oxford University Press, New York.
Peters, R.K., Thomas, D., Hagan, D.G., Mack, T.M., and Henderson B.E. (1986). Risk factors for invasive cervical cancer among Latinas and non-Latinas in Los Angeles County. *J. Nat. Cancer Inst.* **77**, 1063–1077.
Peto, R. (1986). Introduction: Geographic patterns and trends. In *Viral etiology of cervical cancer* (eds R. Peto and H. Zur Hausen). Banbury Report No 21. Cold Spring Harbor Laboratory.
Raymond, L., Obrandovic, M., and Riotton, G. (1984). Une étude cas-témoins pour l'évaluation du dépistage cytologique du cancer du col uterin. *Rev. Epidemiol. Santé Publ.* **32**, 10–15.
Reves, W.C., Brinton, L.A., Brenes, M.M., Quiroz, E., Rawls, W.E., and DeBritton, R.C. (1985). Case-control study of cervical cancer in Herrera Province, Republic of Panama. *Int. J. Cancer.* **36**, 55–60.
Rigoni-Stern (1841). Fatti statistici relativi alle malattie cancerose che servirono di base alle poche cose dette dal dott. Rigoni-Stern il di' 23 Settembre alla Sottosezione di chirurgia del IV Congresso degli scienziati italiani. *G. Servire Prog. Patol. Ter.* **2**, 507–17.
Riotton, G. (1985). Cancer of the cervix: death by incompetence *Lancet* **2**, 603–4.
Rotkin, I.D. (1967). Sexual characteristics of a cervical cancer population. *Am. J. Publ. Hlth* **57**, 815–29.
Smith, P.G., Kinlen, L.J., White, G.C., Adelstein, A.M., and Fox, A.J. (1980). Mortality of wives of men dying with cancer of the penis. *Br. J. Cancer.* **41**, 422–8.
Soutter, W.P., Brough, A.K., and Monaghan, J.M. (1984). Cervical screening for younger women. *Lancet* **2**, 745.
Spriggs, A.I. and Husain, A.N. (1977) Cervical smears. *Br. Med. J.* **1**, 1516–18.
Terris, M., Wilson, F., Smith, H., Sprung, E., and Nelson, J.H. (1967). The relationships of coitus to carcinoma of the cervix. *Am. J. Publ. Hlth* **57**, 840–7.
Vessey, M.P. (1986). Epidemiology of cervical cancer: role of hormonal factors, cigarette smoking and occupation. In *Viral etiology of cervical cancer* (eds R. Peto and H. Zur Hausen). Banbury Report No 21. Cold Spring Harbor Laboratory.
Vonka, V., Kanka, J., Jelinek, J., Subrt, I., Suchánek, A., Havránková, A., Vachal, M., Hirsch, I., Domorázková, E., Závadová, H., Richterová, V., Náprstková, J., Dvoráková, V., and Svoboda, B. (1984). Prospective study on the relationship between cervical neoplasia and herpes simplex type 2 virus. Epidemiological characteristics, and II. Herpes simplex type 2 antibody presence in sera taken at enrollment. *Int. J. Cancer.* **33**, 49, and **61**.
Wakefield, J. and Sansom, C.D. (1966). Profile of a population of women who have undergone a cervical smear examination *Med. Officer* **116**, 145.
Waterhouse, J., Muir, C., Shanmugaratnam, K., and Powell, J. (eds) (1982). *Cancer incidence in five continents.* Vol. IV. IARC Scientific Publications No 42. IARC, Lyon.

19
Breast cancer
Christopher D. Frost

SUMMARY

Screening can reduce mortality from breast cancer. The evidence indicates that a population-based screening programme offering breast examinations on a regular basis to women aged between 50 and 70 years will reduce mortality from the disease in that age group by around 40 per cent. If such screening programmes were introduced in all EEC countries about 15 000 deaths from the disease might be prevented every year. Breast examination by mammography alone is sufficient; a single oblique view of the breast is satisfactory, but either a cranio-caudal or latero-medial view may be taken as well. The ideal interval between successive mammographic examinations relative to the cost of screening is not yet known, but can be most easily determined by incorporating randomization of this interval into the design of screening programmes. Screening should be run on a regional basis, each region under the jurisdiction of a director, skilled in the theory and practice of screening procedures. Screening should be population-based with women individually invited to screening centres that would refer those with positive results to hospital for diagnosis and treatment.

Defining the problem

Breast cancer is the most common cancer in women in Western Europe. As Table 19.1 shows, in the 12 EEC countries alone, 60 000 women die of the disease every year (WHO 1986). This is 18 per cent of the total deaths from cancer and 4 per cent of total deaths among women in the EEC.

Despite advances made in treatment of the disease, notably with the antioestrogen agent tamoxifen and long-term cytotoxic chemotherapy, mortality rates from the disease are still increasing in all EEC countries as they have been over the past 40 years (Kurihara *et al.* 1985) (Figure 19.1).

Table 19.1 Breast cancer deaths in the EEC.

Country	Year	Total deaths from breast cancer
FRG	1985	13 701
UK: England and Wales	1984	13 310
France	1984	9 269
Italy	1981	9 042
Spain	1980	3 629
The Netherlands	1984	2 898
Belgium	1984	2 269
UK: Scotland	1985	1 252
Denmark	1984	1 240
Portugal	1985	1 236
Greece	1984	1 188
Ireland	1983	536
UK: Northern Ireland	1985	308
Luxembourg	1985	95
Total		59 973

Source: *World Health Statistics Annual* (1986).

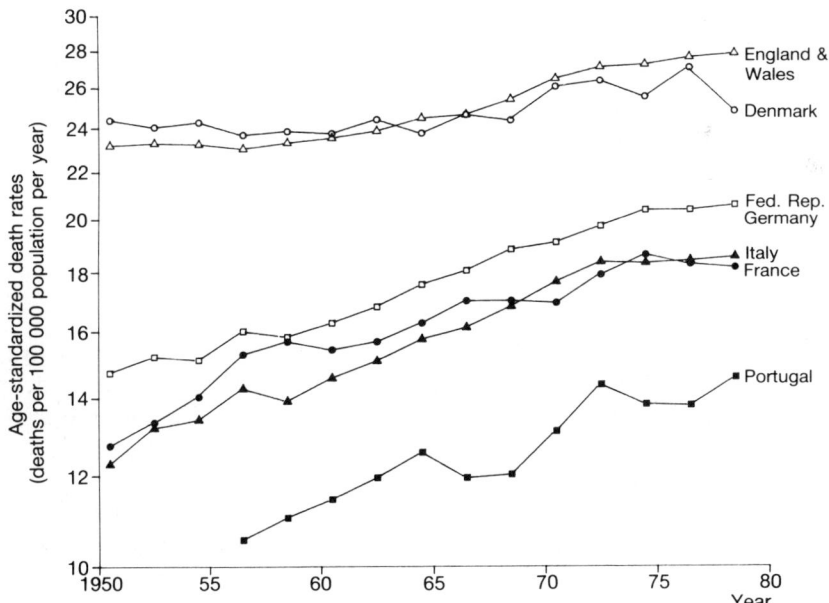

Fig. 19.1 Breast cancer mortality in Europe. (Source: Kurihara *et al.* 1985.)

Table 19.2 Age-standardized mortality rates from breast cancer.

Country	Year	Age-standardized mortality rate from breast cancer (Standard world population) Deaths per 100 000 population
EEC Countries		
Luxembourg	1985	29.9
UK: England and Wales	1984	29.3
UK: Northern Ireland	1985	27.6
UK: Scotland	1985	27.3
Denmark	1984	27.1
Belgium	1984	25.8
The Netherlands	1984	25.5
Ireland	1983	25.4
FRG	1985	22.4
Italy	1981	19.4
France	1984	19.2
Portugal	1985	16.6
Greece	1984	15.4
Spain	1980	13.8
International comparisons		
Israel	1984	23.9
United States of America	1983	22.1
Australia	1984	20.3
Japan	1985	5.8
Peru	1982	4.9

Source: *World Health Statistics Annual* (1986).

Size of the problem

International variation: mortality, incidence, and survival

Western Europe has the highest mortality rates from breast cancer in the world. Rates are also high in America, Canada, Australia, New Zealand, and Israel; they are intermediate in Eastern and Southern Europe; and low in Africa and Asia. Japanese mortality rates are about one-fifth of those in the United Kingdom (WHO 1986) (Table 19.2).

Within Europe, mortality rates increase from south to north and from east to west, the highest rates being accordingly in the United Kingdom, Luxembourg, The Netherlands, Denmark, Belgium, and Ireland. In all the EEC countries mortality rates from the disease have been increasing over the past 30 or 40 years. Mortality rates have increased to a different extent in different countries. Those countries in which the mortality rate was relatively low in 1950 have seen the greatest increases, and this suggests that rates may be tending towards some standard 'European' rate. In Denmark (highest rate in 1950), the age-standardized mortality rate has risen by only 2 per cent between 1950–51 and 1978–79 whereas those in France and Italy have increased by 42 and 51 per cent, respectively, over the same period (Kurihara et al. 1985) (Figure 19.1).

It is surprising that the mortality rate in many European countries is higher than that in the United States where the incidence of breast cancer appears to be higher (Waterhouse et al. 1982). Survival times in Britain (CRC 1982) and the United States (US Department of Health, Education and Welfare 1976) appear similar (5-year survival rate: 57 per cent in England and Wales for cases registered in 1971–73; 58 per cent among whites and 72 per cent among blacks in the United States for cases registered in 1967–73), which tends to suggest that this apparent discrepancy between incidence and mortality rates in Europe and the United States is the result mainly of differences in cancer registration and death certification practices between the countries.

Risk factors

Breast cancer screening must be regarded as a long-term strategy, starting with the selection of women at sufficiently high risk to justify a breast examination and then repeating that examination at intervals. Screening cannot confer lifetime protection. It can only indicate the probable occurrence or absence of the disease during the few years after an examination. This makes age the most important risk factor since breast cancer is primarily a disease of older women. In all EEC countries only 1–2 per cent of total breast cancer deaths occur in women under the age of 35 years (WHO 1986). In those countries where mortality rates are relatively low such as Spain, Portugal, and Greece, a higher proportion of deaths occur in younger women than in other countries where rates are higher. Twelve per cent of deaths from the disease in Spain occur in women under the age of 45 years compared with 6 per cent in the United Kingdom (Figure 19.2).

The first stage of any screening procedure must, therefore be, to identify women above a certain age. All screening programmes have employed a lower age limit of between 35 and 50 years.

The international variation in breast cancer rates in Europe is not big enough to justify restricting screening to EEC countries with the highest rates. Neither are other demographic factors (variation of risk with race, social class, and between urban and rural populations) of sufficient discriminatory power to be used as screening enquiries.

A woman who has already had breast cancer has a four to five-fold increased chance of developing a second breast cancer (Schoenberg 1977).

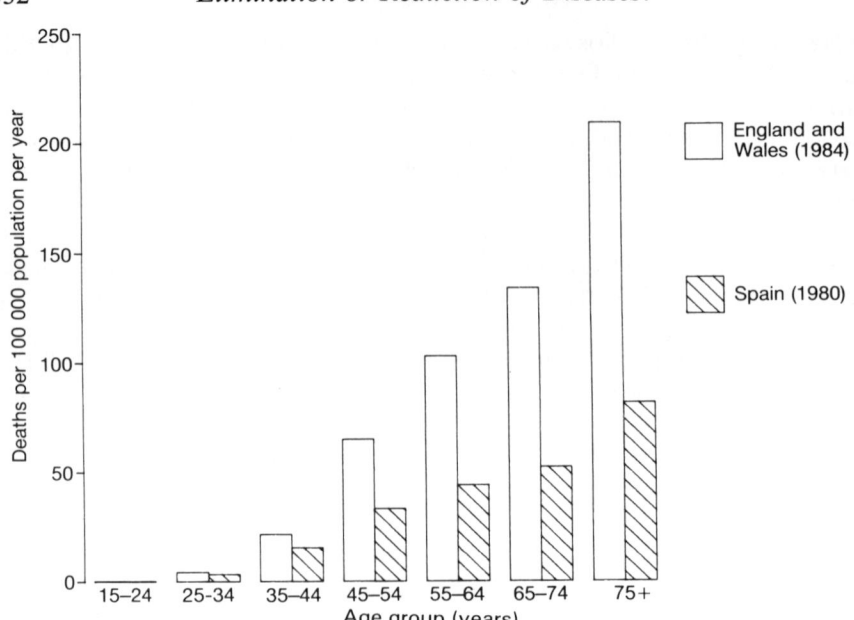

Fig. 19.2 Age-specific death rates from breast cancer in England and Wales, and Spain. (Source: *World Health Statistics annual* (1986).)

Therefore any screening programme must continue to examine detected cases after successful treatment.

The relative risk of breast cancer for a woman with a mother, sister, or daughter who has the disease is about 2–3 (Macklin 1959; Lilienfeld 1963; Papadrianos *et al.* 1967). It is reported (Anderson 1976) that the first-degree relatives of patients with bilateral disease have three times the risk of similar relatives with unilateral disease which is equivalent to a relative risk of 6–9. Lynch (1981) shows that disease resulting from a familial relationship will usually be manifested 15–20 years earlier than normally expected. The examination of relatives of breast cancer cases might therefore be beneficial from a young age. However it has not yet been demonstrated that breast examination (whether by palpation or mammography) is effective in diagnosing breast cancer in women under the age of 40 years.

The possible impact of a screening programme may also be dependent on risk factors if they are related to the uptake of screening. Acceptors of screening, because of some self-selection bias, may have a different risk from the disease than refusers. Age, family history, and educational status are likely to be relevant.

Age is important because older women are less likely to accept screening if it is offered to them than younger women. The Swedish breast cancer trial in

Kopparberg and Östergötland counties had a 93 per cent acceptance rate among women aged 40–70 years, but only a 52 per cent acceptance rate in women over 75 years (Tabár and Gad 1981). In terms of woman-years of life saved, a screening programme aimed at identifying 60–70-year-olds for a breast examination is likely to be more successful than one aimed at 70–80-year-olds even though mortality from the disease is slightly higher in the older age group in most European countries.

Women who have a relative with breast cancer are likely to be specially motivated to accept screening if it is offered to them. Such women are also at high risk from the disease. Similarly, women in the higher social groups are more likely to accept screening if it is offered than women in the lower social groups, and they too are at somewhat higher risk than women in the lower social groups (Coggon and Acheson 1981). Both these factors will tend to make the group of acceptors of screening in a particular age group have a somewhat higher risk than the refusers. Indeed in the Health Insurance Plan of New York (Shapiro *et al.* 1982), refusers of screening had a higher mortality rate from diseases other than breast cancer than the control group but a breast cancer incidence rate 20 per cent lower than that in the control group.

Kalache and Vessey (1982), in a review of other breast cancer risk factors, concluded that none are of sufficient discriminatory power to merit consideration when targeting a population for screening or seem likely to affect markedly the uptake of screening.

Nature of intervention

Primary prevention

Risk factors, such as the decreased risk associated with oophorectomy and the increased risk associated with early age at menarche, late age at menopause, late age at first pregnancy, and nulliparity, strongly suggest that the amount of biologically available oestrogen is a key factor in the aetiology of the disease. Changing circulating oestrogen concentrations in a population has not been investigated and is therefore unevaluated. The role of other risk factors remains to be clarified, but there is little prospect that primary presentation will significantly reduce the incidence in the near future.

Treatment

Advances have been made in the treatment of breast cancer both with the anti-oestrogen agent tamoxifen and long-term cytotoxic chemotherapy. A pooling of some 80 trials involving 16 000 women in randomized trials of tamoxifen and 10 000 women in randomized trials of chemotherapy indicated that both forms of adjuvant therapy increased survival over the short duration of these trials by 10–20 per cent (*Lancet* 1984). Cytotoxic chemotherapy appears to be particularly effective among women diagnosed before age 50 years.

Screening for breast cancer

Mortality from breast cancer can be reduced by screening for the disease and detecting it in its early stages when it is more susceptible to treatment than when it presents clinically.

Screening involves identifying women of the appropriate age and offering them a breast examination consisting of an X-ray of the breast (mammography) (Kopans *et al.* 1984) or a physical examination (to detect palpable breast lumps and other signs of the disease) or both. In order to be fully effective, breast examination by either mammography or physical examination must be repeated at intervals because a single examination is only predictive of the absence or presence of the disease for, at most, a few years.

Evaluation of screening programmes

Sensitivity, false-positive rate, and positive predictive value

The usual parameters quoted for any screening test are its sensitivity (detection rate) and false-positive rate. The evaluation of these parameters is not straightforward in the case of breast cancer screening.

Usually the sensitivity of a test, such as a mammographic examination, is defined as the proportion of 'affected' individuals detected by that test. The definition of 'affected' in the context of mammography needs consideration. It could be said that a woman is 'affected' if she has a pre-clinical lesion. However, from a treatment standpoint, interest centres only on those cancers which reach the clinical stage of the disease, so that the definition is usually modified to involve only those pre-clinical lesions which will in time progress to clinical disease (Day *et al.* 1984). However, sensitivity defined in such a way is not directly calculable because it is not possible to determine whether a cancer appearing say three years after an examination is a cancer 'missed' at that examination or one which was not then present in the pre-clinical stage, only entering that stage after that examination. A potential complicating factor here is the proportion of borderline lesions detected at a mammographic examination and operated upon which, had they been left, would have never reached the clinical stage of the disease. This proportion is not likely to be large since in the Health Insurance Plan study the cumulative incidence in the screened group was not materially higher than in the control group beyond five years from randomization.

What is important is not so much sensitivity, but the ratio of interval cases (screened individuals whose cancers present symptomatically in the interval between examinations) to cases detected at an examination in a screening programme. This ratio depends on the interval between examinations and will tend to be lower for the first examination. Its value for different intervals can help to determine the optimal interval between examinations.

The false-positive rate is the proportion of unaffected individuals screened positive. In practice, detection of the latter results in unnecessary surgery, although operations on benign breast disease may prevent cancer developing in the next few years.

Another useful concept here is the proportion of individuals found positive on examination who are diagnosed as having breast cancer at biopsy. This value, the positive predictive value, has important consequences for the cost of a screening programme.

It is important to know the sensitivity and false-positive rate of the mammographic examination, but this is only one component of the screening process. A screening programme has a sensitivity and false-positive rate dependent not only on the predictive qualities of mammography, but also on other factors such as the age at which mammographic examinations start and the time interval between successive examinations.

Survival comparisons

The effectiveness of different methods of treating clinically presenting breast cancer is usually assessed by comparing survival times. This approach is not valid in assessing the merits of breast cancer screening because of two well-documented biases that favour the survival of women with screen detected cancers (Feinleib and Zelen 1969).

First, slow-growing cancers spend longer in the pre-clinical phase of the disease and so are more likely to be detected than fast-growing cancers. Hence cancers detected by screening tend on average, to be slower growing than those missed by screening and slower growing cancers have a better prognosis. This is *length bias*.

The aim of screening is the early diagnosis of the disease. All cancers detected by screening have, by definition, been detected earlier than they would have been had there been no screening, hence increasing the interval between diagnosis and death, even if the date of death is unaltered. This is *lead time bias*.

Mortality comparisons

An unbiased assessment of screening is provided by considering the breast cancer mortality in two randomized sections of a population, one section being offered screening and the other acting as control subjects.

Comparison of the breast cancer mortality rates in the two groups effectively bypasses the problem of lead time bias. If screening increases the diagnosis to death period only by advancing diagnosis, and not by delaying death, the mortality rate in the two groups will remain the same (within the boundaries of chance).

Length bias would suggest that cases detected on screening have a better prognosis than interval cases. In the analysis of a randomized trial, this problem is surmounted by comparing mortality in the control group with mortality in the whole group offered screening—that is, interval cases and cases among women who refused screening are included with screen-detected cases.

Comparison of mortality in the group offered screening as a whole (whether or not screening is accepted) with that in the control group, together with randomization, completely removes self-selection bias.

Although other effects of screening—such as the longer period of morbidity of cases whose prognosis is unaltered and the overtreatment of borderline abnormalities—need consideration when assessing a trial, the primary measure of the success of the trial is the effect that it has on mortality from the disease.

Evidence of the effectiveness of screening for breast cancer

Benefits of screening

The first randomized trial of breast cancer screening was the Health Insurance Plan of New York (HIP study) started in 1963 (Shapiro 1977). Sixty-two thousand women aged 40–64 years were allocated at random to either a study group or a control group. The women in the study group were offered mammographic and physical examination, and the 65 per cent who accepted the initial examination were offered three additional examinations at annual intervals.

Seven years after entry to the trial, cumulative breast cancer mortality in the study group was two-thirds that in the control group (81 deaths as opposed to 124) (Shapiro *et al.* 1982). This difference of 40–50 deaths between the two groups was maintained up to the tenth year after randomi-

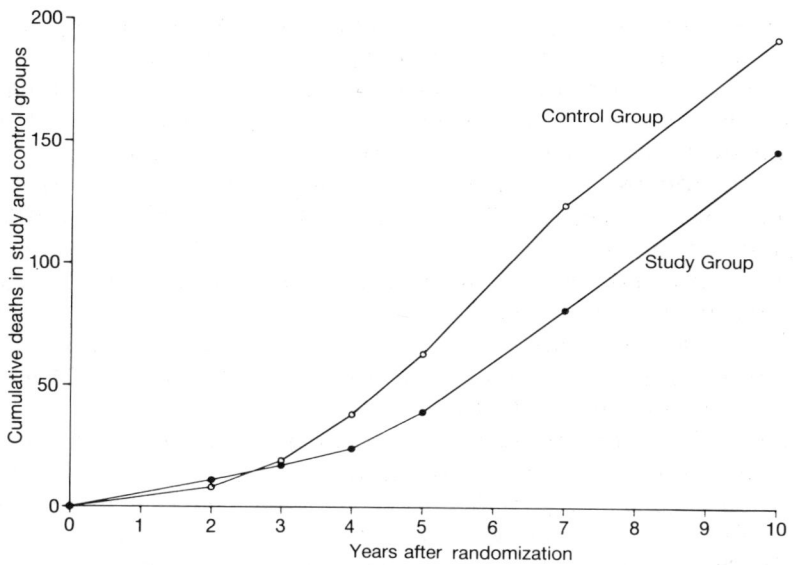

Fig. 19.3 Breast cancer mortality in the HIP study. (Sources: Shapiro (1978); Shapiro *et al.* (1982).)

zation (Figure 19.3) and, for cases diagnosed in the first 10 years, up to the fourteenth year after entry.

Figure 19.3 shows that the percentage difference in mortality between the two groups became smaller (38 per cent after 5 years, 24 per cent after 10 years) with increasing duration from entry. This is caused, in part, by the fact that examinations stopped after an average of 3.5 years so that many cancers in the study group presented well after they could have been detected by mammography or by physical examination. Indeed the data suggest that mortality from breast cancer among cases detected more than 3–4 years after the last examination was similar in both the study and control groups. Shapiro *et al.* (1982) estimate that, had examinations been on an annual basis up to year 10, then the reduction in cumulative mortality seen in years one to 10 would have been 32 per cent compared with the observed reduction over 10 years of 24 per cent and the reduction over 5 years of 38 per cent.

To assess the results of the HIP study, other randomized trials were set up in the two Swedish counties of Kopparberg and Östergötland (Tabár and Gad 1981) and in Malmö (Andersson *et al.* 1979), Edinburgh (Roberts *et al.* 1984), and Canada (Miller *et al.* 1981).

All of these trials are still in progress but interim results from the Swedish Two Counties trial have been published. A total of 163 000 women aged 40 years or more at randomization entered the study. Randomization took place at a community level, the two counties being divided into 19 blocks to give relative socio-economic homogenity within each block. In Östergötland each block was divided into two units of roughly equal size and in one of these units (randomly allocated) screening was offered to the population. In Kopparberg each block was divided into three units and in two of them (randomly chosen) screening was offered to the population: there were therefore about two women in the screened group for every control subject. Women over the age of 50 years in the screened group were offered examinations on average every 33 months while those under 50 years were offered examinations every 24 months. The examination was single oblique view mammography without breast palpation.

After 7 years, mortality in the group randomized to screening was 31 per cent lower than that in the control group in those women aged 40–74 years at randomization (Figure 19.4) (Tabár *et al.* 1985).

This result is felt to be slightly disappointing considering the high acceptance rate (over 90 per cent in women under 70 years, in Sweden and the improved mammographic technique compared with that used in the HIP study. Such comparisons may not be valid since there are considerable differences in the design of the two studies. The interval between successive examinations was longer in the Swedish study (2–3 years dependent on age at randomization) than in the HIP study (annual examination). It might be expected that a higher proportion of cancers detected in the Swedish study

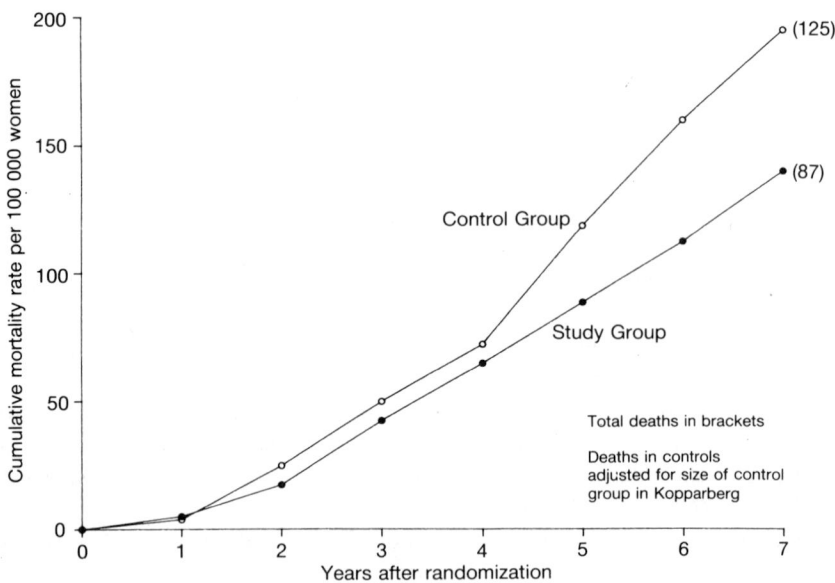

Fig. 19.4 Breast cancer mortality in the Swedish Two Counties study. (Source: Tabár *et al.* (1985).)

group would have been interval cancers (cancers presenting symptomatically between examinations) than would be the case if examinations had been done annually. There were 77 interval cancers between the first two examinations of which only 13 were diagnosed during the 12 months after the first examination. This suggests that the number of interval cancers could be reduced by 60 per cent or so if screening had been done annually (Tabár et al. 1984). Both in Sweden (Holmberg et al. 1986) and New York (Shapiro et al. 1982) interval cases in the study groups appeared to have similar prognosis to control cases, implying that a reduction in the number of interval cases in a screening programme should improve the effectiveness of screening.

Two Dutch non-randomized programmes assessed the efficacy of screening using a case-control approach. The Nijmegen project (Verbeek et al. 1984) involved selecting women aged 35 years and above for breast examinations every two years while that in Utrecht (Collette et al. 1984) involved selecting women aged 50 to 64 years for an initial examination and then seeing them subsequently at increasing intervals of 12, 18, and 24 months. Breast examination was by mammography alone in Nijmegen and by mammography and physical examination in Utrecht.

A case-control analysis of screening compares the screening history of a woman who dies from breast cancer (a case) with the screening histories of age-matched control subjects without breast cancer drawn from the same population, all of whom have been offered screening. In Nijmegen there were five age-matched control subjects for each case while in Utrecht there were three.

In both studies breast cancer mortality was substantially lower in women who accepted screening than in those who did not. The reduction in breast cancer mortality demonstrated in Nijmegen was 52 per cent (95 per cent confidence interval 0–77 per cent) while that in Utrecht was 70 per cent (95 per cent confidence interval 30–87 per cent).

Mortality from breast cancer is the endpoint in case-control studies and so they are not subject to lead time bias. Neither are such studies subject to length bias since a case is classified as having a positive screening history if she had a mammogram between the start of the study and the diagnosis of the disease (not only if the cancer was diagnosed by mammography, but also if it presented clinically in the interval between two examinations).

Such case-control studies of screening are not randomized. Essentially they permit comparison of mortality in acceptors of screening with mortality in refusers of screening and so are open to self-selection bias. The major self-selection bias could have been age but both studies controlled for this by matching control subjects for age. Other selection factors such as the presence of lumps in the breast, a family history of breast cancer, and high social class would all probably have tended to make the women who accepted screening at higher risk of breast cancer than those who refused screening.

This effect would have tended to bias the study against screening thus masking any effect rather than exaggerating it. In fact the incidence of breast cancer was similar in those who refused screening to that in the population as a whole before screening was introduced in Utrecht, and in the case of the Nijmegen study was similar to a control city, Arnhem. It is therefore unlikely that self-selection biased the results of the trials.

Another potential bias was avoided by considering only the breast examination history of the control subjects before the diagnosis of the disease in their respective cases. If this had not been done, control subjects would have had a longer period of time in which to have been examined than cases thus spuriously associating screening with a low risk of breast cancer.

The two Dutch studies demonstrated greater reductions in mortality than did the HIP and Swedish randomized trials. This is not in itself surprising since the Dutch case-control studies compare breast cancer death rates in women who accepted an invitation for a breast examination with those who did not. The randomized trials, however, compare breast cancer mortality in a group invited for breast examination (regardless of whether the invitation was accepted) with that in control subjects and so the demonstrated effect will be diluted because compliance is less than 100 per cent.

The Dutch studies provide evidence to reinforce the conclusions of the HIP and Swedish Two Counties studies that screening for breast cancer can, in practice, reduce mortality from the disease in a population by anything from 30 per cent to, perhaps, 50 per cent depending on considerations discussed in detail later.

Radiation risk from screening

In 1977, based on extrapolation from data on women exposed to multiple fluoroscopic examinations, X-ray treatment for post-partum mastitis, and atomic bomb irradiation, the NCI *Ad Hoc* Working Group on the Risks Associated with Mammography in Mass Screening for the Detection of Breast Cancer, estimated the incremental risk of breast cancer in women aged 35 years at exposure to be about 3.5 to 7.5 cases per million per year per cGy to both breasts, the risk beginning at the end of a 10-year latent period (Upton *et al.* 1977). This figure agrees closely with those estimated by Boice *et al.* (1979) under different models of disease incidence after radiation exposure.

The NCI Working Group concluded that a screening programme such as the HIP study would increase the incidence of cancer in the screened population by 1–2 per cent over a period of 40 years. As a result the Working Group to Review the National Cancer Institute—American Cancer Society Breast Cancer Detection Demonstration projects (BCDDP) recommended that screening in women under 50 years be restricted to those at high risk for familial reasons (Beahrs *et al.* 1979).

However, the radiation doses necessary to achieve good imaging have been markedly reduced since the HIP study which involved an average dose to the breast of around 2 cGy per examination. Current doses are around 0.1 cGy per examination making the risk from screening minute. Feig (1984) estimates that the risk from a mammographic examination is comparable with that of travelling 15 miles in a car, smoking one-third of a single cigarette, or living for 5 minutes at age 60 years.

Issues in maximizing the effect of screening

Age at which to start breast examinations

Breast cancer is primarily a disease of older women. Incidence and mortality rates rise sharply from about age 30 years up to the age of 50 or so and then continue to rise less steeply. The pattern is the same in all Western European countries. No study has attempted to screen women by selecting those under the age of 35 years for breast examination because the potential for saving life is small. Also the effect of breast examination on women under the age of 50 years is uncertain. Both in Sweden (Tabár *et al.* 1985) and Nijmegen (Verbeek *et al.* 1985) no benefit has been demonstrated for women aged under 50 years at the start of the trial, but the number of deaths in this age group is small and consequently the analyses are subject to considerable random variation.

The HIP study showed no benefit after 5 years of follow-up, but after 14 years of follow-up the mortality reduction seen in those who entered the trial aged 40–49 years was similar to that in those aged 50 years or more. There is still speculation as to whether the reduction in mortality seen in those admitted to the trial aged 40–49 is the result primarily of the examinations they received after age 50 years (see, for example, Shapiro *et al.* 1982; Day *et al.* 1985; Habbema *et al.* 1986). The answer will come from a study in which a group of women aged 40–49 years are randomized into two groups, one to receive immediate screening and the other screening from age 50 years. In the Swedish Two Counties study screening of the control group has just started, effectively realizing this aim.

Frequency of examinations

Decreasing the time interval between breast examinations must increase the proportion of cancers found by screening and therefore, by implication, decrease the mortality from the disease. All current screening is done first by selecting women above a certain age and then offering breast examinations at an interval of between 1 and 3 years. Tabár and colleagues (1984) argue that pre-menopausal females should be examined every 12 to 18 months and post-menopausal females every 18 to 24 months, since the mean detection lead time in pre-menopausal females is shorter than in post-menopausal females. The expected benefits of a shortened interval must be judged in the context of cost and feasibility.

Importance of physical examination

In the HIP study physical examination (palpation) was a very important component of the breast examination: indeed more cancers were detected in this way than by mammography. Over the years this situation has changed as a result of advances in mammography. In the BCDDP study involving a quarter of a million American women, only 9 per cent of the cancers detected were found by clinical examination alone, compared with 40 per cent found by mammography alone, and 50 per cent by both mammography and physical examination (Baker 1982). Other large studies (Table 19.3) show a similar marginal benefit in the number of cancers detected by adding physical examination to mammography. Among women under the age of 50 years a higher percentage of cancers are detected by clinical examination than among women over 50 (see for example, Baker 1982). But this may be an artefact of the reduced sensitivity of mammography as opposed to an increased sensitivity of physical examination among younger women.

Table 19.3 Value of adding physical examination to mammography in screening programmes.

	Breast cancer detection		
Study	Mammography No. of cases (a)	Physical examination alone No. of cases (b)	Ratio (a):(b)
Self-referral			
BCDDP (Baker 1982)	1829	186	10:1
Thomas Jefferson (Patchesfsky *et al.* 1977)	107	24	4:1
Invited population			
Utrecht (Rombach 1980)	110	1	110:1
Guildford (Thomas *et al.* 1984)	84	7	12:1
Randomized trial			
HIP (Shapiro *et al.* 1982)	73	59	1:1
Surgical series			
Gävle (Lundgren 1978)	281	21	13:1

Physical examination also has a lower specificity than mammography (see, for example, Chamberlain *et al.* 1984). Its use, therefore, involves prolonged anxiety for a larger proportion of the screened population and heavier costs. In the light of these results many screening programmes (for example, the Swedish Two Counties, Malmö and Nijmegen) do not incorporate a full physical examination.

Mammographic view

One or more of three mammographic views of the breast have been used in studies, the cranio–caudal and the latero–medial, used in the HIP study, and the oblique view, developed by Lundgren (1977) and used as the sole screening test in the trials in Kopparberg and Östergötland.

The relative performance of these three views have been assessed from both screening and surgical series. The single oblique view has a better detection rate than either the cranio–caudal or latero–medial views. The addition of either of the latter views improves the detection rate by about 5 per cent (Table 19.4).

Table 19.4 Detection according to mammographic view. Data from four series.

Study	Number of cancers	Mammographic view	Breast cancers detected
Screening programme cases			
Andersson (1981)	117	CC	104
		O	107
		Either	117
Hospital cases			
Hendriks (1982)	100	CC	89
		IM	94
		Either	94
Andersson *et al.* (1978)	491	CC	441
		IM	437
		O	440
		CC or IM	462
		IM or O	463
		O or CC	457
		Any	467
Lundgren (1977)	392	CC	319
		IM	317
		O	372
		CC or IM	347
		IM or O	373
		O or CC	373
		Any	374

CC = cranio–caudal   IM = latero–medial   O = oblique

Organization of screening programmes

Population-based screening within a particular country would have to be done on a regional basis with programme directors, skilled in screening procedures, responsible for their own defined geographical area. In order to be effective, screening has to operate on a call–recall basis from a population list. Ideally, this list should specify a person's sex and date of birth together with their address and should be updated regularly. Usually the electoral roll in a country will be the list of choice although some will need to be enhanced with data on sex and age.

Screening can, but need not necessarily, be carried out in hospitals as is the case at the Thomas Jefferson University Hospital (Patchefsky *et al.* 1977) and in the Canadian Randomized Trial (Miller *et al.* 1981). The HIP, Swedish Two Counties, and Dutch studies all operated from non-hospital based screening centres and referred cases to hospital after a positive examination. Studies should endeavour to keep biopsy rates as low as possible. A positive predictive value of between one-half and one-third, as achieved in Utrecht (de Waard *et al.* 1984) and at Reading (Cuckle and Wald, 1988, in press), can be achieved if sufficient care in defining positive cases is exercised. A powerful argument in favour of non-hospital based screening centres is that those screened are healthy, non-symptomatic women who should not be treated as patients. In the United Kingdom the acceptance by the government of the Forrest report (1986) will lead to nationwide screening by 1990.

Cost of screening

The four population-based studies of screening in which mortality was the endpoint have differences in study design which makes it difficult to put a single value on the reduction in mortality from breast cancer that can be achieved by screening. They do, however, indicate that breast cancer mortality can be reduced by 30–50 per cent in women invited for a mammographic examination. Since all studies achieved their greatest reductions in breast cancer mortality among women aged 50 years or more at the start of the programme it seems reasonable to assume, from the point of view of approximate costing, that screening will reduce breast cancer mortality by 40 per cent in women over 50 years.

Within the EEC, because age-specific life-expectancy above age 50 years is similar in all countries, the cost per year of life saved by screening will vary from country to country approximately in inverse proportion to mortality rates from breast cancer in older women.

In an arbitrary population of 100 000 women aged 50 years with the same age-specific mortality for breast cancer experienced by 50-year-old women in England and Wales (highest mortality rate within the EEC, excluding

Luxembourg whose rates are subject to considerable random variation,) around 2500 will die of breast cancer before age 75 years (figure based on World Health Statistics Annual 1986). Assuming that mammographic examinations on average every two years from age 50 to age 75 years with a compliance of 70 per cent can reduce mortality among women aged 50–75 years by 40 per cent; 1000 of these 2500 lives could be saved at a cost of 700 000 mammographic examinations (70 per cent × 10 × 100 000). It is estimated that the cost of screening is around £12 per mammographic examination (Forrest 1986), so the cost per life saved is around £8400 and the cost per year of life saved around £500 (average life-expectancy assumed to be 17 years).

In Spain (lowest breast cancer mortality rates in the EEC) mortality rates in older women are about one-third those in England and Wales (Figure 19.2) so the cost per year of life saved of a similar programme will be around £1500.

Screening programmes such as these if implemented can save around one-quarter of total deaths from breast cancer. There is thus potential for saving up to 15 000 lives a year in the EEC through population-based screening programmes.

Conclusions and recommendations

Screening has great potential for reducing mortality from breast cancer throughout the EEC. The evidence suggests that a screening programme offering mammographic examinations on a regular basis to women aged 50–70 years will reduce mortality from breast cancer in this age group by about 40 per cent and accordingly by 20–25 per cent in the whole population.

The great variation in risk with age makes it necessary that determination of a woman's age be the first component of screening, and doubts about the efficacy of breast examination in women under the age of 50 years suggest that regular breast examinations should start at age 50. Follow-up of patients over longer time intervals in the current trials and further larger studies may lead to the recommendation that examinations start at an earlier age.

The ideal interval between examinations relative to the cost of implementation is as yet unknown but this need not hinder the establishment of national screening programmes in Europe. The answers to questions about the interval between examinations will come from studies where those screened are randomized to have examinations at differing intervals varying from perhaps one to five years. This design has been used at the Reading Screening Centre in England and of 2500 women screened so far none have objected to randomization of the interval between examinations (Cuckle and Wald, 1988, in press). There seems to be no reason why such randomization of individuals should not be done on a national basis, allowing the ideal interval between examinations to be discovered relatively quickly while not delaying the introduction of screening.

The second component of screening is mammography. The high false-positive rate of physical examination makes its inclusion in a screening programme of dubious value. Single oblique view mammography is a satisfactory method of breast examination, but since the cost of mammography is not greatly increased by a second view, and the risks of such a view are negligible, it would be acceptable to also take a cranio–caudal or latero–medial view.

Screening must be population-based and involve a call–recall system within each region. Ideally, screening should be based on well-women screening centres referring positive patients to clinical breast cancer units, usually in hospitals, for further assessment, diagnosis, and treatment. This is the third component of screening.

A breast cancer screening programme is not, judged by cost per year of life saved, expensive. Giving women aged 50–70 years breast examinations on average every two years is likely to reduce mortality from the disease by typically 25 per cent in the population at a cost of around £500 to £1500 in different countries in the EEC for every year of life saved.

The fourth component of screening is monitoring which should form an integral part of every programme. Every screening centre must monitor its acceptance rate, the proportion of women having a biopsy, the stage distribution of the lesions detected, and the ratio of malignant to benign lesions detected, to ensure that all these measures of screening are satisfactory. A flagging system similar to the Southport system which monitors all deaths together with all moves from one region to another, is useful in the calculation of age-specific mortality rates within a regional population, rates which are important in determining the overall value of a screening programme in influencing breast cancer mortality.

Acknowledgements

I should like to thank Professor Nicholas Wald and Dr Howard Cuckle for their help in developing the argument in this chapter, both of them together with Dr Nick Day, Ms Kiran Nanchahal, and Mr Simon Thompson for providing helpful comments on various drafts of the chapter, and Ms Jane Folwell for carefully typing those drafts.

References

Anderson, D.E. (1976). Genetic predisposition to breast cancer. In *Risk factors in breast cancer* (ed. B. Stoll), Vol. 2, Ch. 1, p 6. Heinemann, London.

Andersson, I. (1981). Radiographic screening for breast carcinoma. III. Appearance of carcinoma and number of projections to be used at screening. *Acta. Radiol. (Diagn.)* **22**; 407.

——, Hildell, J., Mühlow, A., and Pettersson, H. (1978). Number of projections in mammography: influence on detection of breast disease. *Am. J. Radiol.* **130**, 349.

——, Andrén, L., Hildell, J., Linell, F., Ljungqvist, U., and Pettersson, H. (1979). Breast cancer screening with mammography. *Radiology* **132**, 273-6.

Baker, I.H. (1982). Breast Cancer Detection Demonstration Project: five-year summary report. *CA* **32**, 194-225.

Beahrs, O.H., Shapiro, S., Smart, C., and McDivitt, R.W. (1979). Summary report of the Working Group to Review the National Cancer Institute-American Cancer Society Breast Cancer Detection Demonstration Projects. *J. Nat. Cancer Inst.* **62**, 647-709.

Boice, J.D., Land, C.E., Shore, R.E., Norman, J.E., and Tokunaga, M. (1979). Risk of breast cancer following low-dose radiation exposure. *Radiology* **131**, 589-97.

Cancer Research Campaign (1982). *Trends in cancer survival in Great Britain*. Cancer Research Campaign, London.

Chamberlain, J., Clifford, R.E., Nathan, B.E., Price, J.L., and Burn, I. (1984). Repeated screening for breast cancer. *J. Epidemiol. Comm. Hlth.* **38**, 54-7.

Coggon, D. and Acheson, E.D. (1981). Trends in cancer morbidity in England and Wales. *Hlth Trends* **13**, 89-92.

Collette, H.J.A., Day, N.E., Rombach, J.J., and De Waard, F. (1984). Evaluation of screening for breast cancer in a non-randomised study (the DOM Project) by means of a case-control study. *Lancet* **1**, 1224-6.

Cuckle, H. and Wald, N. (1988). Breast cancer screening in the UK. *New Scientist* (in press).

Day, N.E., Tabár, L., and Fajerberg, G. (1985). Breast cancer screening. *Lancet* **1**, 94-5.

——, Walter, S.D., and Collette, H.J.A. (1984). Statistical models of disease natural history: their use in the evaluation of screening programmes. In *Screening for cancer—general principles on evaluation of screening for cancer and screening for lung, bladder and oral cancer* (eds P.C. Prorok and A.B. Miller), pp 55-70. International Union Against Cancer, Technical Report Series No 78. Geneva.

de Waard, F., Collette, H.J.A., Rombach, J.J., Baanders-van Halewijn, E.A., and Honing, C. (1984). The DOM Project for the early detection of breast cancer, Utrecht, The Netherlands. *J. Chron. Dis.* **37**, 1-44.

Feig, S.A. (1984). Hypothetical breast cancer risk from mammography. In *Recent results in cancer research* (eds S. Brünner, B. Langfeldt, and P.E. Andersen). Springer-Verlag, Berlin.

Feinleib, M. and Zelen, M. (1969). Some pitfalls in the evaluation of screening programmes. *Arch. Environ. Hlth* **19**, 412-5.

Forrest, P. (1986). *Breast cancer screening*. Report to the Health Ministers of England, Wales, Scotland and Northern Ireland. Department of Health and Social Security. HMSO, London.

Habbema, J.D.F., van Oortmarssen, G.J., van Putten, D.J., Lubbe, J.T., and van der Maas, P.J. (1986). Age-specific reduction in breast cancer mortality by screening: an analysis of the results of the Health Insurance Plan of Greater New York Study. *J. Nat. Cancer Inst.* **77**, 317-20.

Hendriks, J.H.C.L. (1982). *Population screening for breast cancer by means of mammography in Nijmegen 1975-1980*. G.J. Thieme, Nijmegen.

Holmberg, L.H., Tabár, L., Adami, H.O., and Bergström, R. (1986). Survival in breast cancer diagnosed between mammographic screening examinations. *Lancet* **2**, 27-30.

Kalache, A. and Vessey, M. (1982). Risk factors for breast cancer. *Clin. Oncol.* **1**, No. 3.

Kopans, D.B., Meyer, J.E., and Sadowsky, N. (1984). Medical Progress: Breast Imaging. *New Engl. J. Med.* **310**, 960-7.

Kurihara, M., Aoki, K., and Tominaga, S. (eds.) (1985). *Cancer mortality statistics in the world*. University of Nagoya Press, Nagoya.

Lancet. (1984). Review of mortality results in randomised trials in early breast cancer. *Lancet* **2**, 1205.

Lilienfeld, A.M. (1963). The epidemiology of breast cancer. *Cancer Res.* **23**, 1503-13.

Lundgren, B. (1977). The oblique view at mammography. *Br. J. Radiol.* **50**, 626-8.

—— (1978). Malignant features of breast tumours at radiography. *Acta Radiol. Diagn.* **19**, 623-33.

Lynch, H.T. (1981). Introduction to breast cancer genetics. In *Genetics and breast cancer* (ed. H.T. Lynch), pp. 1-13. Van Nostrand Reinhold, New York.

Macklin, M.T. (1959). Comparison of number of breast cancer deaths observed in relatives of breast-cancer patients and the number expected on the basis of mortality rates. *J. Nat. Cancer Inst.* **22**, 929-51.

Miller, A.B., Howe, G.R., and Wall, C. (1981). The National Study of Breast Cancer Screening. Protocol for a Canadian randomised controlled trial of screening for breast cancer in women. *Clin. Invest. Med.* **4**, 227-58.

Papadrianos, E., Haagensen, C.D., and Cooley, E. (1967). Cancer of the breast as a familial disease. *Ann. Surg.* **165**, 10-19.

Patchefsky, A.S., Shaber, G.S., Schwartz, G.F., Feig, S.A., and Nerlinger, R.E. (1977). The pathology of breast cancer detected by mass population screening. *Cancer* **40**, 1659-70.

Roberts, M.M., Alexander, F.E., Anderson, T.J., Forrest, A.P.M., Hepburn, W., Huggins, A., Kirkpatrick, A.E. Lamb, J., Lutz, W., and Muir, B.B. (1984). The Edinburgh randomised trial of screening for breast cancer: description of method. *Br. J. Cancer.* **50**, 1-6.

Rombach, J.J. (1980). Breast cancer screening: results and implications for diagnostic decision making. Dissertation Utrecht 1980. Staflev Scientific Publishing Company, Utrecht.

Schoenberg, B.S. (1977). *Multiple primary malignant neoplasms: the Connecticut experience 1935-64*. Springer-Verlag, New York.

Shapiro, S. (1977). Evidence on screening for breast cancer from a randomised trial. *Cancer* **39**, 2772-82.

—— (1978). Efficacy of breast cancer screening. In *Screening for cancer*. A Report of the UICC International Workshop, Canada (ed. A.B. Miller). UICC Technical Report Series—**40**, 133-57.

——, Venet, W., Strax, P., Venet, L., and Roeser, R. (1982). Ten to fourteen year effect of screening on breast cancer mortality. *J. Nat. Cancer Inst.* **69**, 349-55.

Tabár, L. and Gad, A. (1981). Screening for breast cancer: the Swedish trial. *Radiology* **138**, 219-22.

——, Åkerlund, E., and Gad, A. (1984). Five-year experience with single-view mammography. Randomised controlled screening in Sweden. In *Recent results in cancer research* (eds S. Brünner, B. Langfeldt, and P.E. Andersen), pp. 105-14. Springer Verlag, Berlin.

Tabár, L., Gad, A., Holmberg, L.H., Ljundquist, U., Fagerberg, C.J.G., Baldetorp, L., Gröntoft, O., Lundström, B., Månson, J.C., Eklund, G., Day, N.E., and Pettersson, F. (1985). Reduction in mortality from breast cancer after mass screening with mammography. *Lancet* **1**, 829-32.

Thomas, B.A., Price, J.L., Boulter, P.S., and Gibbs, N.M. (1984). The first three years of the Guildford Breast Screening Project. In *Recent results in cancer research* (eds S. Brünner, B. Langfeldt, and P.E. Andersen), pp. 195-9. Springer Verlag, Berlin.

United States Department of Health, Education and Welfare. Report No. 5. (1976). *Cancer surveillance, epidemiology and end results (SEER) program. Cancer patient survival.* US Department of Health, Education and Welfare, Washington.

Upton, A.C., Beebe, G.W. Brown, J.M., Quimby, E.H., and Shellaburger, C. (1977). Report of the NCI *Ad Hoc* Working Group on the risks associated with mammography in mass screening for the detection of breast cancer. *J. Nat. Cancer Inst.* **59**, 481-92.

Verbeek, A.I.M., Hendriks, J.H.C.L., Holland, R., Mravunac, M., Sturmans, F., and Day, N.E. (1984). Reduction of breast cancer mortality through mass screening with modern mammography. First results of the Nijmegen project 1975-1981. *Lancet* **1**, 1222-24.

——, ——, ——, ——, ——, (1985). Mammographic screening and breast cancer mortality: age-specific effects in Nijmegen Project, 1975-82. *Lancet* **1**, 865-6.

Waterhouse, J., Muir, C., Shanmugaratnam, K., Powell, J., Peacham, D., and Whelan, S. (1982). *Cancer incidence in five continents.* Volume IV. International Agency for Research on Cancer, Lyon.

World Health Organization. (1986). *World health statistics annual, 1986.* WHO, Geneva.

Appendix I

Summary of main conclusions for the topics considered

Chapter	Topic	Suggested intervention	Main target groups	Realistic community health goal	Comments
1	Congenital rubella	Immunization	(i) Mass strategy—all children OR (ii) Selective strategy pre-pubertal females	Elimination of congenital rubella syndrome (CRS)	Unlikely to be achieved for a number of reasons. Elimination of 90% of cases of CRS is feasible
2	Whooping cough	Immunization with whole cell vaccines, perhaps to be replaced by new component vaccines	Newborns, three doses completed by 6 months	Containment as defined by each country	Anxieties about vaccine toxicity. Limited success. Benefit–risk ratio greatest in high incidence area
3	Measles	Immunization at 12 months (new aerosol vaccine may be effective at 4 months)	Total population at 12 months	Containment by achieving vaccine uptake of 90–95%	Elimination probably not feasible in countries without compulsory immunization

4	Mumps	Immunization in combination with measles (+/– rubella)	Total population at 12 months	Containment as for measles	Only cost-effective when combined with measles. Immunization repeated at age 12 may be necessary to protect older susceptibles
5	Hepatitis B	Immunization	Homosexuals. Drug abusers. High risk areas.	Reduction of disease incidence and carrier status in high risk groups	Vaccine expensive— newer types may be cheaper. Current publicity on AIDS may lead to reduction in disease in high risk groups
6	Tuberculosis	(i) Case-finding and adequate chemotherapy (ii) BCG immunization	(i) Contacts of infected people, migrants from high prevalence countries (ii) Mass BCG immunization in high-prevalence countries, and in migrants and health service workers in low-prevalence countries	Below one new case per million	Elimination achieved by 2025 at the earliest in countries with the lowest risk of infection. Other countries should follow within 25–75 years. Extensive migration from high-prevalence countries might delay achievement of this target.

Chapter	Topic	Suggested intervention	Main target groups	Realistic community health goal	Comments
7	Vitamin D deficiency	Fortification of food, especially flours, bread and milk with vitamin D	Housebound elderly and other social and ethnic groups with low exposure to sunlight	90% reduction in vitamin D deficiency diseases	There are no data nor are trials feasible to suggest whether intervention is beneficial. Suggestion is to intervene in an absence of this proof
8	Iodine deficiency and goitre	Iodine supplementation of salt	More relevant to countries with low soil-iodine e.g. FDR, Belgium, France, Italy	Elimination of moderate or severe endemic goitre	Health education drive to reduce salt intake might affect programme adversely
9	Iron deficiency	Fortification of food with iron, particularly flour or bread	Whole population	A substantial reduction in iron deficiency however defined is possible	Evidence in favour of intervention comes mainly from Sweden and is limited to changes in circulatory haemoglobin concentrations alone. Current views on iron deficiency probably greatly overemphasize morbidity

10	Dental caries	Use of fluoride toothpaste combined with either fluoride in water or fluoride tablets, and/or fluoride mouth rinsing programmes plus integrated health education programmes	50–60% reduction in countries with moderate to high caries prevalence. Less than 50% reduction in countries with low caries prevalence	As more cost-effective methods of utilizing fissure sealants are developed, higher percentage reductions in dental caries levels will be achieved, especially in countries now experiencing low prevalence
11	Occupational cancers	Identification of carcinogens and workers at risk, removing and not introducing carcinogens in industrial processes, specific policies to protect workers at risk	Possible to quantify only for time and place specific targets	Identification of hazards from human studies and from results of long- and short-term tests is a priority to avoid human exposure to new suspected and known carcinogens
12	Down syndrome	Amniocentesis followed by termination of affected pregnancies	All mothers aged over 35 years	Maximum likely reduction of 40%
				No intervention feasible for the majority of cases born to younger mothers. Success of strategy dependent on trend in age-specific fertility

Chapter	Topic	Suggested intervention	Main target groups	Realistic community health goal	Comments
12	Neural tube defects	Serum alpha fetoprotein screening or ultrasound followed by termination if defect diagnosed	All mothers	75% reduction in open spina bifida at birth	Ultrasound if available and in skilled hands may increase sensitivity but at greater cost and may therefore be limited to countries of relatively lower prevalence
13	Thalassaemia	Public education and community involvement in: carrier screening genetic counselling prenatal diagnosis	Population of reproductive age in high prevalence population groups	Elimination of homozygous births	Community participation is essential
14	Congenital hypothyroidism	Screening for low T4 or raised TSH in neonatal period	All neonates	Less than 1–2 children with mental retardation due to congenital hypothyroidism per 100 000 livebirths	Benign transient hypothyroidism detected as false-positive while rarer causes of congenital hypothyroidism may be missed
15	Congenital hip dislocation	Routine evaluation of all newborns by better trained professionals	All neonates particularly breech deliveries	No data from which a realistic goal can be set	Criteria for introduction of screening not met, though mainly through lack of data

Appendix I

16	Perinatal mortality	Antenatal screening Antenatal care Intra-partum care Neonatal intensive care	Single mothers Lower socio-economic groups Ethnic minorities	Elimination of geographical, social class, and ethnic differentials to rates of the most advantaged (8 per 1000)	The avoidance of high-risk conceptions offers the best opportunity for reducing perinatal mortality without increasing handicap rates in survivors
17	Post-neonatal mortality	Scoring system to identify target groups for increased surveillance	Particularly those in most socially disadvantaged groups	Reduction of rates in target groups to 2 per 1000	Only achievable with countries with a positive commitment to infant welfare policies
18	Cervical cancer	Cervical cytology at age 25 years and then every 3 years	Female population 25–65 years	80% reduction in incidence of invasive cancer	This is extrapolated from results in Nordic countries
19	Breast cancer	Screening by mammography Optimal interval between examination awaits results of randomized trials	Female population 50–70 years	Reduction of mortality by up to 40% in target group screened	Extrapolation from clinical trials difficult. Reduction in general population mortality may be substantially less

Appendix II

Theoretical prerequisites for elimination

Listed in this table are what we believe to be prerequisites for elimination of the disorders discussed in this book. These prerequisites are based on a theoretical assumption that for the suggested programmes there is near perfect organizational efficiency and no financial, political, or ethical barriers to their implementation.

Chapter	Topic	Theoretical prerequisites
1	Congenital rubella	(i) immunization programme for young infants with a sustained coverage of 90% or more and/or an immunization programme for teenage girls with a sustained coverage close to 100%
		(ii) systematic screening for immunity in women of childbearing age and vaccine administration to those found susceptible
		(iii) surveillance of susceptible pregnant women and therapeutic abortion in case of acute rubella infection during the first trimester
		(iv) since elimination is feasible, any CRS in a newborn should be considered as a case of malpractice
2	Whooping cough	(i) improved vaccine efficacy
		(ii) very high levels of immunization coverage (over 95 per cent) required to completely halt transmission of *B. pertussis*. To compensate for waning of immunity, at least one booster immunization required. Coverage unlikely to be sufficiently high without making immunization compulsory
		(iii) routine recording of full details of all immunizations and side-effects, and all cases of whooping cough required in order to monitor individual vaccines for efficacy and safety, and to monitor programmes for effectiveness. Some

Chapter	Topic	Theoretical prerequisites
		form of compulsion required for complete notification
3	Measles	(i) 97% immunization rate required to achieve 99% reduction in disease with current vaccine efficacy of 95%
		(ii) improved vaccine efficacy would allow a slightly lower uptake rate. Uptakes of this level presuppose compulsion.
		(iii) effective immunization programmes world-wide to minimize importation of cases
4	Mumps	(i) 95% immunization rate is required to achieve a 95–99% reduction in disease
		(ii) compulsory immunization is a prerequisite for achieving a substantial reduction in disease incidence
5	Hepatitis B	(i) detection of carrier status particularly in groups likely to be responsible for transmission
		(ii) availability of an effective treatment for carrier status.
		(iii) programmes directed towards interruption of transmission, including provision of clean needles and syringes to drug addicts, and condoms to homosexual men
		(iv) immunization of all at-risk groups. This will require novel approaches to reach some of the most alienated groups of society
6	Tuberculosis	(i) active case-finding in high-risk groups (e.g. new immigrants, the homeless, alcoholics)
		(ii) legislation may be necessary to ensure adequate compliance with chemotherapy for newly discovered cases
		(iii) identification and chemoprophylaxis of tuberculin converters in high-risk groups (tested regularly) and in the general population (compulsory testing, for example, on leaving school or entering military service)
7	Vitamin D deficiency	(i) compulsory fortification of appropriate food-stuffs sufficient to prevent deficiency. The specific foods fortified

Chapter	Topic	Theoretical prerequisites
8	Iodine deficiency and goitre	would need to be altered in the face of changing dietary habits (i) legislation on the introduction of iodized salt; international co-operation to co-ordinate legislation and surveillance (ii) alternative strategy required for areas where sea salt is major source of salt
9	Iron deficiency	(i) it is likely that if sufficient iron is added to foodstuffs such as flour and bread, iron deficiency could be virtually eliminated in the general population (ii) the elimination of iron deficiency may be undesirable for two reasons: the danger of masking serious diseases which present as an unexplained anaemia; the association between haemoglobin concentration and ischaemic heart disease (IHD) needs further investigation lest supplementation with iron lead *inter alia* to an increase in IHD
10	Dental caries and peridontal disease	(i) reduce per capita consumption of sugar from present European average of 37.6 kg per head to 10 kg per head. (ii) daily use of fluoride toothpaste by the whole population (iii) mandatory fluoridation of the piped water supply where feasible (iv) fluoride tablets and/or fluoride mouth rinsing programmes to school children (v) fissure sealant programmes for all permanent molar teeth soon after eruption
11	Occupational cancers	(i) elimination of occupational cancer from specific exposures necessitates a) identification of hazard b) avoidance of contact by change in work process or substitution of chemicals (ii) use of long- and short-term tests to predict carcinogenicity in humans
12	Down syndrome	(i) amniocentesis of all pregnancies with no false negatives (ii) termination of all affected pregnancies
12	Neural tube defects	(i) for all pregnancies, high quality ultrasound performed and interpreted by highly trained staff. Likely false-negative

Appendix II 359

Chapter	Topic	Theoretical prerequisites
		rate 15%. Amniocentesis as an alternative strategy for AFP measurement could reduce false negative rate to 0.2%
		(ii) termination of all affected pregnancies
13	Thalassaemia	(i) 100% screening of males before reproductive age to detect carrier status
		(ii) 100% detection of carriers in subsequent female partners of proven male carriers
		(iii) either avoidance of conception by carrier couples or prenatal diagnosis of all pregnancies of such couples and termination of any affected pregnancies
14	Congenital hypothyroidism	(i) 100% coverage of neonatal population by screening
		(ii) improvement of current test sensitivity beyond 97%
		(iii) 100% early recall and treatment of screening positive children
		(iv) secondary and tertiary hypothyroidism cannot be detected and, until an effective prenatal screening test is introduced, some cases of primary hypothyroidism with residual mental deficiency cannot be prevented
15	Congenital hip dislocation	(i) congenital hip dislocation cannot be eliminated as the sensitivity of current screening tests results in significant false-negative rates of up to 50%
16	Perinatal mortality	(i) identification before conception or early in fetal life of individual genes or combinations of genes that predispose to perinatal death. If such genes or their markers could be identified, this would have to be followed by termination or gene therapy. This is clearly not a realistic option for the foreseeable future yet such genetic factors are likely to be responsible for a significant proportion of perinatal deaths
		(ii) programmes to improve maternal health and eliminate the difference in perinatal mortality between the most advantaged and the most disadvantaged groups.

Chapter	Topic	Theoretical prerequisites
		Such programmes would require major political and economic action and are outside the scope of health services
		(iii) secondary prevention specifically by high technology obstetric and neonatal care available at all at-risk pregnancies. A reduction in mortality may be associated with an increased rate of handicap
17	Post-neonatal mortality	(i) congenital malformations are responsible for up to 40% of all post-neonatal deaths. Elimination requires identification before conception or early in fetal life of individual genes or combinations of genes that predispose to congenital malformations and other genetic disorders lethal in the post-neonatal period. The identification of such genes, or their markers, would have to be followed by termination or gene therapy. This is clearly not a realistic option for the foreseeable future.
		(ii) programmes to improve infant health could eliminate the difference in post-neonatal mortality between the most advantaged and the most disadvantaged groups. Such programmes would in part rely on improvement in child health services but to a large extent would necessitate major political and economic action and would thus be outside the scope of health services
18	Cervical cancer	(i) every adult woman should be screened every three years
		(ii) there should be quality control of smear collection and reading
		(iii) treatment protocols should be established to avoid over-treatment of non-invasive lesions
		(iv) effectiveness of the programme should be monitored
		(v) women should be actively invited and reminded to participate, and those who do not participate should be traced and obstacles to participation should be removed

Chapter	Topic	Theoretical prerequisites
19	Breast cancer	(i) since primary prevention does not appear feasible at present, mammography should have the ability when offered at the appropriate time intervals—perhaps related to age—to detect all cancers at a treatable stage

Index

accidents, post-neonatal mortality from 228, 296-8
acetabular dysplasia 243
age
 breast cancer risk and 331, 334
 for cervical cancer screening 324
 compliance with screening procedures and 322, 332-3
 maternal, *see* maternal age
 paternal, Down's syndrome and 187
agriculture, occupational cancers 162
AIDS (acquired immune deficiency syndrome) xv, 72, 95
alcoholism, iron overload in 134-5
alpha-fetoprotein (AFP)
 in congenital hypothyroidism 233
 in Down's syndrome 188, 191, 194, 195, 206
 in neural tube defects (NTD) 200-2, 206-7
amniocentesis 270
 Down's syndrome 188, 191, 192
 neural tube defects (NTD) 200-1
 thalassaemia 221
anaemia
 Cooley's 221, 213-14; *see also* thalassaemia
 iron deficiency
  clinical importance 132-4
  definition 126
  prevalence rates 127-8, 131
  see also iron deficiency
 in thalassaemia 212-13, 214
anencephaly 196-9; *see also* neural tube defects (NTD)
antenatal care 269-72
 general care 271-2
 late attendance 268
 routine interventions 270-1
 screening for abnormalities 269-70
antenatal diagnosis, *see* prenatal diagnosis
army recruits, screening for thalassaemia carriers 219-20
asbestos, cancer induced by 162, 163, 164, 170, 172-4
Asians
 attendance for antenatal care 268
 vitamin D deficiency 104, 105, 106, 107

barbiturate use, vitamin D deficiency and 105
BCG vaccination 88, 94
benzidine 165, 170, 171, 172
benzo(a)pyrene 162, 163, 165
beta-naphthylamine 165, 170, 172
birth injury, perinatal mortality caused by 260
birthweight
 birth notifications and 258
 post-neonatal mortality and 295-6
 relationship to perinatal mortality 262-4
 very low, *see* very low birthweight infants (VLBW)
bis-chloromethylether (BCME) 163, 164
bladder cancer 159, 165, 169, 170, 171-2
blood and blood products, hepatitis B transmission 69
boot and shoe manufacture, occupational cancers 162-3, 172, 173, 174
brain damage
 associated with whooping cough vaccines 37-9
 diagnosis in neonates 277-8
 in survivors of neonatal intensive care 274-6
bread, iron fortification 136
breast cancer 328-46, 355
 mortality, incidence, and survival rates 330-1
 prerequisites for elimination 361
 primary prevention 333
 risk factors 331-3
 screening xiv, 334-46
  benefits 336-40
  compliance 332-3
  costs 344-5
  evaluation of programmes 334-6
  mammographic views 343
  optimal age 341
  organization of programmes 344
  radiation risk 340-1
  recommendations 345-6
  role of physical examination 342-3
  time intervals 341-2
 treatment 333-4
breast-feeding, protection against rickets 107, 108

breasts, physical examination 334, 342–3, 346

Caesarian section, risks of 273
cancer
  haemoglobin concentrations and 134
  occupational, *see* occupational cancers
  screening to reduce morbidity 311–46
carbon tetrachloride 172, 173
carcinogens
  occupational 160–4
  testing for 167–8
cardiovascular disease, haemoglobin concentrations and 133–4
cerebral palsy in survivors of neonatal intensive care 276
cervical cancer 311–25, 355
  carcinoma *in situ* (CIS) 315
  occurrence 311–13
  prerequisites for elimination 360
  risk factors 315–17
  screening xiv, 317–25
    efficacy 317–18
    ethical considerations 324
    optimal age 324
    outcome of specific programmes 319–21
    population compliance 322
    recommendations 325
    strategies 318–19
    test sensitivity 322–3
  time trends 313–14
cervical intraepithelial neoplasia (CIN) 315
chappatti flour 107, 108, 109
chemical industry, occupational cancers 163
child health clinics 300–1
child health services, improvements in 303
children, iron deficiency in 132, 133, 135
chorionic villus biopsy 221, 223
colorectal cancer screening xv
community care
  antenatal 271–2
  prevention of post-neonatal mortality 300–2
community involvement in thalassaemia screening 216–18
congenital anomalies 181–2
  in congenital rubella syndrome 9–10
  perinatal mortality caused by 260
  post-neonatal deaths caused by 288, 295, 296, 297
  potential risk factors 205
construction industry, occupational cancers 163
containment of disease 5
contraceptives, oral, cervical cancer and 318

Cooley's anaemia 211, 213–14
cot death, *see* sudden infant death syndrome
cretinism 226–7; *see also* hypothyroidism, congenital
cytotoxic chemotherapy of breast cancer 333–4

deafness 10, 60–1
dental caries 140–52, 353
  current trends 142, 143–4
  historical changes in prevalence 140–2
  pathology 147
  prerequisites for elimination 358
  preventive measure 146–52
    fissure sealants 148, 149
    health education 148–9
    immunization 150
    nutrition policies 148, 149
    problems in maximizing effectiveness 150–2
    recommendations 153
    use of fluorides 120, 147–8
dental health, global goals for 142, 144
diabetes, juvenile onset 61
diet
  neural tube defects (NTD) and 199–200
  sugar (sucrose) in 141, 148, 149
  vitamin D content 107
disabled, vitamin D deficiency 106
disease
  containment 5
  elimination, *see* elimination of disease
  eradication 5
diuretics, in pregnancy 270
DNA sequencing xv
Doppler ultrasonography 278
Down's syndrome 181–94, 353
  interventions 188–94
    costs and benefits 194
    evidence for effectiveness 188–91
    problems of maximizing population effectiveness 191–2
    recommendations 204–6, 207
    techniques 188
  occurrence 182–3
  prerequisites for elimination 358
  risk factors 186–8
  trends 183–5
drug abusers, hepatitis B transmission 69, 71–2, 73
dry cleaners, carbon tetrachloride exposure 172, 173
dye workers, occupational cancers 163, 165, 171–2

education, health, *see* health education
elderly
  iron deficiency 131-2
  vitamin D deficiency 103, 104-5, 106
elimination of disease xi, 5
  reasons for failure xii
  targets xii-xiv
  theoretical prerequisites 356-61
encephalitis
  measles 47
  rubella 9
encephalocele 196-9; *see also* neural tube defects (NTD)
epilepsy, vitamin D deficiency 105
eradication of disease 5
ethnic groups
  perinatal mortality and 267-8
  thalassaemia in 215-16, 222, 223
  vitamin D deficiency 104, 105, 106
  see also immigrants
Eurocat Project 182, 183, 245

family history, breast cancer risk and 332
femoral neck fracture, relationship to vitamin D deficiency 103, 104-5, 108, 109
ferritin, serum 127, 128-30
fertility, relationship to perinatal mortality 265-7
fetal diagnosis, *see* prenatal diagnosis
fetal hypoxia, *in utero* assessment 270
fetal monitoring, continuous electronic (CEFM) 272
fetus, growth retarded 262, 270
fissure sealants 148, 149, 151
flour
  chappatti 107, 108, 109
  iron fortification 136
fluoridated toothpastes 147, 148, 153
fluoridation
  of salt 120, 121, 147, 148
  of water 122, 147-8, 150, 151-2, 153
fluorides 147-8
  mouth rinses 147, 148
  tablets 147, 148
  topical applications 147
foods
  iodination 121, 122-3
  iron fortification 135-6
  vitamin D fortification 108-9, 110
furniture manufacture, occupational cancers 163

gas industry, occupational cancers 162

gastrointestinal infections, post-neonatal mortality from 295, 296
genetic counselling
  in Down's syndrome and neural tube defects (NTD) 207
  in thalassaemia 214, 220, 221-2, 223
gingivitis 152
glaucoma screening xv
goitre, endemic 115-23, 352, 358; *see also* iodine deficiency
gum disease 152

haemochromatosis 134-5
haemoglobin A 212, 213
haemoglobin concentrations
  clinical importance 132-5
  in iron deficiency 126, 127
  in pregnancy 270
  variations in 127-32
haemoglobin F 212, 213
haemoglobinopathies 212, 218; *see also* thalassaemia
haemolytic disease of newborn 260
haemorrhage, brain, in premature infants 278
handicap
  national registers 279-80
  parental experience of 277
  prediction of, in neonates 277-8
  in survivors of neonatal intensive care 274-6
  see also Down's syndrome *and* neural tube defects
Hashimoto's thyroiditis, iodine supplementation and 123
health care workers, hepatitis B infection 70, 72
health education xii
  on dental caries 148-9
  oral hygiene 152
  thalassaemia screening 216-18
  vitamin D consumption and 108
health visitors, prevention of sudden infant death syndrome 301-2
heart disease, ischaemic, haemoglobin concentrations and 133-4
hepatitis A virus (HAV) 65-6
hepatitis B 65-74, 351
  carriers 66, 67-8, 70, 71, 72, 74
  high risk groups 68-71
  immune globulin 72-3
  interventions 71-4
    elimination of reservoirs 71
    immunization 72-4
    interruption of transmission 71-2

hepatitis B (*cont.*)
  carriers (*cont.*)
    recommendations 74
    outcomes of infection 66
    prerequisites for elimination 357
    prevalence rates 67–8
    vaccines 73–4
    virus (HBV) 66
hepatitis non-A, non B 65
herpes virus type 2 (HSV2) 316
hip, congenital dislocation of
    (CDH) 243–52, 354
  occurrence 244, 245
  prerequisites for elimination 359
  results of treatment 249
  risk factors 245
  screening xiv, 246–52
    clinical diagnosis 246
    constraints in maximizing
      effectiveness 249–50
    efficacy 247–9
    population effectiveness 249
    radiological diagnosis 247
    recommendations 251–2
    ultrasound 247
homosexual men, hepatitis B
    transmission 69–70, 72, 73
human papilloma viruses (HPV) 316
hygiene
  cervical cancer and 316, 318
  transmission of hepatitis B and 70, 71
hypertension, effectiveness of treatment xiii
hyperthyroidism, *see* thyrotoxicosis
hypopituitarism, hypothyroidism in 232
hypothyroidism, congenital (CH) 116,
    226–39, 354
  neonatal screening 229–39
    efficacy and effectiveness 231–7
    limitations 237
    methodology 230–1
    procedural problems 236–7
    recommendations 237–9
    validity of screening tests 233–6
  occurrence 227–9
  prerequisites for elimination 359
hypothyroidism, transient neonatal 116,
    118–19, 227, 236

immigrants
  from high prevalence tuberculosis
    areas 86–7, 92–4
  iron deficiency in 132
  prevention of thalassaemia 223
  see also ethnic groups
immunity, cell-mediated, in hepatitis B
    carriers 70

immunization
  dental caries 150
  effectiveness 6
  hepatitis B 72–4
  measles 49–58
  mumps 61–3
  rubella 11–22
  tuberculosis 88
  whooping cough 28–42
infant mortality 287–8; *see also* post-
    neonatal mortality
intellectual development
  in transient hypothyroidism 116, 119
  in treated congenital hypothyroidism 227,
    231–3
intra-partum care 272–3
intra-uterine growth retardation 262, 270
iod-Basedow (iodine-induced
    thyrotoxicosis) 119, 122
iodinated water 121–2
iodine deficiency 115–23, 352
  clinical effects 115–16
  interventions 119–23
    alternatives to iodization of salt 121–2
    constraints and
      recommendations 122–3
    efficacy and effectiveness 120
    iodization of salt 119–20
  prerequisites for elimination 358
  prevalence 116–19
iodization of salt 119–20
iodized oil 121, 122
iron deficiency 126–37, 352
  definition 126–7
  interpretation of measures of iron
    status 132–5
  interventions 135–6
    food fortification xiv, 136–7
    treatment and follow-up 136
  prerequisites for elimination 358
  prevalence rates 127–30
  risk factors and vulnerable groups 131–2
  trends over time 130–1
iron overload 134–5
iron supplementation in pregnancy 270

job exposure matrices 69

labour
  difficult, perinatal mortality caused
    by 260
  optimal management 272–3
leucomalacia 277–8

mammography 334, 342-3, 346
  evaluation of sensitivity 334-5
  radiation risks 340-1
  radiographic views 343
Mantoux (tuberculin) test 86, 96
maternal age
  Down's syndrome and 186-7, 188-92, 194, 205, 206
  neural tube defects (NTD) and 199
  post-neonatal mortality and 296
measles 46-58, 350
  complications 47-8
  containment 54-5, 57
  diagnosis 47
  elimination 51-4, 57-8, 357
  eradication 50-1, 57
  history 46
  immunization programmes 49-58
    cost-benefit analysis 56-7
    effectiveness 50-5
    epidemiological side-effects 55-6
    recommendations 57-8
    target population 49-50
  occurrence and trends 48
  vaccines 49
meningitis, mumps 60
mental performance in iron deficiency 133
mental retardation in congenital hypothyroidism 226-7, 231
metal industry, occupational cancers 162
military recruits, screening for thalassaemia carriers 219-20
milk, vitamin D fortification 108, 109
mining industry, occupational cancers 162, 165
mumps 60-3, 351
  clinical features and complications 60-1
  history 60
  immunization programmes 61-2
    cost-benefit analyses 62-3
    effectiveness 62
    recommendations 63
    target population 61-2
  prerequisites for elimination 357
  vaccines 61
    combined with measles and rubella (MMR) 61, 62, 63
    efficacy and safety 62
Muslims, vitamin D deficiency in 104, 106

near infrared spectrophotometry 278
neonatal intensive care (NIC) 273, 274-8
  costs 278, 279
  health problems in survivors 276-7
  increased survival, handicap and morbidity 274-6

  prediction of outcome 277-8
neonatal mortality 287-8, 289; see also post-neonatal mortality
neonatal screening
  congenital dislocation of hips 246-52
  congenital hypothyroidism 229-39
  for haemoglobinopathies 218
neonates
  hepatitis B infection 68, 70
  resuscitation 273
  thyroid disorders 228
neural tube defects (NTD) 181, 182, 194-207, 354
  interventions
    evidence for effectiveness 200-3
    primary prevention 199-200
    problems in maximizing population effectiveness 203-4
    recommendations 204, 206-7
    secondary prevention 200
  occurrence 194-6
  prerequisites for elimination 358-9
  recurrence rate 203
  risk factors 199
  trends 196-9
neurological disorders, associated with measles 47-8, 49
nickel refining, occupational cancers 162, 171
nuclear magnetic reasonance spectroscopy 278
nutrition policies, on sugar consumption 148, 149

occupational cancers 157-75, 353
  carcinogenic agents 160-4
  categories of occupations or substances 166-7
  constraints and problems of elimination 174
  control measures 170-4
  detection of new carcinogens 167-9
  occupations with evidence of increased risk 162-3
  patterns in discovering new carcinogens 164-6
  prerequisites for elimination 358
  quantitative estimates 158-60
  recommendations 174-5
occupational hazards, hepatitis B 70, 72
oestrogen, aetiology of breast cancer and 333
oil, iodized 121, 122
oral health, global goals for 142, 144
Ortolani technique 246
osteoarthritis of hips 244

osteomalacia 101, 103, 104, 104–5; *see also* vitamin D deficiency
osetoporosis 103
otitis media
  in measles 47
  secretory (glue ear) xv

panencephalitis
  progressive rubella 10
  subacute sclerosing (SSPE) 47, 48
papilloma viruses, human (HPV) 316
parity
  cervical cancer and 317
  neural tube defects (NTD) and 199
  post-neonatal mortality and 296
paternal age, Down's syndrome and 187
perinatal mortality 257–80, 355
  causes 260–1
  current trends 261–2
  definition of perinatal period 258
  distinction between stillbirth and live birth 258–60
  factors affecting 262–8
    birthweight 262–4
    cigarette smoking 268
    social class and ethnic group 267–8
  intervention strategies 269–78
    antenatal care 269–72
    intra-partum care 272–3
    neonatal care 273–8
    recommendations 279–80
  prerequisites for elimination 359–60
periodontal disease 140, 152, 358
pertussis, *see* whooping cough
phenylketonuria 230
post-neonatal mortality 287–303, 355
  causes 288, 296–8
  interventions 300–2
  prerequisites for elimination 360
  recommendations 302–3
  risk factors 293–6
    low birthweight 295–6
    maternal age and parity 296
    sex 295
    social class 293–5
  trends 288–93
  see also sudden infant death syndrome
pregnancy
  antenatal care 269–72
  osteomalacia in 104, 105, 106
  screening for thalassaemia 218–19
  termination of, *see* termination of pregnancy
  see also prenatal diagnosis
prematurity
  bed rest for prevention of 271
  perinatal mortality caused by 260, 262
  see also very low birthweight infants
prenatal diagnosis
  Down's syndrome 182, 183, 188–94, 204–6, 207
  neural tube defects (NTD) 200–4, 206–7
  routine screening 269–70
  thalassaemia 218, 220–1, 222, 223
prevention, primary xiii
'prevention paradox' 39
printing industry, occupational cancer risk 172, 173

radiation exposure from mammography 340–1
radiography
  diagnosis of congenital dislocation of hips 247
  mass miniature 86
registers
  Down's syndrome 182–3
  national handicap 279–80
  of workers exposed to occupational carcinogens 168
registration systems for births and perinatal deaths 262
religious attitudes, thalassaemia prevention and 217, 222, 223
respiratory diseases
  complicating measles 47–8
  post-neonatal deaths caused by 288, 295, 296, 297
rickets 101, 104; *see also* vitamin D deficiency
rubber industry, occupational cancers 162, 172, 173
rubella 8–22, 350
  congenital rubella syndrome (CRS) 9–10
  elimination of 20–1, 356
  risks of 10–11
  epidemiology of infection 8–9
  eradication 12–14
  immunization programmes
    cost-benefit anaylses 12–13, 16, 17, 19
    effectiveness 14–19
    objectives 12–14
    recommendations 21–2
    strategies 14, 15
  size of problem 10–11
  vaccines 11–12

salt
  fluoridated 120, 121, 147, 148
  iodization of 119–20
screening xiii

Index

antenatal 269-70, 271
  breast cancer 334-46
  cervical cancer 317-25
  occupational cancers 174
  for thalassaemia carriers 218-20
  see also neonatal screening *and* prenatal diagnosis
sex differences
  in congenital dislocation of hips 245
  in iron deficiency 131-2
  in post-neonatal mortality 295
sexual contact, hepatitis B transmission via 69-70, 71-2
sexual practices, cervical cancer and 316-17
shipbuilding, occupational cancers 163
sickle cell (HbS) syndromes 212, 218, 224
skin pigmentation, vitamin D deficiency and 104, 106
smallpox eradication 5, 6, 7
smoking, cigarette xii
  perinatal mortality and 268
socio-economic status
  cervical cancer incidence and 315
  compliance with screening procedures 192, 322
  congenital hypothyroidism and 233
  dental caries and 143
  hepatitis B infection and 70
  neural tube defects (NTD) and 199
  perinatal mortality and 267-8
  post-neonatal mortality and 292, 293-5, 303
soot, carcinogenic effects 165
spina bifida 196-9; *see also* neural tube defects (NTD)
stillbirths 258-60
stress, perinatal mortality and 268
subacute sclerosing panencephalitis (SSPE) 47, 48
sucrose (sugar), dietary 141, 148, 149
sudden infant death syndrome (cot death) 288, 298-300
  prevention 301-2
  risk-scoring system 301
sugar (sucrose), dietary 141, 148, 149
surfactant, administration at birth 274

T4 (thyroxine) 227, 231, 234, 235
tamoxifen therapy 333-4
termination of pregnancy
  Down's syndrome 188, 192
  perinatal mortality and 266, 267
  in thalassaemia 220-1
thalassaemia 211-24, 354
  carriers or heterozygotes 212, 214, 218-20
  clinical classification 212-13

clinical and laboratory diagnosis 213-14
current trends in prevalence 216
genetic classification 212
homozygotes 212, 213-14
occurrence and risk factors 214-16
prerequisites for elimination 359
preventive measures 216-24
  efficacy 221
  genetic counselling 220
  population effectiveness 221-4
  prenatal diagnosis 220-1
  public education and community involvement 216-18
  recommendations 224
  screening for carriers 218-20
thrombocytopenic purpura, in rubella 9
thyroid hormone replacement therapy 227, 231-3
thyrotoxicosis
  iodine-induced (iod-Basedow) 119, 122
  iodine supplementation and 122-3
toothbrushing, improvements in 152
toothpastes, fluoridated 147, 148, 153
toxaemia of pregnancy, screening for 269
TSH (thyroid stimulating hormone) 227, 230-1, 223-4, 235, 237
tuberculin coverters 88-9
tuberculin (Mantoux) test 86, 96
tuberculosis 77-96, 351
  annual risks of infection 81
  control programmes 85-9
    case-finding and chemotherapy 86-7
    chemoprophylaxis 88-9
    mass BCG vaccination 88
  elimination 89-95
    definition 89
    feasibility 89-91
    problems 91-4
    recommendations 94-5
  endogenous reactivation 79, 91, 95-6
  glossary of terms 95-7
  high risk groups 86-7
  limitations of chemotherapy 78-9
  occurrence and trends 81-5
  post-primary 79-80
  prerequisites for elimination 357
  primary 79
  transmission characteristics 80-1

ultrasonography, Doppler 278
ultrasound
  antenatal screening 200, 202, 206-7, 269
  congenital dislocation of hips 247
  in leucomalacia 277-8
ultraviolet radiation, vitamin D deficiency and 104, 106, 108

umbilical cord blood, *in utero* sampling 270
unemployment, post-neonatal mortality and 295

vaccines, efficacy and acceptability 6; *see also specific vaccines*
vegetarians, vitamin D deficiency in 104, 106, 107
ventilation, artificial, for neonates 274
very low birthweight infants (VLBW) 258, 264, 274
  costs of intensive care 278, 279
  health problems in survivors 276–7
  increased survival, handicap and morbidity 274–6
  prediction of outcome 277–8
vinyl chloride, carcinogenicity 163, 164, 170
vitamin D 101
  metabolism 102
  oral supplements 108–9
vitamin D deficiency 101–10, 352
  diagnosis 102
  effects 101
  interventions 107–10
    constraints 109–10
    effectiveness 109
    fortification of foodstuffs 108–9
    recommendations 110
  prerequisites for elimination 357–8
  prevalence 103–5
  relationship to femoral neck fractures 103, 104–5, 108, 109
  risk factors 104–5, 106–7
  trends in incidence 105
vitamin supplementation, prevention of neural tube defects (NTD) 199–200

water
  fluoridation of 122, 147–8, 150, 151–2, 153
  iodinated 121–2
weight gain in pregnancy, limitation of 270
whooping cough (pertussis) 26–42, 350
  clinical features 26–7
  immunization programmes 28–32
    boosters 36
    cost-benefit ratio 40–1
    effectiveness 31–2, 33–6
    high-risk groups 31
    problems in maximizing effectiveness 36–41
    recommendations 41–2
    target population 30–1
  occurrence and trends 27–8, 29
  prerequisites for elimination 356
  vaccines 28
    acceptability 40
    acellular 32, 42
    contraindications 39–40
    efficacy 31, 32–3
    toxicity 37–9
    variability 28–30
work output, haemoglobin concentrations and 132–3